# PRACTICAL
# Radiation
# Oncology
# Physics

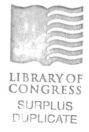

# PRACTICAL Radiation Oncology Physics

A Companion to
**GUNDERSON&TEPPER'S**
**CLINICAL RADIATION ONCOLOGY**

**Sonja Dieterich, PhD, DABR**
Associate Professor
Department of Radiation Oncology
University of California
Davis, California

**Eric Ford, PhD, DABR**
Associate Professor
Department of Radiation Oncology
University of Washington School of Medicine
Seattle, Washington

**Dan Pavord, MS, DABR**
Chief Medical Physicist
Radiation Oncology
Health Quest
Poughkeepsie, New York

**Jing Zeng, MD, DABR**
Assistant Professor
Department of Radiation Oncology
University of Washington School of Medicine
Seattle, Washington

ELSEVIER

# ELSEVIER

1600 John F. Kennedy Blvd.
Ste 1800
Philadelphia, PA 19103-2899

PRACTICAL RADIATION ONCOLOGY PHYSICS:
A COMPANION TO GUNDERSON & TEPPER'S
CLINICAL RADIATION ONCOLOGY

ISBN: 978-0-323-26209-5

---

### Notices

Knowledge and best practice in this field are constantly changing. As new research and experience broaden our understanding, changes in research methods, professional practices, or medical treatment may become necessary.

Practitioners and researchers must always rely on their own experience and knowledge in evaluating and using any information, methods, compounds, or experiments described herein. In using such information or methods they should be mindful of their own safety and the safety of others, including parties for whom they have a professional responsibility.

With respect to any drug or pharmaceutical products identified, readers are advised to check the most current information provided (i) on procedures featured or (ii) by the manufacturer of each product to be administered, to verify the recommended dose or formula, the method and duration of administration, and contraindications. It is the responsibility of practitioners, relying on their own experience and knowledge of their patients, to make diagnoses, to determine dosages and the best treatment for each individual patient, and to take all appropriate safety precautions.

To the fullest extent of the law, neither the Publisher nor the authors, contributors, or editors, assume any liability for any injury and/or damage to persons or property as a matter of products liability, negligence or otherwise, or from any use or operation of any methods, products, instructions, or ideas contained in the material herein.

---

Library of Congress Cataloging-in-Publication Data
Dieterich, Sonja, author.
  Practical radiation oncology physics: a companion to Gunderson & Tepper's Clinical radiation oncology / Sonja Dieterich, Eric Ford, Daniel Pavord, Jing Zeng.
    p. ; cm.
  Per publisher's web site, this book is a companion to the fourth edition of Clinical radiation oncology, by Drs. Leonard Gunderson and Joel Tepper.
  ISBN 978-0-323-26209-5 (pbk. : alk. paper)
  I. Ford, Eric (Radiation oncologist), author.   II. Pavord, Daniel, author.   III. Zeng, Jing (Radiation oncologist), author.   IV. Clinical radiation oncology (Gunderson). 4th ed. Supplement to (expression):   V. Title.
  [DNLM: 1. Radiation Oncology.  2. Physics. QZ 269]
  RC270.3.R33
  616.99'40757—dc23

2015013608

*Senior Content Strategist:* Suzanne Toppy
*Senior Content Development Specialist:* Dee Simpson
*Publishing Services Manager:* Hemamalini Rajendrababu
*Senior Project Manager:* Beula Christopher
*Design Manager:* Amy Buxton
*Illustrations Manager:* Karen Giacomucci
*Marketing Manager:* Deborah Davis

Printed in China

Last digit is the print number:   9  8  7  6  5  4  3  2  1

Working together
to grow libraries in
developing countries

www.elsevier.com • www.bookaid.org

# Dedications

*For Sigrid "Witzi" Dieterich, 1950–1996.*
*—Sonja Dieterich*

*To my wife, Elisa. Your support and love is everything.*
*—Eric Ford*

*To my family—Anna, Craig, Lillian, and Scott.*
*To my friends and mentors—Mitch, Kris, and Peggy.*
*—Dan Pavord*

*For my husband, parents, and mother-in-law who made this possible.*
*—Jing Zeng*

# FOREWORD

There are few fields in medicine for which the role of the radiation physicist is as important as it is in radiation oncology. Our machines are designed by engineers based on sophisticated physical principles, machines are commissioned in individual institutions by physicists and engineers to ensure that they meet exacting tolerance, and daily treatments are designed by dosimetrists and implemented by the entire treatment team. As new clinical approaches are developed they need to be implemented in individual clinics, with modifications necessary for the idiosyncrasies of the equipment and needs of each department. For this to be done well, the physics team must have a strong knowledge of the basic principles involved as well as the design of the hardware and software packages.

As radiation therapy has become far more complicated, the expectations that the physicians have of the physics team have escalated accordingly. The days are long past when central axis dose calculations were sufficient, and when imaging was never more than a weekly port film and computer software was rudimentary. Thus, quality control has become critical in all areas of radiation therapy delivery because there is so much more that can go wrong. Systems need to be put in place in each institution to ensure, prior to treatment delivery, that the treatment that the physician intended is indeed what was delivered to the patient.

The critical nature of this work is made even harder by the very small margin of error that is routine in radiation therapy treatment delivery. The physician is usually prescribing radiation doses that are at the edge of what the normal tissues will tolerate, and at the edge of what is needed for best tumor control. Any substantial deviation from those doses is likely to lead either to complications or loss of tumor control.

Thus, a book such as this that covers these areas well is important to the radiation oncology community. This new handbook is intended to provide a concise and practical summary of current standards of practice in radiation therapy physics and is appropriate for medical physicists, radiation oncologists, and residents. This book covers the topics needed for high-quality physics support at any contemporary institution in a practical and understandable manner. It provides far more than texts that limit themselves to simply describing the physical aspects of radiation therapy delivery, but also has a strong emphasis on the quality and safety issues that have come to the forefront in the past number of years.

The fact that this book is written by four individuals allows for consistency in terms of writing style and approach and helps avoid duplication or missing topics of importance. It will be a valuable resource to allow patient care to proceed at the highest level.

*Joel E. Tepper, MD, FASTRO*
*Hector MacLean Distinguished Professor of Cancer Research*
*Department of Radiation Oncology*
*University of North Carolina Lineberger Comprehensive Cancer Center*
*University of North Carolina School of Medicine*
*Chapel Hill, North Carolina*

# PREFACE

Every so often, an email lands in our inboxes asking for help in getting started with a new clinical program; often these are questions about radiosurgery, brachytherapy, prone breast, use of CBCT, and many other new clinical procedures. As medical physicists responsible for implementing new technologies, we have many questions: Are the vendor recommendations sound? What professional society guidance documents are available, and are they still describing the current best practices? Is the method described in the recent paper by a major research university something I can follow with the resources I have at my smaller clinic, or is it not quite ready for prime time yet?

At present there are no standard resources available to answer these questions. We looked at our bookshelf of great didactic works and wished there was a book out there we could use to convey the basic overview of current best clinical practice and a curated reference list of guidance documents and publications to deepen the knowledge. The medical residents all carry such a book for radiation oncology in their coat pockets; why do we not have one for medical physics?

Each of us approached the others about finding solutions to these questions. We quickly realized that we were focusing on the same topic, and thus the idea of this book was formed. And then came Hurricane Sandy. Trapped in Boston with the ASTRO meeting temporarily suspended, we pitched the book proposal, and in Elsevier found a publisher who also saw the need and was ready to support our idea.

The goal of this book is to promote the safe and effective treatment of patients by providing an easily accessible distillation of all the current background and recommendations for best practices in the field. We have drawn from society recommendations, high-impact papers, and our own clinical experience absorbed from our mentors and learned in the trenches.

Of the many ways to organize the material, we chose the following approach. The first twelve chapters cover the technical basics of the major clinical areas. Roughly, those are all the tasks physicists perform on phantoms, without a patient being in the room. The second half of the book covers major clinical treatment modalities. The work done in those areas directly involves patients and requires teamwork from the multiple professions that make up the patient care team. There are often several valid approaches to achieve the treatment goals, and the standard of care is changed and improved as new publications provide evidence for changing practice.

Each book chapter provides a short introduction, followed by several sections providing an overview of the current best clinical practice(s). Recommendations from the various guidance documents published by IAEA, ACR, ASTRO, AAPM, ABS, and other professional organizations or regulatory bodies are summarized and referenced as applicable. A "For the Physician" section concludes each chapter. This section summarizes the most important points with the goal to enable physicians to quickly check whether the physics work performed under their supervision is in agreement with safety and quality standards.

How should you use this book? Physics residents and junior physicists just entering the clinic will find the chapters to be introductions to their clinical rotations. Medical residents might want to focus on the clinical chapters to gain insight on the technical and process components of patient treatments. Physicists setting out to implement a new procedure can focus on the applicable chapters of both the technical and the clinical sections of the book. Departments preparing for accreditation and physicians/physicists working on practice quality improvement projects will find the references in each chapter to be good starting points to evaluate their own practice against best practices recommended by their peers. And if none of the above apply, we the authors hope that in reading this book you will still find a few new pieces of information to expand your knowledge. As authors, we found the experience of learning and discovery while writing this book so rewarding that it well made up for the occasional difficult task of writing.

We hope that this book will prove to be a valuable investment of your time and money. Finally, we would love to hear from you. Do you know of a good guidance document we have missed? A clinical practice standard that should have been mentioned? What did we do well? After all, the best learning often does not come from books, but in the face-to-face discussion of ideas and concepts.

*Sonja Dieterich, PhD, DABR (sdieterich@ucdavis.edu)*
*Eric Ford, PhD, DABR (eford@uw.edu)*
*Dan Pavord, MS, DABR (dpavord@health-quest.org)*
*Jing Zeng, MD, DABR (jzeng13@uw.edu)*

# CONTENTS

# PART I

# Building Blocks

# Reference Dosimetry for Ionizing Radiation

## 1.1 Introduction

The key to the accurate delivery of radiation is the ability to establish the absolute dose delivered. In radiation therapy clinical practice the primary tool used to measure absorbed dose is the ion chamber. The use of ion chambers has been well described by international codes of practice. While some of the details may differ slightly, the basic concepts of the various codes of practice are the same. The ionization measured by the chamber (typically filled with air) is converted to absorbed dose by applying a calibration factor (determined by an accredited calibration lab) and other correction factors based on the chamber design. The calibration factor may be a direct calibration in water (megavoltage (MV) photons, MV electrons, protons) or a calibration based on air kerma (kilovoltage (kV) photons, brachytherapy sources). The end goal is to determine absorbed dose to water in either case.

The starting point for these calibrations is the absorbed dose standard developed at a primary standard dosimetry laboratory (PSDL). End users obtain a calibration factor for their equipment at a secondary standard dosimetry laboratory (SSDL), also known as an accredited dosimetry calibration lab (ADCL). The SSDL applies the standard developed by the PSDL using the available radiation sources at that lab. All SSDLs have $^{60}$Co sources available for calibration but may not have linac-generated beams. Some labs do have other high energy photon beams available and can provide a calibration at multiple beam qualities. In the absence of this, correction factors must be applied to the calibration determined at $^{60}$Co energy to determine the calibration for the beam quality of interest. Further corrections are needed if the beam of interest is protons or other heavy ions. For a more complete discussion of the interaction between PSDLs, SSDLs, and the end user, the reader is referred to section 2.1 of International Atomic Energy Agency (IAEA) TRS-398, Absorbed Dose Determination in External Beam Radiotherapy: An International Code of Practice for Dosimetry Based on Standards of Absorbed Dose to Water.[1]

The regulations on the frequency of a full calibration in water may vary from country to country but are generally required at least once per year. The suggested regulations by the Conference of Radiation Control Program Directors (CRCPD) and implemented by many states in the United States require full calibrations at intervals not to exceed 12 months (section X.7.iii). More frequent constancy checks are required but can be done using solid phantoms and dosimetry equipment that is not calibrated by a calibration laboratory. These constancy devices should be compared with the calibrated system immediately after the annual full calibration. The equipment used for the full calibration should be sent for recalibration every 2 years. A constancy check should be performed before sending equipment to the calibration lab and after receiving it back to ensure that nothing happened during the process to change the response of the chamber. For new radiation therapy treatment machines, a second check of the absolute dose calibration should be obtained prior to treating patients.[2] This could be accomplished by using a mail-order reference dosimetry service or a second check by a colleague using an independent dosimetry system.

## 1.2 Standard Megavoltage Photon Beams

Several international codes of practice are used to determine absorbed dose for MV photon beams, the American Association of Physicists in Medicine (AAPM) TG-51, Protocol for Clinical Reference Dosimetry of High-Energy Photon and Electron Beams,[3] IAEA TRS-398, Absorbed Dose Determination in External Beam Radiotherapy,[1] Deutsche Industrie-Norm (DIN) 6800-2, Dosimetry Method for Photon and Electron Radiation—Part 2 Dosimetry of High Energy Photon and Electron Radiation with Ionization Chambers,[4] Institute of Physics and Engineering in Medicine (IPEM) 1990, Code of Practice for High-Energy Photon Therapy Dosimetry,[5] and others. An addendum to AAPM TG-51 has been published containing new $k_Q$ values.[6] They are all based on absorbed dose in water calibrations of cylindrical ion chambers. The charge reading obtained from the ion chamber is corrected for temperature, pressure, ion recombination, and polarity. Corrections are then made to account for the perturbation to the medium (water) caused by the presence of the ion chamber. The calibration factor is then used to convert charge to absorbed dose. All of the protocols use a reference field size of 10 cm × 10 cm but the depth and source-to-surface distance (SSD) can vary among them. It is important to note that the reference depth for the calibration protocol is likely not the depth of absorbed dose specification in the clinic. For example, the protocol may specify measurement at 10 cm depth but the output of the machine is adjusted to 1.0 cGy/MU at depth of dose maximum ($d_{max}$). This will require the use of accurate percent depth dose to correct the readings taken at 10 cm depth to $d_{max}$ depth. The general equation to calculate absorbed dose from a charge reading of an ion chamber measured with an electrometer is:

$$D_w(z) = M \, N_{D,w} \, k_p \, k_s \, k_\rho \, k_Q(z)$$

where $D_w(z)$ = absorbed dose to water at depth z

    M = the ion chamber reading corrected for the electrometer calibration

    $N_{D,w}$ = calibration factor for absorbed dose to water for $^{60}$Co energy

    $k_p$ = polarity correction. The value is generally less than 1% from unity. The value should be stable from year to year and any deviation greater than 0.5% from the running average should be investigated. For new chambers, it should be measured several times to establish consistency.

    $k_s$ = ion recombination factor. The value is generally less than 1.01 and AAPM TG-51 recommends not using a chamber if the correction is greater than 5%. The same recommendation regarding year-to-year stability applies.

    $k_\rho$ = air density correction factor (often formulated as a temperature/pressure correction)

    $k_Q(z)$ = beam quality correction factor for the measured beam versus the $^{60}$Co beam (in which $N_w$ is determined). $k_Q$ is specific to the beam energy being measured and the ion chamber used to make the measurement. Typical values range from 1 to approximately 0.96 for MV photon beams.

A comparison of the four codes of practice is shown in Tables 1.1 to 1.5. Comparisons among the codes of practice show variations within the expected uncertainty levels of 1% to 1.5%.[8-10] Standards labs are moving toward offering calibrations at beam qualities other than $^{60}$Co. This has the advantage that the $k_Q$ factor determined will be for the specific chamber used in the clinic, not a generic $k_Q$ for a given chamber model. There are two possibilities for implementing this strategy:

## TABLE 1.1 ▪ Polarity Correction ($k_p$) Determination for the Various Protocols

| | |
|---|---|
| AAPM TG-51 | $\left\lvert \dfrac{(M_{raw}^+ - M_{raw}^-)}{2M_{raw}} \right\rvert$ |
| IAEA TRS-398 | $\left\lvert \dfrac{(M_{raw}^+ - M_{raw}^-)}{2M_{raw}} \right\rvert$ |
| DIN 6800-2 | $(M_1 + M_2)/M_1/[(M_1 + M_2)/M_1]_{Co}$ |
| IPEM 1990 | none |

When determining polarity corrections and comparing among systems, care should be taken to understand the bias configuration used. This can vary among manufacturers. The value can either be less than or greater than 1 depending on which polarity is used for the final output determination but should not exceed 1%. In general $k_p$ is a smaller effect with increasing energy. It should be noted that if $k_p$ is known for the calibration beam quality ($Q_0$), $k_p$ will then be determined as $k_p = k_{p,Q}/k_{pQ0}$. It follows from this that if the user beam quality (Q) is the same as the calibration beam quality ($Q_0$), $k_p = 1$. This must be done if $k_p$ exceeds 0.3% for 6 MV or $^{60}$Co energies.

## TABLE 1.2 ▪ Ion Recombination ($k_s$) Determination for the Various Protocols for Pulsed Beams

| | |
|---|---|
| AAPM TG-51 | $\dfrac{1 - V_H/V_L}{M_{raw}^H/M_{raw}^L - V_H/V_L}$ |
| IAEA TRS-398 | $k_s = \dfrac{M_1/M_2 - 1}{U_1/U_2 - 1}$ <br> or <br> $k_s = a_0 + a_1\dfrac{M_1}{M_2} + a_2\left(\dfrac{M_1}{M_2}\right)^2$ |
| DIN 6800-2 | $\dfrac{U_1/U_2 - 1}{U_1/U_2 - [(M - M_0)k_p k_p]_1/[(M - M_0)k_p k_p]_2}$ |
| IPEM 1990 | 1+X% for an X% decrease in reading when chamber voltage is halved |

Since $M_{raw}^H > M_{raw}^L$, the value is always >1. It should be noted that ion recombination is mostly dependent on dose per pulse and therefore will be different for flattening filter free beams.[7]

## TABLE 1.3 ▪ kρ Determination for the Various Protocols

| | |
|---|---|
| AAPM TG-51 | $\dfrac{273.2+T}{273.2+22.0} \times \dfrac{101.33}{P}$ where $T$ = water temperature in °C and $P$ = pressure in kPa. Humidity must be between 20% and 80%. |
| IAEA TRS-398 DIN 6800-2 IPEM 1990 | Standard temperature is 20 instead of 22. Therefore the denominator is 273.2 + 20.0 in the temperature term. |

1. The calibration lab determines $N_{D,w}$ for the chamber along with a series of $k_Q$ values across the range of beam qualities including electrons. This has the advantage that because the beam energy dependence for the chamber is not expected to change, future calibrations will only require determination of $N_{D,w}$ at the reference quality, $Q_0$.
2. The calibration lab determines a series of $N_{D,w}$ values, eliminating the need for $k_Q$.

**TABLE 1.4 ■ Photon Beam Quality Correction Factors for the Various Protocols**

| AAPM TG-51 | Table of values for various ion chambers across a range of beam energies. Beam quality is specified by the percent depth dose (PDD) at 10 cm depth, 100 cm SSD with electron contamination removed or PDD(10)$_x$ for energies ≥10 MV. To measure the photon component PDD, a thin lead foil (1 mm) is placed at 50 cm from the source to eliminate electron contamination from the beam at energies of 10 MV or greater. This lead foil is used for measurement of the PDD only and must be removed for the output measurement. |
|---|---|
| IAEA TRS-398 | Table of values for various ion chambers across a range of beam energies. Beam quality is specified by the ratio of the TPR at 20 cm depth and the TPR at 10 cm depth for the reference field size or TPR$_{20,10}$. This can be measured directly or calculated from PDD measurements using the equation 1.2661* (PDD(20)/PDD(10)) − 0.0595. Recommend using a measured value rather than a generic value. |
| DIN 6800-2 | Same as IAEA. |
| IPEM 1990 | Beam quality is specified by the ratio of the TPR at 20 cm depth and the TPR at 10 cm depth for the reference field size or TPR$_{20,10}$. |

**TABLE 1.5 ■ Ion Chamber Location for the Various Protocols**

| AAPM TG-51 | Reference point (center of chamber) at measurement depth. |
|---|---|
| IAEA TRS-398 | Reference point at measurement depth. |
| DIN 6800-2 | Reference point 0.5 $r$ below measurement depth. DIN 6800-2 also explicitly uses a perturbation correction to account for the difference in chamber position at the calibration lab (reference point at measurement depth) and the local dose measurement. Factor = 1 + |δ| $r$/2, where δ is the relative gradient of the depth dose curve at the point of measurement (about 0.006 mm$^{-1}$ for $^{60}$Co) and $r$ is the inner radius of the chamber. |
| IPEM 1990 | Reference point at measurement depth. |

## 1.3 Nonstandard Megavoltage Photon Beams

There are photon delivery machines that cannot produce the required 10 × 10 cm reference field and/or the SSD required by the codes of practice, including TomoTherapy, CyberKnife, Gamma Knife, and Vero. Furthermore, the geometry of some treatment units such as Gamma Knife do not readily accommodate the use of water phantoms for primary dose calibration, and so an air/medium protocol such as AAPM TG-21, A Protocol for the Determination of Absorbed Dose from High Energy Photon and Electron Beams, is sometimes used.[11] The forthcoming AAPM TG-178, Gamma Stereotactic Radiosurgery Dosimetry and Quality Assurance, will address the topic of dose calibration of stereotactic radiosurgery beams for Gamma Knife. Some beams are not compliant with standard protocols because they do not have a flat dose profile (e.g., TomoTherapy or flattening filter free beams), which complicates reference dosimetry.[12]

In addition, the size of the detector must be appropriate for the beam. The detector size should be small enough so that the gradient across detector volume is less than a few percent. Kawachi et al. showed that the relatively flat portion of the beam for a CyberKnife cone does not exceed 1 cm, as shown in Figure 1.1.[13] The gradient can be caused by the inherent gradient created by beams without flattening filters. References are available that describe the additional corrections that must be made for these units to accurately calculate absorbed dose. The corrections are made by adjusting the value of k$_Q$ to account for the lack of charged particle equilibrium.

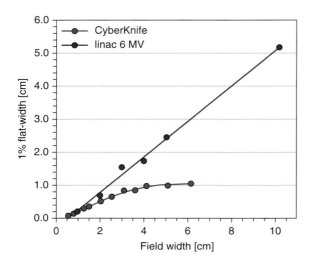

**Figure 1.1** A comparison of the 1% flat widths at 10 cm of depth in water between the CyberKnife and an ordinary 6 MV linac (Clinac 21EX, Varian, ME). The SCD is 80 cm for the CyberKnife and 100 cm for the linac. *(Adapted from Kawachi T, Saitoh H, Inoue M, et al. Reference dosimetry condition and beam quality correction factor for CyberKnife beam. Med Phys 2008;35(10):4591.)*

The correction is about 1% for a TomoTherapy unit[14] to as much as 10% for small cones on a CyberKnife unit.[13] For flattening filter free beams there may be a slight correction needed for the quality factor if the Tissue-Phantom Ratio $(TPR)_{20}^{10}$ is used to specify beam quality.[12] There are several treatment machines either in early clinical use or in development that use MR imaging. Ion chamber readings will need a correction factor that may depend on the magnetic field strength.[15,16]

# 1.4 Megavoltage Electron Beams

The measurement of absorbed dose for megavoltage electrons is similar to that of megavoltage photon beams. AAPM TG-51 and AAPM TG-70, Recommendations for Clinical Electron Beam Dosimetry, describe the methodology in detail. AAPM TG-70 is a supplement to AAPM TG-25, Clinical Electron Beam Dosimetry, and describes many clinical issues related to electron beams in addition to reference dosimetry.[17,18] Again the primary reference dosimeter is an ion chamber. For electrons, however, parallel plate ion chambers can be used and are in fact recommended for lower energy electron beams. AAPM TG-51 requires a parallel plate chamber for ≤6 MeV and recommends using one for <10 MeV beams. IAEA TRS-398 and DIN 6800-2 recommend parallel plate chambers for all energies but allow cylindrical chambers for beams with $R_{50} > 4$ cm in water. The same corrections are applied for air density, polarity, recombination, and electrometer calibration as for megavoltage photon beams. If a cylindrical ion chamber is used an additional gradient correction factor, $P_{gr}^{Q}$, must be measured and included.

Beam quality is specified by the depth of the 50% depth dose in water. If a cylindrical ion chamber is used to measure the depth dose, the curve must be shifted upstream by 0.5 $r_{cav}$ to account for the effective point of measurement, and the resulting depth ionization curve must be converted to depth dose by using stopping power ratios. AAPM, IAEA, and DIN all specify the same equations to convert depth ionization to depth dose at the depth of 50% ionization:

$$R_{50} = 1.028 * I_{50} - 0.06 \text{ cm} \quad \text{for } I_{50} \leq 10 \text{ cm in water}$$

$$R_{50} = 1.059 * I_{50} - 0.37 \text{ cm} \quad \text{for } I_{50} > 10 \text{ cm in water}$$

It is also possible to derive $R_{50}$ more directly from a measurement with a diode, which does not require the shift or stopping power corrections described for ion chambers.

The reference depth for all of the protocols is calculated as 0.6 $R_{50}$ − 0.1 (cm). The absorbed dose at $d_{max}$ is then determined using the measured percent depth dose.

If using a parallel plate chamber without a calibration factor from a standards lab, the calibration factor can be obtained through cross calibration with a calibrated cylindrical chamber. The cross calibration should be performed using a high energy electron beam. Details are given in AAPM TG-51 in section X.C and in TRS-398 in section 7.6.1.

## 1.5 Kilovoltage Photon Beams

Beams in the kV range may be handled differently, depending on the actual beam energy and on the protocol. Superficial, orthovoltage, and electronic brachytherapy units are included in this section.

AAPM TG-61, AAPM Protocol for 40-300 kV X-ray Beam Dosimetry in Radiotherapy and Radiobiology,[19] and IAEA TRS-398[1] describe the methodology used to measure absorbed dose for kV photon beams. AAPM TG-61 is based on an air kerma calibration of an ion chamber. It covers the range from 40 kV to 300 kV. Either parallel plate or cylindrical chambers can be used for beams >70 kV, with the effective point of measurement being the center of the air cavity. A parallel plate chamber with a thin entrance window must be used for beams <70 kV. Thin plastic plates may be needed to remove electron contamination and provide adequate build-up. For beams <100 kV the measurement must be made in air, and a backscatter factor used to account for phantom scatter. A table of backscatter values based on SSD and beam quality is given. Beam quality is based on half value layer (HVL) in Al or Cu. Beams >100 kV are measured in water at a reference depth of 2 cm.

Corrections for ion recombination, polarity, electrometer calibration, and air density are made as described in Section 1.2. In addition, corrections for timer end effect and chamber stem effect are made. The beam quality correction factors for kV beams in IAEA TRS-398 uses an absorbed dose to water methodology. Because absorbed dose in water calibrations is not readily available at standards labs, the calibration factor is usually calculated from an air kerma calibration factor. This is described in Appendix A.2 of IAEA TRS-398. TRS-398 has a section for low energy kV and medium energy kV beams. For low energy kV beams a parallel plate chamber is recommended. The reference point is the outer surface of the parallel plate chamber or the outer surface of the plastic plates if they are used to ensure adequate build-up. Because the reference point is at the outer surface of the chamber (or plates) and must be flush with the phantom surface, plastic phantoms are recommended due to the difficulty of doing this in a water phantom. HVL is used as the beam quality index, although there is discussion that this is not entirely accurate and introduces up to about 1.5% uncertainty. For medium energy kV beams a cylindrical chamber with a volume between 0.1 and 1.0 cm$^3$ must be used. The reference point is at the center of the volume and should be placed at 2 cm depth in water.

Both AAPM TG-61 and IAEA TRS-398 recommend that the calibration be obtained by matching kV and HVL of the clinical beam if possible. If not possible, then multiple calibration points should be obtained and the clinical calibration factor is then determined by interpolation. The method of interpolation (ln based) is described in the absorbed dose calculation worksheet. A comparison of kV dosimetry protocols showed good agreement, with the exception of the IPEM and AAPM TG-61 protocols at 120 kV where differences on the order of 5% to 7% were seen.[20] The differences may be due to the accuracy of the backscatter factors used or use of HVL as the sole beam quality specification.

## 1.6 Brachytherapy Sources

Brachytherapy sources are generally calibrated using an air-filled well chamber. AAPM TG-43, Dosimetry of Interstitial Brachytherapy Sources, and the following updates[21-23] describe a general method to calculate absorbed dose at any point from an air kerma strength value, $S_k$, which has units of $\mu Gy\ m^2\ hr^{-1}$, which is given the symbol U. The well chamber is calibrated in terms of this air kerma strength by obtaining a calibration factor to convert the current reading from the well chamber to air kerma strength from an ADCL.

The well chamber can either be open to the air or pressurized to increase the signal of the chamber. If a pressurized well chamber is used, it is very important to perform constancy measurements to ensure that there has not been a leak in the chamber. The response of the well chamber is dependent on the position of the source within the well. A source holder is used to reproducibly position the source in the center of the well. For low dose rate (LDR) seeds the source is simply dropped into the holder, which is designed to position the seed at the area of uniform response. If possible, there should be a visual indication that the seed is in the correct position to ensure reproducibility. Figure 1.2 shows a typical well chamber and source holder. For high dose rate (HDR) remote afterloading systems the source is usually stepped through the length of the well by inserting a thin catheter connected to the HDR unit into the holder to find the position of maximum reading. This position should be consistent from measurement to measurement, but the stepping process ensures that the correct reading is obtained. Figure 1.3 shows a typical well chamber response versus source position. The point of maximum reading is generally referred to as the "sweet spot". It should be noted that usually the LDR seed holder is different from the HDR holder. In either case, the holder used in the clinic must be sent with the well chamber when it is calibrated so that the exact conditions can be repeated in the clinic. For low energy sources such as $^{125}I$ or $^{103}Pd$, the calibration must be obtained for the specific model of seed used clinically. This is due to the fact that the energy spectrum is greatly affected by the seed construction. For higher energy sources such as $^{192}Ir$, a generic value can be used.[24] The IPEM has published a protocol for $^{192}Ir$ using reference air kerma rate (RAKR).[25] The RAKR is given as $Gy\ s^{-1}$ at 1 m. A conversion to air kerma strength is given so that it can be compared with AAPM TG-43 formalism.

When calibrating an $^{192}Ir$ source, the well chamber should be 1 m from any wall or scattering material and placed on a plastic cart. The well chamber should be left in the room for sufficient time to allow for thermal equilibrium, which could be up to 7 hours for a $4\,^{\circ}C$ temperature difference using a Standard Imaging HDR 1000 Plus well chamber. It has been shown that the well chamber reading can change by as much as 1.1% as it is moved toward a scattering surface and that without the Styrofoam insert thermal changes can be 0.15%.[26] The protocol also mentions that a source geometry factor may be included in the future that would account for different source models. This factor is currently assumed to be unity. Air density, ion recombination, and

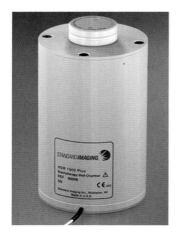
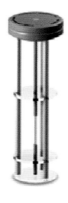

**Figure 1.2** A typical well chamber and source holder.

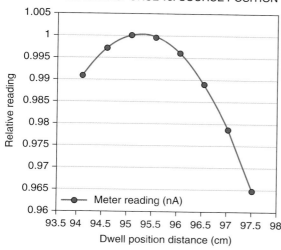

WELL CHAMBER RESPONSE vs. SOURCE POSITION

**Figure 1-3** Sample well chamber response versus source position for an $^{192}$Ir HDR source.

electrometer calibration corrections are applied. This protocol and AAPM TG-56, Code of Practice for Brachytherapy Physics,[27] recommend the use of a tertiary system to confirm the constancy of the secondary system used for the calibration. This can either be another well chamber or a farmer chamber placed in a jig at 10 cm distance. There is also an older AAPM Report, TG-41, Remote Afterloading Technology, that describes HDR source calibrations.[28] A useful review of international protocols for $^{192}$Ir HDR sources has been published by Azhari et al.[29]

Calibration of sterilized seeds for interstitial implants presents a challenge to the clinical user. The AAPM TG-56 has recommended that at least 10% or 10 sources, whichever is greater, must be assayed by the on-site physicist for loose seeds.[30] For stranded products the recommendation is 5% or 5 seeds, whichever is fewer. To meet this requirement, extra sources from the same batch may be ordered for calibration purposes, which will increase the cost. Alternatively, the calibration seeds could be ordered nonsterile and then assayed on site and resterilized. In addition, methods for calibrating the seeds while maintaining sterility have been proposed.[31,32]

When calibrating a brachytherapy source, a comparison is made to the manufacturer's calibration certificate. AAPM TG-56 recommends that the values should match within 3%. Deviations between 3% and 5% should be investigated. Having a tertiary dosimetry system will aid in this investigation and is recommended as mentioned previously. Differences greater than 5% should be reported to the manufacturer. If the source is part of a batch to be used for seed implantation, the mean of the batch should agree with the manufacturer's calibration within 3% and all sources should be within 5% of the mean.

## 1.7 Proton Radiotherapy Beams

IAEA TRS-398[1] describes the determination of absorbed dose in proton beams. Parallel plate chambers can be used for all beam energies, but cylindrical chambers can be used only for beam qualities at reference depth $R_{res} > 0.5$ g cm$^{-2}$. Cylindrical chambers are preferred when appropriate. $R_{res}$ is the residual range and is defined as the distance from the center of the spread out Bragg peak (SOBP) to the distal 10% depth. $R_{res}$ is used as the beam quality index in the protocol and is determined from depth dose measurements made with a parallel plate chamber. The depth ionization is converted to depth dose by applying stopping power ratios. If $P_{ion}$ and $P_{pol}$ vary with depth, these corrections should also be used. The reference point for the absorbed dose measurement is the center of the SOBP. One of the factors affecting accuracy is the ripple in the SOBP, which should be $<\pm3\%$. The protocol has tables for the values of $k_{Q,Q_0}$ which are all calculated values with $Q_0$ equal to $^{60}$Co. Air density, ion recombination, and polarity corrections are used when calculating the absorbed dose. For small fields that are less than twice the diameter of the parallel plate chamber air cavity, a more suitable dosimeter such as a diode or microchamber should be used. It must be validated against the parallel plate chamber at a larger field size.

## 1.8 Potential Errors in Reference Dosimetry

The Radiological Physics Center (RPC; now called IROC-Houston) published a report describing common errors encountered when switching to AAPM TG-51.[33] These included incorrect use of parallel plate chambers, mixing of phantom materials, inconsistent use of depth dose factors to transfer dose to $d_{max}$, incorrect use of the lead foil used to measure $PDD(10)_X$, incorrect chamber shifts, and the use of outdated stopping power data. In addition, an error of approximately 5% could be introduced if the lead foil required for determination of $PDD(10)_X$ is not removed before measuring absorbed dose. Polarity and ion recombination effects vary with depth and should be measured at the reference depth. TRS-398[1] makes many references to the errors introduced by using non-water phantoms (with the exception of low energy kV beams). There have been several instances of large calibration errors made due to using an inappropriately large chamber for small fields. Examples include a stereotactic radiosurgery beam at a facility in Springfield, MO, commissioned with a detector that was too large, which resulted in 76 patients receiving an overdose of 50% from 2004 to 2009.[34] In these instances, the chamber appropriate for the calibration of the standard field ($10 \times 10$) was also used when determining the absolute dose for add-on devices such as a stereotactic cone or multi-leaf collimator (MLC).

## 1.9 Dosimetric Uncertainties

Accurate reference dosimetry is the key to delivering accurate doses in Radiation Oncology, and this is vitally important because an error will affect every patient treated with the beam in question. Use of incorrect equipment or procedure has led to multiple reports of clinical misadministration of radiation therapy to patients. Many times in this book we refer to the goal of achieving $\leq5\%$ combined error in dose delivery. To achieve this, the reference dosimetry must contribute a small uncertainty because there are also other contributing factors to the 5% combined error. Dosimetry protocols should be adhered to and measurements should be documented. Best practice is to perform absolute dose calibration measurements in water on a yearly basis with reference dosimetry equipment that receives an outside calibration. Before treating patients, calibration should be audited with an independent measurement.

When reviewing an annual calibration report, multiple factors contribute to the measurement uncertainty. Typical values are shown in Table 1.6 for external beam therapy.

A similar analysis for brachytherapy sources was performed by AAPM TG-138, A Dosimetric Uncertainty Analysis for Photon-Emitting Brachytherapy Sources.[35] They concluded that the determination of air kerma strength has an overall uncertainty of less than 3%. Table 1.7 shows the different sources of uncertainty and their magnitude. It should be noted that this uncertainty applies only to the determination of air kerma strength. Uncertainties in the determination of AAPM TG-43 dosimetric parameters and delivery issues are not included.

It is instructive to read the explanation of uncertainties given by the calibration lab in their report. This provides an idea of the types and magnitudes of uncertainties in the calibration process. Along with the calibration factor itself, the greatest sources of errors can come from the determination of the beam quality correction factor and the electrometer reading.

TABLE 1.6 ■ Impact of Various Uncertainties in External Beam Reference Dosimetry[36]

| Parameter | Uncertainty | Resulting % Error |
|---|---|---|
| SSD | ±1 mm | ±0.02 |
| Depth | ±1 mm | ±0.03 |
| Field size | ±1 mm | ±0.03 |
| Temperature | ±1 degree | ±0.18 |
| Pressure | ±1 mm Hg | ±0.09 |
| Electrometer reading | Meter reproducibility, stability, linearity, and leakage | ±0.29 |
| Beam quality correction factor | Measurement reproducibility, different methodologies for measurement | ±0.5 |
| Ion recombination correction factor | Measurement reproducibility, different methodologies for measurement | ±0.06 |
| Polarity correction factor | Measurement reproducibility, different methodologies for measurement | ±0.2 |
| Calibration factor | Measurement reproducibility | ±1.0 |
| Overall uncertainty | | ±1.5 |

TABLE 1.7 ■ Estimated Uncertainty in the Calibration of Air Kerma Strength

| Measurement Description | Quantity (units) | Relative Propagated Uncertainty (%) |
|---|---|---|
| NIST WAFAC calibration | $S_{K,NIST}$ | ±0.8 |
| ADCL well chamber calibration | $S_{K,NIST}/I_{ADCL}$ (U/A) | ±0.9 |
| ADCL calibration of source from manufacturer | $S_{K,ADCL}$ (U) | ±1.1 |
| ADCL calibration of clinic well chamber | $S_{K,ADCL}/I_{clinic}$ (U/A) | ±1.2 |
| Clinic measured source air kerma strength | $S_{K,clinic}$ (U) | ±1.3 |
| Expanded uncertainty | $S_{K,clinic}$ (U) | ±2.6 |

**FOR THE PHYSICIAN**

The initial reference dosimetry of a radiation source, either external beam or brachytherapy, must be performed with a high degree of accuracy because an error at this step will affect every patient treated with that source. To standardize this dosimetry, various professional societies, government agencies, and international agencies have established protocols for determining the absolute absorbed dose for the types of radiation sources used in Radiation Oncology.

At the core of a dosimetry protocol is the establishment of a dose standard at a primary standard dose laboratory. The dosimetry equipment used in a clinic is sent to a secondary standard dosimetry laboratory to obtain a calibration factor. This is repeated at a minimum of 2-year intervals to ensure that the response of the equipment remains unchanged.

For megavoltage photon and electron beams there are many national calibration protocols as well as an international protocol. Comparisons among the various protocols have shown agreement on the order of 1% to 1.5%. They all use the common methodology of converting the charge collected by an air-filled ion chamber in a water phantom to absorbed dose to water for a reference field, 10 cm × 10 cm. Various corrections to account for air density, chamber response, and perturbation of the radiation beam due to the replacement of the medium (water) by the ion chamber are applied to the charge reading. The corrected reading is then multiplied by the calibration factor to obtain the absorbed dose. There are several units that cannot produce the standard reference field, and special corrections are needed in those cases (e.g., TomoTherapy, CyberKnife, Gamma Knife, and Vero).

Low energy kilovoltage beams have the maximum dose at or very near the surface, and the measurements can be made in air instead of water. The chamber is calibrated in air at the standards laboratory, and corrections are applied to convert to dose in water. Kilovoltage beams can have very different beam spectra even for beams with the same accelerating potential. Because of this, calibration should be made by matching the accelerating potential and half-value layer of the beam as closely as possible. It may be necessary to obtain multiple calibration points and then interpolate to obtain the calibration factor for the clinical beam.

Brachytherapy sources are calibrated using a well chamber. The calibration factor from the standards laboratory converts the current reading from the well chamber to air kerma strength. Sources that are delivered in sterile packaging for interstitial implants present a particular challenge. Either a method to calibrate the seeds while maintaining sterility must be developed or an appropriate number of nonsterile seeds from the same batch can be ordered for calibration purposes.

For any radiation source, the reference dosimetry protocol should be well understood to minimize the chance for errors. Errors of 50% or more have been reported, with severe consequences to the patients. To further minimize the potential for error, reference dosimetry should be carefully reviewed by another physicist prior to clinical use; in the case of a new external beam unit, the reference dosimetry should be verified using a remote dosimetry service or peer review.

## References

1. IAEA TRS-398 (V.11b), Absorbed dose determination in external beam radiotherapy: An international code of practice for dosimetry based on standards of absorbed dose to water. Vienna: The International Atomic Energy Agency; 2004.
2. ASTRO. Safety is no accident. 2012. p. 34. https://www.astro.org/uploadedFiles/Main_Site/Clinical_Practice/Patient_Safety/Blue_Book/SafetyisnoAccident.pdf.
3. Almond PR, Biggs PJ, Coursey BM, et al. AAPM's TG-51 protocol for clinical reference dosimetry of high-energy photon and electron beams. Med Phys 1999;26(9):1847–70.
4. DIN 6800-2, Dosimetry method for photon and electron radiation: Part 2, Dosimetry of high energy photon and electron radiation with ionization chambers. National Standard Dosimetry Protocol, Germany, 2008.
5. Lillicrap SC, Owen B, Williams JR, et al. Code of practice for high-energy photon therapy dosimetry based on the NPL absorbed dose calibration service. Phys Med Biol 1990;35(10):1355–60.
6. McEwen M, DeWerd L, Ibbott G, et al. Addendum to the AAPM TG-51 protocol for clinical reference dosimetry of high-energy photon beams. Med Phys 2014;41:041501-1-20.
7. Lang S, Hrbacek J, Leong A, et al. Ion-recombination correction for different ionization chambers in high dose rate flattening filter free photon beams. Phys Med Bio 2012;57:2819–27.
8. Zakaria A, Schuette W, Younan C. Reference dosimetry according to the new German protocol DIN 6800-2 and comparison with IAEA TRS-398 and AAPM TG-51. Biomed Imaging Interv J 2011;7(2):e15.
9. Castrillon SV, Henriquez FC. Comparison of IPSM 1990 photon dosimetry code of practice with IAEA TRS-398 and AAPM TG-51. JACMP 2009;10(1):136–46.
10. Zakaria A, Schuette W, Younan C. Determination of absorbed dose to water for high-energy photon and electron beams—comparison of the standards DIN 6800-2 (1997), IAEA TRS-398 (2000) and DIN 6800-2 (2006). J Med Phys 2007;32(1):3–11.
11. McDonald D, Yount C, Koch N, et al. Calibration of the Gamma Knife Perfexion using AAPM TG-21 and the solid water Leksell dosimetry phantom. Med Phys 2011;38(3):1685–93.
12. Xiong G, Rogers DW. Relationship between %dd(10)x and stopping power ratios for flattening filter free accelerators: A Monte Carlo study. Med Phys 2008;35(5):2104–9.
13. Kawachi T, Saitoh H, Inoue M, et al. Reference dosimetry condition and beam quality correction factor for CyberKnife beam. Med Phys 2008;35(10):4591.
14. Duane S, Palmans H, Sephton J, et al. Alanine and ion chamber dosimetry in helical TomoTherapy. Radiother Oncol 2006;81:S45.

15. Reynolds M, Fallone BG, Rathee S. Dose response of selected ion chambers in applied homogeneous transverse longitudinal magnetic fields. Med Phys 2013;40(4):042102-1-7.
16. Meijsing I, Raaymakers BW, Raaijmakers AJE, et al. Dosimetry for the MRI accelerator: The impact of a magnetic field on the response of a Farmer NE2571 ionization chamber. Phys Med Biol 2009; 54(10):2993–3002.
17. Gerbi BJ, Antolak JA, Deibel FC, et al. Recommendations for clinical electron beam dosimetry: Supplement to the recommendations of Task Group 25. Med Phys 2009;36(7):3239–78.
18. Khan FM, Doppke KP, Hogstrom KR, et al. Clinical electron beam dosimetry: Report of AAPM radiation therapy committee task group 25. Med Phys 1991;18:79–103.
19. Ma C-M, Coffey CW, DeWerd LA, et al. AAPM protocol for 40-300 kV x-ray beam dosimetry in radiotherapy and radiobiology. Med Phys 2001;28(6):868–93.
20. Munck PM, Nilsson P, Knöös T. Kilovoltage x-ray dosimetry—an experimental comparison between different dosimetry protocols. Phys Med Biol 2008;53(16):4431–42.
21. Rasmussen BE, Davis SD, Schmidt CT, et al. Comparison of air-kerma strength determinations for HDR ¹⁹²Ir sources. Med Phys 2011;38(12):6721–9.
22. Nath R, Anderson LL, Luxton G, et al. Dosimetry of interstitial brachytherapy sources: Recommendations of the AAPM radiation therapy committee Task Group No. 43. Med Phys 1995;22:209–34.
23. Rivard MJ, Coursey BM, DeWerd LA, et al. Update of AAPM Task Group No. 43 Report: A revised AAPM protocol for brachytherapy dose calculations. Med Phys 2004;31(3):633–74.
24. Rivard MJ, Butler WM, DeWerd LA, et al. Supplement to the 2004 update of the AAPM Task Group No. 43 report. Med Phys 2007;34(6):2187–205.
25. Bidmead AM, Sander T, Locks SM, et al. The IPEM code of practice for determination of the reference air kerma rate for HDR ¹⁹²Ir brachytherapy sources based on the NPL air kerma standard. Phys Med Bio 2010;55:3145–59.
26. Podgorsak MB, DeWerd LA, Thomadsen BR, et al. Thermal and scatter effects on the radiation sensitivity of well chambers used for high dose rate ¹⁹²Ir calibrations. Med Phys 1992;19(5):1311–14.
27. Nath R, Anderson LL, Meli JA, et al. Code of practice for brachytherapy physics: Report of the AAPM radiation therapy committee task group No. 56. Med Phys 1997;24(10):1557–98.
28. Glasgow GP, Bourland JD, Grigsby PW, et al. AAPM Report No. 41, remote afterloading technology. New York, NY: The American Association of Physicists in Medicine; 1993.
29. Azhari HA, Hensley F, Schütte W, et al. Dosimetric verification of source strength for HDR afterloading units with ¹⁹²Ir and ⁶⁰Co photon sources: Comparison of three different international protocols. J Med Phys 2012;4:183–92.
30. Butler WM, Bice WS Jr, DeWerd LA, et al. Third-party brachytherapy source calibrations and physicist responsibilities: Report of the AAPM low energy brachytherapy source calibration working group. Med Phys 2008;35(9):3860–5.
31. Otani Y, Yamada T, Kato S, et al. Source strength assay of iodine-125 seeds sealed within sterile packaging. JACMP 2013;14(2):253–63.
32. Butler WM, Dorsey AT, Nelson KR, et al. Quality assurance calibration of ¹²⁵I rapid strand in a sterile environment. Int J Radiat Oncol Biol Phys 1998;41(1):217–22.
33. Tailor RC, Hanson WF, Ibbott GS, et al. AAPM TG-51: Experience from 150 institutions, common errors, and helpful hints. JACMP 2003;4(2):102–11.
34. Bogdanich W, Ruiz RR. Radiation errors reported in Missouri. New York Times 2010. Available from: http://www.nytimes.com/2010/02/25/us/25radiation.html.
35. DeWerd LA, Ibbott GS, Meigooni AS, et al. A dosimetric uncertainty analysis for photon-emitting brachytherapy sources: Report of AAPM Task Group No. 138 and GEC-ESTRO. Med Phys 2011; 38(2):782–801.
36. Castro P, García-Vicente F, Minguez C, et al. Study of the uncertainty in the determination of the absorbed dose to water during external beam radiotherapy calibration. JACMP 2008;9(1):70–86.

CHAPTER *2*

# Relative Dosimetry for MV Beams

## 2.1 Introduction

Since the basic physics of dosimetry for radiation beams is extensively covered in textbooks on radiotherapy physics, this chapter will focus on the measurement of dosimetry data in clinical practice. There are two main goals in measuring relative dosimetry data: (1) confirming the accurate technical functionality of the accelerator to produce a symmetric beam of correct energy and known relative output as specified at acceptance testing and (2) characterizing the available beams of a specific treatment device for input in treatment planning software (TPS).

### (1) ACCURATE TECHNICAL FUNCTIONALITY

Relative dosimetry is very sensitive to technical changes in the accelerator itself. For example, changes in the steering coils or ion chamber can cause the beam symmetry to deviate above the limits specified by acceptance testing and American Association of Physicists in Medicine (AAPM) recommendations. Relative dosimetry is used during installation and acceptance testing to fine-tune accelerator technical parameters. Subsequently, relative dosimetry measurements are used as part of periodic accelerator QA to verify accurate and consistent functioning of the accelerator. AAPM Task Groups (TG)-40[1] and TG-142[2] provide detailed tables of the relative dosimetry measurements, frequencies, and tolerances recommended for clinical practice in standard linear accelerators. AAPM TG-135[3] and TG-148[4] provide additional information for CyberKnife and TomoTherapy, respectively.

### (2) CHARACTERIZING BEAMS FOR TPS

Measurements of relative dosimetry data during commissioning are used as input in TPS and secondary monitor unit (MU) calculation. **It is therefore essential for the data to be of high quality, because they provide the basis for treating thousands of patients during the lifetime of the treatment delivery machine.** The relative dosimetry data set taken during annual QA serves two purposes. First, it is a more stringent check on accelerator technical performance than the monthly or daily relative dosimetry measurements. Second, the annual dosimetry data are used to confirm that the machine is still accurately characterized by the data set used in the TPS. Therefore, it is important to use the baseline TPS data after commissioning as the basis for comparison. For example, if a measured value was originally 2% different from the TPS value and changed to 3.5% different in subsequent years, a comparison to measurement baseline would show only a 1.5% difference, which occludes the actual mismatch between TPS and beam data.

Vendors of TPS generally do provide a list of required relative dosimetry measurements for TPS commissioning. There are several main approaches to commissioning TPS:

1. The TPS requires a set of relative dosimetry data to be measured and entered by the user. Some of these types of TPS do provide standard beam data sets for delivery machines for comparison purposes but use the measured data set for treatment planning. An example for this approach is the CyberKnife MultiPlan TPS.

2. The TPS is delivered with a standard data set for a delivery machine. The measured relative dosimetry data set could be used for verification that the machine is "sufficiently matched" to the standard data set to be used for treatment planning. An example of this approach is the Varian Eclipse TPS. There are currently no manufacturer-independent recommendations on the tolerance for the measured versus standard data set match. While this use of pre-existing beam data is not in agreement with the recommendations of AAPM TG-106[5], it follows established clinical practice for TomoTherapy and Gamma Knife (see item 4 below). If this approach is taken, the vendor-provided data must be very carefully compared against measured data and any deviations thoroughly assessed.

3. The relative dosimetry measurement data are used to generate parameters for one or more beam models. Examples of this approach are the Philips Pinnacle, Elekta XIO, and RaySearch RayStation planning systems. Modeling beam sizes from 40 cm × 40 cm maximum down to small fields of 0.5 cm × 0.5 cm size with one parameter set may require compromise on model accuracy that may not be acceptable in clinical practice. In those cases, it may be prudent to generate two beam models for one beam energy to match the relative dosimetry across all field sizes.

4. The TPS is part of a treatment delivery system and comes precommissioned from the manufacturer. The relative dosimetry measurements are used only to verify the manufacturer-generated data. An example for this approach is the TomoTherapy system and Leksell Gamma Knife.

The rapid development of technology has had an impact on the requirements for relative dosimetry measurements as well. Accelerator dose rates have increased by a factor of 10 or more due to improvements in accelerator design and the adoption of flattening filter free (FFF) beam delivery across almost all delivery systems. The introduction of intensity-modulated radiation therapy (IMRT) and volumetric modulated arc treatment (VMAT) has heightened the importance of accurate penumbra dosimetry measurements to correctly model steep dose gradients at the field edge in the TPS. Improvements in multi-leaf collimator (MLC) design have reduced the leaf width to 2.5 mm in some cases, allowing the treatment of targets as small as 5 mm using the rule of thumb of 2× the minimum leaf width. This development requires the use of small-field relative dosimetry techniques, which previously were restricted to dedicated stereotactic radiosurgery/stereotactic body radiotherapy (SRS/SBRT) devices. The increased use of SRS, SBRT, and hypofractionated treatment regimens has increased the demands on relative dosimetry accuracy, because the impact on systematic errors introduced by uncertainties in relative dosimetry on clinical plan delivery accuracy is increased compared to conventional fractionation schemes.[6,7] The Institute of Physics and Engineering in Medicine (IPEM) report on small field dosimetry[8] provides a very comprehensive introduction to relative dosimetry in small megavoltage (MV) photon beams. In this chapter, we follow the nomenclature of AAPM TG-106[5] to define "small field" as any field equal to or less than 4 cm × 4 cm equivalent square. "Very small field" denotes fields equal to or smaller than 2 cm × 2 cm equivalent square.

Chapter 4 deals in more depth with the topic of commissioning and QA of new treatment equipment (a TPS being one of them). Standard references are AAPM TG-53[9] (QA for Clinical Radiotherapy Equipment) and International Atomic Energy Agency (IAEA) Report 430 (Commissioning and QA of Computerized Planning Systems).

## 2.2 Commissioning Equipment

### WATER TANK

Acquiring a good quality set of relative dosimetry data requires the appropriate equipment. The largest single piece of equipment is the water phantom, which should have the following features:

- Size appropriate to measure the largest required field, plus several centimeters of additional depth/width to create backscatter at the edges of the field
- A phantom stand allowing alignment of the tank itself
- 2D or 3D motion axes that can be adjusted such that the detector moves parallel to the water surface
- An automated central axis (CAX) function to compensate for minor deviations of the beam CAX to the detector vertical motion

In addition to the traditional large water tanks, there are specialized small water tanks available for measuring tissue-phantom ratios (TPR) in small beams, or performing monthly QAs. Details on commissioning a water tank are covered in Chapter 4 of this book, as well as AAPM TG-106.[5]

For monthly and especially daily dosimetry measurements, solid phantoms are used in place of water tanks. These materials should have an electron density as closely matched to water or muscle tissue as possible. Because these materials are not electric conductors, there is a concern that charge build-up could potentially lead to erroneous readings if extended measurement times or very high doses are used.

## 1D DOSIMETERS

Dosimeters measuring a point dose, or rather the dose in a relatively small volume, fall into two categories: single-measurement detectors that need to be processed for readout (TLD, OSLD, Metal–oxide–semiconductor field-effect transistor (MOSFET), alanine pellets) and detectors that can be operated with continuous readout to take either multiple readings at one location or consecutive readings along a trajectory (chambers, diodes, diamond detectors).

Ion chambers have been the gold standard for measuring relative dosimetry data. For fields down to 4 cm × 4 cm, Farmer-type chambers are the gold standard for point dose measurements. In fields smaller than 4 cm × 4 cm, especially in FFF beams, the length of the Farmer chamber leads to volume averaging, which lowers the measured point dose compared to the actual point dose.[8,10-12] Therefore, small volume ion chambers must be used for small fields. These chambers with volumes of approximately 0.006 cm³ are often characterized as "stereotactic" chambers. Several physical issues pertinent to small chambers need to be studied before using them in relative dosimetry measurements: signal-to-noise ratio, leakage current, increased stem effect relative to chamber size, increased energy dependence, and stability of current. See Table I in Low et al.[12] for a useful list of ion chambers and their characteristics. Low et al. recommend that ion chambers not be used for scanning profile measurements of relative dosimetry.

Diodes are increasingly used to complement chambers, especially for dosimetry measurements in small fields. Dedicated stereotactic diodes with active detector size diameters of 0.8 mm to 1 mm allow for highly accurate penumbra measurements. Diodes are available as shielded and unshielded models; unshielded models are more sensitive to low energy components of the radiation beam. Diodes are also useful for measuring percent depth doses (PDDs) in an electron beam (since no ionization-dose conversion is needed), but they should not be used for PDD measurements in a photon beam due to their energy response. Special diode designs are also available for measurements in electron beams. Diamond detectors[13] are very similar to diodes both in size and in their physical characteristics as solid state semiconductor radiation detectors. The major reason diamond detectors have not been adopted into widespread clinical use compared to diodes is limited commercial availability and price. Another type of solid-state detector, the MOSFET, is not useful for commissioning due to its short lifetime.

Point dose measurements to measure output factors can also be performed using alanine gel pellets.[14] Alanine gel is nearly water equivalent and can therefore be used over a wide range of x-ray energies. Like thermoluminescence dosimeters (TLD) and optically stimulated luminescence dosimeters (OSLD), alanine pellets can be used for dosimetry verification by accredited dosimetry laboratories.[13] Because of the well-known energy response and low energy dependency in the therapeutic range, alanine dosimetry is often used as the "gold standard" for studying energy-dependent detector response.

The uncertainty of alanine dosimetry is on the order of 1.7%.[15] TLD and OSLD detectors are used by Accredited Dosimetry Calibration Laboratory (ADCL)-accredited dosimetry labs, the Imaging and Radiation Oncology Core (IROC) QA Center Houston, and the IAEA for dosimetric verification of beam calibration. Because of their small size, they can be used to measure output factors as well. The measurement uncertainty for a well-maintained and calibrated TLD/OSLD system is around 3%. While TLDs and OSLDs are typically not used for commissioning measurements per se, they can be very useful as an in-house secondary dosimetry system to perform a cross-check of reference dosimetry calibrations on output factor measurements in small fields. AAPM TG-191 (in progress) will provide recommendations on the use of OSLD for dosimetry.

## 2D AND 3D DOSIMETERS

Radiographic and radiochromic film are the highest resolution 2D dosimeters available. AAPM TG-69[16] contains information and recommendations on the use of radiographic film. Because many applications for film imaging have been replaced by electronic portal imaging devices (EPIDs), the maintenance of a dark room and film processor for radiographic film processing has increased the cost of radiographic film QA, and most institutions no longer have a functioning processor. Availability of radiographic film from manufacturers is becoming increasingly limited. Therefore, many clinical physicists have or are in the process of switching relative dosimetry measurements to radiochromic film.

AAPM TG-55[17] is an older publication describing the properties, use, and handling of radiochromic film for clinical dosimetry. This will be updated by the forthcoming AAPM TG-235.[18] Chapter 23 of the 2009 AAPM Summer School Conference Proceedings[13] contains more recent information on radiochromic film. AAPM TG-235 will update the recommendations published in AAPM TG-55. Radiochromic film offers the distinct advantage of easy handling, since short exposure to visible light is acceptable and film can easily be cut to the desired size and shape. The disadvantages include relatively high cost, nonuniformity of response across the film caused by nonuniformity of the scanner light at the scan edges, and dose dependence based on film orientation. Accurate dosimetry using radiochromic film requires the following steps:

1. Shipping, handling, and storage within the manufacturer's recommended temperature range and shielded from light sources.
2. A high-end document flatbed scanner capable of scanning in the appropriate spectral range defined by the film. Commissioning includes establishing the equal light intensity area to avoid introduction of systematic offsets due to changes in the light field at the edges of the scan area.
3. Establishing the background density for each film batch by scanning a nonirradiated film. Though, see below for a three-color channel technique that may eliminate the need for this.
4. For each film batch, a step-wedge or multiple film irradiation scan to establish the optical density curve.
5. Film should be scanned at a defined time interval after irradiation to avoid introducing systematic errors due to postirradiation color change.

A protocol has been reported for using radiochromic film that relies on the relative response of three color channels, thereby minimizing the effects of film variations and artifacts and eliminating the need to scan film prior to irradiation.[19]

An alternative to film is 2D detector arrays, which consist of chambers or diodes arranged in a symmetric pattern. They are often used for relative dosimetry measurement as part of a daily or monthly QA to check field flatness and symmetry, as well as wedge factors. Because of the physical distance between detectors, 2D arrays do not yet have the resolution to accurately measure the beam penumbra for relative dosimetry during commissioning. However, they can be used in the commissioning of dynamic deliveries such as dynamic wedges. A recent study[20] using liquid-filled ionization chambers in the array shows the possibility of increasing the resolution of arrays. A summary of commonly used detector arrays is found in Chapter 5, Table 5.6.

The use of EPID dosimetry and plastic scintillators is a more recent development in 2D dosimetry, promising to resolve the resolution issue of other 2D arrays. EPID dosimetry is at this time the more developed technology of those two detector types. Commercially available EPIDs typically have pixel sizes of around 0.4 mm, with active areas of up to 40 cm$^2$. While EPID use is actively being developed and used for transit dosimetry in pretreatment IMRT QA, its use in relative dosimetry has not been established. Reasons for this are issues with support arm back-scatter, pixel sensitivity, and the lack of or limited panel position flexibility to change SSD.

3D dosimetry can be performed using polymer gels. However, no society recommendations exist on the use of polymer gels for relative dosimetry measurements. Since the detector has potential for rapid acquisition of multiple beam parameters (OF (output factor), PDD, and OARs (off-axis ratios) in one exposure), an increase in use can be expected for routine relative dosimetry QA measurements (Table 2.1).

## 2.3 Best Practice for Beam Scanning

Raw beam data contain artifacts created by water ripples caused by detector/mechanical move-ment near the surface, detector noise, and mechanical uncertainties. Beam data processing is intended to remove these artifacts. Because data processing such as smoothing and making data symmetric can in turn introduce uncertainties, it is best practice to keep the processing to the absolute minimum necessary. To acquire high quality raw beam data, time and attention must be dedicated to the setup of the beam scanning system.

For all measurements, the gantry must be level to the water surface prior to making measure-ments. The machine is aligned as vertically as possible first using a scale, then optical beam CAX indicators if available. In the next step, the radiation CAX alignment is verified by scanning cross-beam profiles at two different depths (e.g., 5 cm and 30 cm). Modern water scanner soft-ware often has a built-in tool for the CAX vertical check. Figure 7 in AAPM TG-106 (Figure 2.1) demonstrates the effects of scanning arm tilt on beam profiles.

For defining the surface position by using the detector reflection at the water surface (Figure 2.2), it is important to move the detector toward the water surface from below to minimize the effect of surface tension. A drop of liquid soap or dishwashing detergent can aid in minimiz-ing water tension. When taking beam data over an extended timeframe, such as the days or weeks required for commissioning, water evaporation is not negligible and can be as large as 1 mm/day. It is therefore required to check the setup on at least a daily basis to verify that the water surface, source-to-surface distance (SSD), and other parameters relative to the water surface are still within the desired tolerance levels.

An often overlooked part of the water tank setup process is ensuring that the motion axes move the detector in parallel to the water surface and that the axes of motion are orthogonal. This can be accomplished by setting the detector to water surface level at one side of the tank and scanning across the width of the tank. See Figure 2.2 (Figure 6 of AAPM TG-106) for a useful illustration of this.

In summary, the order of water tank and detector setup should be:

1. Carefully align the water phantom and beam gantry with each other. The water phantom motion axes should be aligned to the accelerator $x$ and $y$ axes (in IEC coordinates). The accelerator should be at 0 degrees as accurately as possible.

TABLE 2.1 ■ Dosimeter Summary

| | | Farmer | SRS Chamber | Diode | Diamond | Alanine | TLD/OSLD | Parallel Plate | Extrapolation | Film | Polymer Gel |
|---|---|---|---|---|---|---|---|---|---|---|---|
| **OF (photon)** | Large field | +++ | + | - | +++ | +++ | ++ | - | - | + | - |
| | Small field | - | ++ | + | +++ | +++ | ++ | - | - | + | + |
| | Very small field | - | - | + | +++ | +++ | ++ | - | - | + | + |
| **OF (electron)** | | + | + | + | + | + | + | + | - | + | No data |
| **PDD** | | +++ | - | - (Photons) + (Electrons) | +++ | - | - | - (Photons) + (Electrons) | - | + | - |
| **Buildup Region** | | no | - | + | + | - | - | ++ | - | + | + |
| **Surface Dose** | | - | - | - | - | - | - | + With correction factors | +++ | + | + |

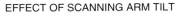

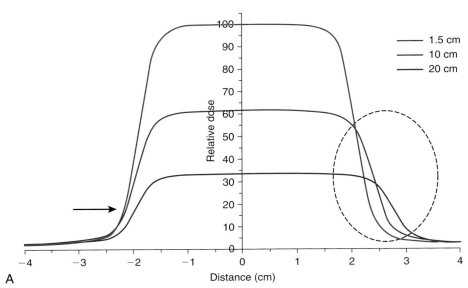

A

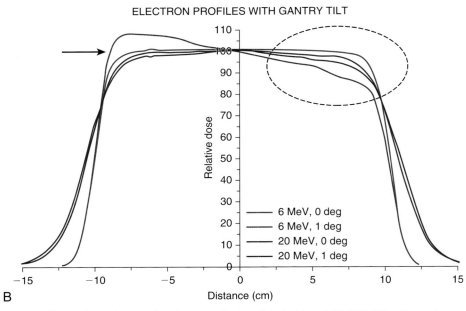

B

**Figure 2.1** Effects of scanning arm tilt on beam profile data. *(Adapted from AAPM TG-106, with permission.)*

2. Verify the accuracy of setup parameters several times, especially if extended time of data acquisition in a water tank is needed. Evaporation can change the location of the water surface on the order of 1 mm or more per day.
3. Accurately set up and level the water tank and mechanical motion axes.
4. Carefully set the locations for water surface, beam central axis, and CAX vertical correction as discussed in the preceding paragraphs.

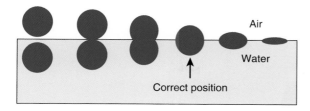

**Figure 2.2** Using the detector reflection at the water surface to define the correct surface position. It is essential to approach the water surface from below to minimize the effect of surface tension. *(Adapted from AAPM TG-106, with permission.)*

5. Use the minimum possible length of cable in the beam.
6. Set the scan speed such that the disturbance of the water surface is kept to a minimum, especially at low scan depths for OARs.
7. Adjust the scan speed to the dose rate such that good detector signal-to-noise ratio is present at the low signal locations of the beam (e.g., PDD at depth, region beyond penumbra for OAR).
8. Set the scan data point spacing small enough to accurately measure high gradient regions of the beam shape.

Scanning technique also influences the data quality in the penumbra region. For best results, the following scan parameters should be set for the penumbra region:

- The scan speed should be slow enough to allow for adequate signal-to-noise ratio through the whole range of dose rates in the penumbra region.
- Scan data points should be spaced closely to well define the shoulders and inversion point (used for FWHM determination).
- The scan must be extended 5-10 centimeters beyond the penumbra.

## 2.4 Relative Dosimetry Measurements

### REFERENCE DETECTOR POSITIONING

For PDD, OAR, and some TPR measurements, a reference detector has been used to eliminate uncertainties caused by instability of the beam output over the time of measurement. While AAPM TG-106[5] still recommends the use of a reference detector, most modern linacs have achieved good enough output stability to ensure that good quality reference data can be acquired without the use of a reference detector (unpublished private communication). Until published data are available, best practice remains for a reference detector to be used. There are four possible locations to place a reference detector, as shown in Figure 2.3. The traditional placement is inside the measured field as shown for Reference Detector 2, either in air or in water toward the surface of the water phantom. For small fields, this placement can introduce perturbation of the field or shadowing of the field detector, which is especially a concern for OAR measurements. The best alternative is to place the reference detector in a dedicated position above the secondary collimators as shown for Reference Detector 1, which requires the linac head to be engineered to provide a space for a reference detector. A good alternative if access to the accelerator head is not available is to place the reference detector at the bottom of the water tank below the field detector, as shown for Reference Detector 4. The divergence of the field creates a larger beam cross-section in which to place the reference detector with easier avoidance of detector overlap or field perturbation compared to Reference Detector 2. AAPM TG-106[5] specifically states that a reference detector should not be placed outside the primary beam (Reference Detector 3) because the low amount of scatter would lead to a low signal-to-noise ratio for the reference detector. The amount of detector cable in the beam should be minimized as much as possible.

The direction of scanning is important. For depth dose scans it is best to scan from the deepest depth up to the surface to minimize water tension effects. Profile scans should typically be acquired using the highest resolution dimension of the detector (the exception being for diodes

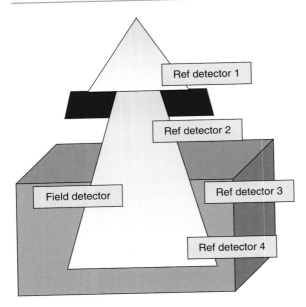

**Figure 2.3** Possible reference detector locations: (1) above secondary collimators, (2) in field, (3) outside of field, (4) at bottom of field.

where angular dependence effects dictate the diode be irradiated "end on"). This will increase the scanning time but will produce more accurate data if required. See Chapter 4 for more details.

## OUTPUT FACTORS/TOTAL SCATTER FACTORS (IN WATER)

The OF or total scatter factor ($S_{cp}$) is defined as the output rate for field size $x$, normalized to the reference field size. In most accelerators, the reference field size is 10 cm × 10 cm; the machine-specific reference field[21] is used in small field dosimetry.

For measuring the output factor, the detector needs to be centered on the CAX of the radiation beam. The clinical procedure is to first visually align the center of the detector with the beam CAX laser or the light field cross-hairs. Because the tolerance of optical CAX indicators to the beam CAX is <1 mm and the active detector volume may vary slightly within the detector housing, this visual alignment has to be fine-tuned by using cross-profile scans. Most water phantoms have the functionality to perform cross-profile scans, determine the beam CAX in each direction, and shift the detector to the measured beam CAX. The cross-profile scan–based detector CAX position adjustment should be iterated until the detector is positioned within 0.1 mm of the beam CAX.

For the choice of detector used to measure output factors, several physical characteristics of the beam have to be considered. The *energy spectrum* of the beam changes as the field size changes. Therefore, the detector response should have low dependency on beam energy. The *smallest field size* to be measured determines the maximum dimensions of the detector that can be used without introducing errors due to volume averaging in the center of the field. This effect is even more important for OF measurements in small FFF beams. The paper published by Araki[11] demonstrates an output factor deviation of 1.3% for a typical Farmer chamber in a 6 cm diameter FFF beam.

There are several possible approaches for OF measurements across a very wide range of beam sizes. Typically, a detector such as a Farmer-type chamber or other ionization chamber is used to measure OF from the maximum field size down to a minimum field size of about 4 cm × 4 cm. Below this field size, smaller detectors such as small volume ionization chambers, diodes, or diamond detectors offer the small detector size needed for small field OF measurements. The 4 cm × 4 cm field size is a good choice for cross-calibrating, or daisy-chaining, the measured OF of the large fields to the small field OF measurements, since the energy change from the 4 cm × 4 cm field to the smallest field size is minimized if diodes are used. Small-volume ionization chambers, on the other hand, may not be suitable for OF measurement in large fields, because the ratio of irradiated stem to detector volume is large.

For very small fields (i.e., fields below 2 cm × 2 cm field size) the energy spectrum changes significantly enough to affect the energy response of both chambers and diodes. Very recently, this has led to Monte Carlo studies and comparisons of OF measured with gel to determine correction factors for detector response to small field size irradiation conditions. Examples of this work are publications by Francescon et al.,[22] Gago-Arias et al.,[15] and Benmakhlouf et al.[23] Detector correction factors are specific to one type of detector used in a specific treatment beam.

Drawing a comparison to the introduction of new sources in brachytherapy,[24] ideally there would be two independent peer-reviewed publications for a detector correction factor that could be averaged before applying it to measured data. At this time, since the field is still in its infancy, these types of data are not available yet. Therefore, the best approach in clinical practice is to measure OF using two different detectors that either have opposite energy dependence or for both of which correction factors have been published. Both AAPM TG-155 on Small Field Dosimetry and the IAEA Working Group on Small Field Dosimetry have documents under preparation to review published detector correction factors and offer recommendations.

Electron output factors are defined as the ratio of the dose per MU at depth $d_{max}$ for the measured field to the dose per MU at $d_{max}$ for the reference field. The reference field is typically chosen to be the 10 cm × 10 cm open cone. Because $d_{max}$ for electrons changes as a function of field size, becoming shallower as the field gets smaller and reaches the range of electronic equilibrium, the PDD for smaller electron fields must be measured to determine the measurement depth for the OF measurement.

Electron OFs are typically measured at commissioning for all energies, all available open cones, all standard clinical square and circular cutouts, and SSDs of 100 cm, 105 cm, and 110 cm. TPS with electron MC capabilities may require additional OF measurements. For custom cutouts that are relatively close in shape to rectangular or square standard cutouts, OF can be interpolated using computational models based on measurements of standard field PDD and OF. AAPM TG-25 covers basic computational methods, while AAPM TG-70 discusses the more recent developments including uncertainties of the OF calculation models. For very irregular custom cutouts, the OF should be measured on a per-patient basis if the field shapes differ too much from the standard cutout shapes that computational models cannot be applied. In addition, the depth of $d_{max}$ should be verified. Since irregularity cannot easily be quantified, in clinical practice it is customary to measure a range of individual patient cutout shapes until a custom library is developed to provide a range of data for comparison.

On occasion, electron fields need to be shaped such that the central axis is blocked. For these fields, the detector should be placed in the center of the open field section of the cutout. For very irregular fields (e.g., fields with a large open area and a long narrow section), at least two sets of measurements should be made: in the center of the large open area and in the narrow area. Film can also be used to obtain a 2D plot of dose variation across the area. It is then a clinical decision for the physician how to adjust the MU to obtain the desired dose distribution for the patient. Figure 2.4 shows examples of a field shape with central axis coverage and a highly irregular field shape.

AAPM TG-70 on clinical electron beam dosimetry provides a rule of thumb for when the electron fields are too small/narrow. A custom measurement must be made if:

$$\text{field radius} \leq 0.88\sqrt{\bar{E}_0} \text{ cm,}$$

where $\bar{E}_0$ denotes the mean incident energy at the surface of the phantom.

| Recommended Field Sizes for Custom Measurements (AAPM TG-70) | | | | | |
|---|---|---|---|---|---|
| $\bar{E}_0$ (MeV) | 6 | 9 | 12 | 15 | 18 |
| Field radius (cm) | 2.2 | 2.6 | 3.1 | 3.4 | 3.7 |

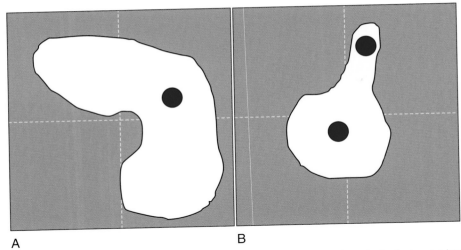

**Figure 2.4** Sample detector locations for electron OF measurements in irregular cutouts. **A** shows a large cutout with the central axis blocked. The OF should be measured at the approximate center of the field. **B** shows a highly irregular field. The OF should be measured at the center of the open sector. A second measurement should be taken in the narrow section to assess the change in OF.

## OUTPUT FACTORS/COLLIMATOR SCATTER FACTORS (IN AIR)

The in-air output factor for photon beams, sometimes also called the "collimator scatter factor," is used in some beam models to better model different contributions of scatter dose in the dose computation models. AAPM TG-74[25] provides a detailed discussion of the theoretical background regarding in-air OFs and develops a protocol to standardize measurement techniques among institutions. Traditionally, build-up caps have been used to increase the detector wall thickness to $d_{max}$ to provide electronic equilibrium. However, this method does not prevent charged particle contamination for higher energy beams. AAPM TG-74 discusses in detail the various mini-phantoms and brass caps that have been developed to find the optimum geometry to generate electronic equilibrium while removing charged particle contamination.

However, some treatment planning systems still use the original method of measuring the in-air OF with $d_{max}$-thickness buildup caps to perform TMR based MU calculations. Therefore, clinical physicists must pay careful attention to the instructions in the TPS manual in determining which experimental setup is required for their respective TPS.

## WEDGE FACTORS AND PROFILES

Dosimetry data acquisition techniques for wedges depend on the type of wedge. For physical wedges and the universal wedges the OARs are measured using the same techniques as for open fields. Profiles are measured along the wedge direction as well as across at the central axes. The across measurement is recommended because increasing angular incidence of the radiation beam on the wedge for large fields may cause "rounding" of the cross-wedge profile. For measuring the wedge transmission factor, the detector is positioned on the central axis, and two sets of measurements are taken with the wedge rotated by 180 degrees between measurements. This technique reduces uncertainties introduced by the uncertainty of aligning the detector to the wedge CAX.

## PDD

For measuring the PDD in FFF, small fields or very small fields, it is essential to get the beam CAX aligned within <0.5° *and* use the water phantom's CAX correction utility. A beam misalignment of 0.5° to the detector vertical motion will cause a deviation of detector versus beam CAX of 0.9 mm at 10 cm depth. Because FFF small fields or very small fields consist predominantly of penumbra, even a small detector CAX to beam CAX misalignment can lead to PDD errors of >5% or more. A misaligned PDD will show as a steeper dose falloff at depth compared to standard data. As the beam hardens with depth, PDD measurements in small fields should be performed with detectors that have low energy dependency.

AAPM TG-51[26] recommends a shift of the PDD curve of $0.6r_{cav}$ for photon beams and $0.5r_{cav}$ for electron beams when the PDD is measured with cylindrical or spherical chambers. No shift is needed for diodes or for parallel plate chamber PDD measurements, because there is no significant beam divergence across the depth of the chamber shifting the effective point of measurement. Several publications[27-29] have studied the effective point of measurement for different chamber types, field sizes, and beam energies both experimentally and using MC simulations. The findings show variability of the effective point of measurement location. Nevertheless, in clinical practice the shift recommended in AAPM TG-51 should be applied until updated recommendations are published. For electron beams the depth-ionization curve must be converted to a depth-dose curve by application of the proper (depth-dependent) stopping power ratios. Most commercial water tank scanners have automatic algorithms for accomplishing this. This correction is not needed if diodes are used.

Special experimental techniques are required to measure the surface dose and PDD for the buildup region accurately. In clinical practice, it is usually well understood that the surface dose as displayed by the TPS carries a large uncertainty. For clinical situations in which accurate dose to superficial structures is required, bolus is typically used to shift the dose distribution toward the skin surface. In addition to increasing the skin dose, this also brings the more accurately measured sections of the PDD toward the skin surface. The exception to this general clinical rule is head and neck patients, where both clinical target and critical structures can be found near the skin surface. Because dose to these superficial structures is a combination of the en-face beam, exit dose from the contralateral beams, and field edge dose from the remaining beam directions, the absolute dose originating from the buildup region of a beam is relatively small. The beam energy used for head and neck patients, as well as for patients in whom bolus is used, is typically the lowest energy photon beam (i.e., 6 MV in most cases). Therefore, if a physicist wishes to perform higher accuracy surface dose and buildup region measurement with a detector different from the one used for the PDD beyond $d_{max}$, the 6 MV beam would be the best choice with regard to clinical impact of the improved accuracy.

Ideally, the surface dose would be measured with an extrapolation chamber. Detector availability and measurement time usually limit this option, especially given the relative clinical significance. The best alternative to using an extrapolation chamber is parallel plate chambers with a small plate separation, thin entrance window, and wide guard ring. The buildup region is characterized by a steep dose gradient, lack of electron equilibrium, and relatively large low energy component of the beam. As always for measurements in steep dose gradient, using a detector with a small dimension in the direction of the gradient will improve the accuracy. The measurement direction for the PDD in the buildup region should always be from $d_{max}$ toward the water surface to avoid issues caused by the water surface tension. For further information on surface dose measurements see AAPM TG-176[30] on the effects of immobilization devices.

To summarize, for PDD measurements, the order of clinical setup is:

1. Vertical alignment of radiation beam using optical CAX indicators and/or mechanical levels
2. Water phantom alignment: overall tank alignment followed by aligning the mechanical axes to the water surface
3. Cross-profile scans to set the detector zero position on the beam CAX at depth
4. Cross-profile scans at two depths (e.g., $d_{max}$ and 20 cm) to determine CAX angle
5. Measure PDD
6. If desired, follow by dedicated surface dose and buildup region measurement for selected energies

According to AAPM TG-70 Recommendations for Clinical Electron Beam Dosimetry,[31] the gold standard for measuring PDD for electrons is an ionization chamber (plane parallel or cylindrical) in a water phantom. The PDD is established by measuring the percent depth–ionization curve and, for cylindrical ion chambers, converting it to a PDD using the equations described in Chapter 1 of this volume. Electron PDDs can also be measured directly using electron diodes, film, or diamond detectors. These detectors should be verified against PDDs measured with ionization chambers first to verify that detector response leads to comparable PDD results. AAPM TG-70[31] provides detailed instructions on the accurate measurement of PDDs using ionization chambers; AAPM TG-25[32] covers PDD measurements using diodes. Film is a very useful dosimeter for clinical PDD measurements in irregular fields. The film is aligned in a solid water phantom with the film parallel to the beam and the edge of the film oriented along the shortest dimension of the field. In addition to PDD, the measurement result will also provide the isodose curves. For matched fields, film can provide PDD information as well as information about the dose overlap in the match region.

The majority of TPS requires PDD beam data, with the exception of TPS for dedicated SRS systems limited to small fields. The reason for this exception is that accurately measuring the PDD is increasingly difficult for small field sizes, especially in FFF beams, because it requires the detector to accurately travel on the radiation beam CAX to depth with a tolerance of <0.2 mm over the whole depth range. **Because of this large uncertainty in PDD measurement for small and very small fields, physicists should not attempt to measure the PDD and then process the beam data using a PDD-to-TPR conversion.** While this method may be acceptable for large field sizes, it will introduce large uncertainty into the TPR data.

Measuring TPR data in a water phantom on a linac is challenging, because it requires both shifting the water tank and the detector very accurately. Therefore, TPR measurements are often done in smaller (i.e., lighter) slabs of water-equivalent material placed on the treatment couch. TPR measurements for the CyberKnife are performed by mounting the detector on a frame fixed to the linac head; the linac can then be driven vertically up and down using the robot to change the detector depth in water. In recent years, special small water phantoms for SRS TPR measurements have become available to make TPR measurements more efficient. Another solution is using water tanks where water can be pumped in or out of the tank automatically; a sensor measuring the water surface position can provide TPR depth.

## OARs

Off-axis ratios (OARs), or beam profiles, are taken at several depths to characterize the beam profile. For square, rectangular, and circular fields, two OARs at a 90-degree angle are usually taken. Other beam shapes (e.g., the hexagonal beam created by the CyberKnife IRIS collimator) require more beam profiles at angles determined by the collimator design. AAPM TG-106 recommends that data NOT be scaled to provide data at different SSDs required in treatment planning systems. This is because the larger projected field size changes scatter conditions and the electron contamination is different at different SSDs. This recommendation does not apply to treatment planning systems that require OARs to be measured under TPR conditions. Clinical physicists should carefully study the specifications for OAR measurement conditions for their respective planning systems.

The most important part of the OAR profile is the 20% to 80% penumbra region, because this section drives the steep dose gradient used for IMRT and SBRT treatments. The penumbra region has several major dosimetric characteristics: steep dose gradient, large change in dose rate, change in beam energy, and lack of lateral electron equilibrium. The detector choice should therefore be focused on small detectors with low dose rate and energy dependence. Several papers and reports discuss the effect of volume averaging as a function of detector resolution for OAR penumbra[5,8,33]; Wuefel[10] shows the effect of volume averaging on the OAR shape of a flattening filter free Guassian-shaped beam. Based on these findings, the detector size should not exceed one third of the 20% to 80% penumbra width.

Even using excellent data acquisition practices, some data processing will still be necessary. Usually this encompasses:

- Smoothing the data to minimize noise; care should be taken in the choice of smoothing parameters to maintain the shape of high dose gradients in the penumbra region.
- Making the OARs symmetric; this reduces the errors introduced by the detector effective measurement point versus beam CAX alignment, or collimator asymmetry.
- For circular fields only, averaging in-line and cross-line OARs; this should not be done for square fields, because the penumbra in particular may be different due to the mechanical differences in the defining collimators.

## 2.5 Safety Considerations

It is essential for reference beam data to be of high quality, because they provide the basis for treating thousands of patients during the lifetime of the treatment delivery machine. An essential safety feature is peer review of relative dosimetry data. AAPM TG-103, Peer Review in Clinical Radiation Oncology Physics,[34] provides guidelines on peer review between two clinical Radiation Oncology physicists; AAPM TG-109 Code of Ethics[35] covers the ethical aspects of the peer-review process.

To facilitate an effective peer-review process, the commissioning report should be completed and available to the reviewing physicist. The commissioning report should contain comparisons of the acquired data sets with published standard data sets. Any deviations from published data by more than 3% should be thoroughly investigated. The complete set of relative dosimetry data should be clearly labeled and saved in a location available to all physicists and can be made available to individuals or organizations involved in peer review. The data must be protected from accidental or intentional changes/modifications and must be securely backed up.

### FOR THE PHYSICIAN

A critical step in accurate radiation treatment of patients is obtaining high quality relative dosimetry data during commissioning. This characterizes the beam data for every patient subsequently irradiated over the lifetime of the treatment machine. AAPM TG-106[5] provides a formula to roughly estimate the time to acquire beam data, but this formula does not include setup and calibration of commissioning equipment, dosimetry data processing for the treatment machine, and other tasks required as part of machine commissioning covered in Chapter 4.

*Equipment*: The physicist will need the appropriate water phantom and measurement detectors to acquire quality data. The equipment should be up-to-date on maintenance, software upgrades, and calibrations as applicable.

*Effort Required*: Because relative dosimetry data acquisition for commissioning is the basis for treatment planning for every patient during the lifetime of a delivery device, this must be done correctly. Especially in smaller clinics with fewer total physics FTE, the physicist must have adequate time to dedicate to relative dosimetry measurements. Because taking commissioning data requires considerable skill, hiring medical physics consultants who perform many relative dosimetry measurements for beam commissioning during a year compared to a resident medical physicist who commissions a new machine only every few years may be the best solution for quality and efficiency.

*Commissioning Report*: An essential safety feature is peer review of relative dosimetry data. The commissioning report should contain comparisons of the acquired data sets with published standard data sets. Any deviations from published data by more than 3% should be thoroughly investigated. The complete set of relative dosimetry data should be clearly labeled and saved in a location available to all physicists and can be made available to individuals or organizations involved in peer review. The data must be protected from accidental or intentional changes/modifications, and must be securely backed up.

*Periodic Dosimetry Measurements*: After commissioning, annual, monthly, and daily QA measurements of a subsection of dosimetry data are used to monitor the consistency of the treatment machine. Statistical process control methods of monitoring data quality can help in discovering and correcting deviations before causing machine downtime or treatment errors. Equipment and time to accomplish these tasks must be available to physicists (monthly, annual) and RTTs (daily) to perform these measurements. The physicist is responsible for designing written procedures and monitoring relative dosimetry measurements for periodic QA as listed in the tables of AAPM TG-40[36] and AAPM TG-142.[2] A review mechanism should be in place to ensure that relative dosimetry measurements are taken in a timely manner, are within tolerance, and any issues discovered during QA are followed up in a timely manner.

## References

1. Kutcher GJ, Coia L, Gillin M, et al. Comprehensive QA for Radiation Oncology: report of AAPM radiation therapy committee task group 40. Medical Physics-Lancaster Pa- 1994;21:581.
2. Klein EE, Hanley J, Bayouth J, et al. Task Group 142 report: Quality assurance of medical accelerators. Med Phys 2009;36(9):4197–212 [Eng]. [Epub 2009/10/09]; PubMed PMID: 19810494.
3. Dieterich S, Cavedon C, Chuang CF, et al. Report of AAPM TG-135: Quality assurance for robotic radiosurgery. Med Phys 2011;38(6):2914–36 [Eng]. PubMed PMID: 21815366.
4. Langen KM, Papanikolaou N, Balog J, et al. QA for helical TomoTherapy: Report of the AAPM Task Group 148. Med Phys 2010;37(9):4817–53 [Eng]. [Epub 2010/10/23]; PubMed PMID: 20964201.
5. Das IJ, Cheng CW, Watts RJ, et al. Accelerator beam data commissioning equipment and procedures: Report of the AAPM TG-106 of the Therapy Physics Committee of the AAPM. Med Phys 2008;35(9):4186–215 [Eng]. [Epub 2008/10/10]; PubMed PMID: 18841871.
6. Herschtal A, Foroudi F, Silva L, et al. Calculating geometrical margins for hypofractionated radiotherapy. Phys Med Biol 2013;58(2):319–33. PubMed PMID: 23257319.
7. van Herk M. Errors and margins in radiotherapy. Semin Radiat Oncol 2004;14(1):52–64. PubMed PMID: 14752733.
8. Aspradakis MM, Byrne JP, Palmans H, et al. Small field MV photon dosimetry. York: Institute of Physics and Engineering in Medicine; 2010. pp. xi, 186.
9. Fraass B, et al. American Association of Physicists in Medicine Radiation Therapy Committee Task Group 53: quality assurance for clinical radiotherapy treatment planning. Med Phys 1998;25(10):1773–829.
10. Wuefel JU. Dose measurements in small fields. Med Phys Int 2013;1(1).
11. Araki F. Monte Carlo study of a CyberKnife stereotactic radiosurgery system. Med Phys 2006;33(8):2955–63 [Eng]. [Epub 2006/09/13]; PubMed PMID: 16964874.
12. Low DA, Moran JM, Dempsey JF, et al. Dosimetry tools and techniques for IMRT. Med Phys 2011;38(3):1313–38.
13. Publishing MP. Clinical dosimetry measurements in radiotherapy (2009 AAPM Summer School). Medical Physics Publishing; 2011.

14. Pantelis E, Moutsatsos A, Zourari K, et al. On the implementation of a recently proposed dosimetric formalism to a robotic radiosurgery system. Med Phys 2010;37(5):2369–79.

15. Gago-Arias A, Rodríguez-Romero R, Sánchez-Rubio P, et al. Correction factors for A1SL ionization chamber dosimetry in TomoTherapy: Machine-specific, plan-class, and clinical fields. Med Phys 2012;39(4):1964–70.

16. Pai S, Das IJ, Dempsey JF, et al. AAPM TG-69: Radiographic film for megavoltage beam dosimetry. Med Phys 2007;34(6):2228–58. PubMed PMID: 17654924.

17. Niroomand-Rad A, Blackwell CR, Coursey BM, et al. Radiochromic film dosimetry: Recommendations of AAPM Radiation Therapy Committee Task Group 55. American Association of Physicists in Medicine. Med Phys 1998;25(11):2093–115 [Eng]. [Epub 1998/11/26]; PubMed PMID: 9829234.

18. Chiu-Tsao ST, et al. Report of AAPM Task Group 235 Radiochromic Film Dosimetry: An Update to TG-55. Med Phys (in review).

19. Micke A, Lewis DF, Yu X. Multichannel film dosimetry with nonuniformity correction. Med Phys 2011;38(5):2523–34.

20. Brualla-González L, Gómez F, Vicedo A, et al. A two-dimensional liquid-filled ionization chamber array prototype for small-field verification: Characterization and first clinical tests. Phys Med Biol 2012;57(16):5221.

21. Alfonso R, Andreo P, Capote R, et al. A new formalism for reference dosimetry of small and nonstandard fields. Med Phys 2008;35(11):5179–86 [Eng]. [Epub 2008/12/17]; PubMed PMID: 19070252.

22. Francescon P, Cora S, Cavedon C. Total scatter factors of small beams: A multidetector and Monte Carlo study. Med Phys 2008;35(2):504–13 [Eng]. [Epub 2008/04/04]; PubMed PMID: 18383671.

23. Benmakhlouf H, Sempau J, Andreo P. Output correction factors for nine small field detectors in 6 MV radiation therapy photon beams: A PENELOPE Monte Carlo study. Med Phys 2014;41(4):041711.

24. Nath R, Anderson LL, Luxton G, et al. Dosimetry of interstitial brachytherapy sources: recommendations of the AAPM Radiation Therapy Committee Task Group No. 43. American Association of Physicists in Medicine. Med Phys 1995;22(2):209–34. No abstract available. Erratum in: Med Phys 1996 Sep;23(9):1579. PubMed PMID: 7565352.

25. Zhu TC, Ahnesjö A, Lam KL, et al. Report of AAPM Therapy Physics Committee Task Group 74: In-air output ratio, Sc, for megavoltage photon beams. Med Phys 2009;36(11):5261–91. PubMed PMID: 19994536.

26. Almond PR, Biggs PJ, Coursey BM, et al. AAPM's TG-51 protocol for clinical reference dosimetry of high-energy photon and electron beams. Med Phys 1999;26(9):1847–70. PubMed PMID: 10505874.

27. Huang Y, Willomitzer C, Zakaria GA, et al. Experimental determination of the effective point of measurement of cylindrical ionization chambers for high-energy photon and electron beams. Phys Med 2010;26(3):126–31. PubMed PMID: 19926506.

28. Looe HK, Harder D, Poppe B. Experimental determination of the effective point of measurement for various detectors used in photon and electron beam dosimetry. Phys Med Biol 2011;56(14):4267 [Eng]. PubMed PMID: 21701053.

29. Wang L, Rogers D. Study of the effective point of measurement for ion chambers in electron beams by Monte Carlo simulation. Med Phys 2009;36(6):2034–42. PubMed PMID: 19610292.

30. Olch AJ, Gerig L, Li H, et al. Dosimetric effects caused by couch tops and immobilization devices: Report of AAPM Task Group 176. Med Phys 2014;41(6):061501.

31. Gerbi BJ, Antolak JA, Deibel FC, et al. Recommendations for clinical electron beam dosimetry: Supplement to the recommendations of Task Group 25. Med Phys 2009;36(7):3239–79. PubMed PMID: 19673223.

32. Khan FM, Doppke KP, Hogstrom KR, et al. Clinical electron-beam dosimetry: Report of AAPM Radiation Therapy Committee Task Group no. 25. Med Phys 1991;18:73–109.

33. Wilcox EE, Daskalov GM. Evaluation of GAFCHROMIC EBT film for Cyberknife dosimetry. Med Phys 2007;34(6):1967–74 [Eng]. [Epub 2007/07/28]; PubMed PMID: 17654899.

34. Halvorsen PH, Das IJ, Fraser M, et al. AAPM Task Group 103 report on peer review in clinical Radiation Oncology physics. J Appl Clin Med Phys 2005;6(4).

35. Serago CF, Adnani N, Bank MI, et al. Code of Ethics for the American Association of Physicists in Medicine: Report of Task Group 109. Med Phys 2009;36(1):213–23.

36. Kutcher GJ, Coia L, Gillin M, et al. Comprehensive QA for Radiation Oncology: Report of AAPM Radiation Therapy Committee Task Group 40. Med Phys 1994;21(4):581–618 [Eng]. [Epub 1994/04/01]; PubMed PMID: 8058027.

CHAPTER 3

# In-Vivo Dosimetry

## 3.1 Introduction

In-vivo dosimetry is used clinically to verify during treatment how accurately the planned dose is delivered to the patient. While American Association of Physicists in Medicine (AAPM) TG-62, Diode In-Vivo Dosimetry for Patients Receiving External Beam Radiation Therapy,[1] sees in-vivo dosimetry as supplementary to a good clinical QA program, more recent developments in understanding failure modes in treatment delivery and adaptive radiotherapy have led to increased attention to the safety and quality gains an in-vivo dosimetry program can generate with relatively low cost per patient.

In-vivo dosimeters can be roughly divided into three categories:

1. **Surface dosimeters** (thermoluminescent dosimeter (TLD), optically stimulated luminescent dosimeter (OSLD), diode, metal-oxide-semiconductor field-effect transistor (MOSFET)) are placed on the patient surface to measure entrance beam dose in 2D and 3D conformal plans. They can also be used more generally to verify skin dose in anatomically critical areas (e.g., above scars or on the contralateral breast). Sometimes these dosimeters have also been used for intracavitary applications.
2. **Implantable dosimeters** were designed to verify dose in situ, both for treatment targets and critical structures. Due to their size, radiographic properties, and the invasive process of placing them, the use of implantable dosimeters has been largely abandoned in favor of transmission dosimetry.
3. **Transmission dosimeters** are fluence detectors that can be placed either immediately downstream of the tertiary collimator or distal to the beam exit from the patient.

In-vivo dosimetry serves four purposes:

1. For patient-specific QA, in-vivo dosimetry is used to confirm the treatment delivery is within the tolerance specified in the policy and procedure (P&P). In-vivo dosimetry can be performed with a diode, an implantable dosimeter, or via a transmission dosimetry system such as an EPID (Electronic Portal Imaging Device). The results of the measurements should be reviewed on a regular basis, usually during weekly chart checks, unless the results are processed and user alerts generated through software analysis. For dosimeters with instant readout (diode, MOSFET) an expected range should be given to the therapists to alert them immediately to any unexpected dose.
2. In addition to patient-specific QA, diodes double up as delivery QA (DQA) for 2D and 3D conformal treatments. Originally, they were intended to find gross errors such as missing or incorrect wedge, setup errors involving source-to-surface distance (SSD) or couch, and errors in manually entered treatment parameters. With the implementation of accessory interlocks, couch tolerance tables, and automated R&V systems using checksum algorithms to verify data transfer as recommended in the International Electrotechnical Commission (IEC) report Medical Electrical Equipment—Requirements for the Safety of Radiotherapy Treatment Planning Systems,[2] the DQA function of diodes has become less safety critical over the past decade.
3. For DQA in intensity modulated radiation therapy (IMRT) or volumetric modulated arc therapy (VMAT) fields, in-vivo dosimetry is performed using transmission dosimetry with

devices downstream of the tertiary collimator. It can be understood as a continuation of the pretreatment DQA, which is customary in IMRT. As such, its use may become more frequent as adaptive planning and rapid dose calculations move into the clinic.

4. In-vivo dosimetry with surface dosimeters is performed where TPS calculations and/or setup uncertainties cause large uncertainties in surface dose that is relevant for clinical outcome.

The European Society for Radiotherapy and Oncology (ESTRO) booklet on methods for in-vivo dosimetry[5] provides a thorough description and references for the surface dosimeters described in Section 2 of this chapter and some detectors used for implantable dosimeters described in Section 4. The International Atomic Energy Agency (IAEA) Human Health Report No. 8, Development of Procedures for In Vivo Dosimetry in Radiotherapy,[6] also gives detailed description of detector technology. It also describes the process of implementing in-vivo dosimetry and reports on results of a pilot program in six countries and four continents.

## 3.2 Clinical Process

### SYSTEM IMPLEMENTATION

The IAEA recommends[6] a qualified medical physicist (QMP) to be the main party responsible for setting up and supervising an in-vivo dosimetry program. To establish a quality clinical process, input from physicians as to setting appropriate clinical action levels is required. In addition, therapy staff should be involved in evaluating the in-vivo dosimetry system for ease and practicality of use in daily clinical practice. The IAEA[6] provides a sample flow chart for setting up the process, which could be adapted into a clinical procedure.

The commissioning process of any in-vivo dosimetry system should characterize the detector performance for the range of parameters encountered in clinical use. The calibration and measurement of correction factors are typically performed in solid water. For the verification process, measurements of standard beams incident on an anthropomorphic phantom should be followed by verification in clinically used patient plans on an anthropomorphic phantom. Table 3.2 provides a short summary of commissioning tests.

### ESTABLISHING ACTION LEVELS/STATISTICAL PROCESS CONTROL

Tolerance levels and action levels need to be defined so that they are clinically as well as technically meaningful. The International Commission on Radiation Units and Measurements (ICRU)[7] defined 5% deviation from the planned dose as an acceptable action limit, which was re-emphasized by AAPM TG-40, Comprehensive QA for Radiation Oncology.[8] With this in mind, the IAEA[6] set 5% as the action limit for their pilot study of in-vivo dosimetry. It is established clinical practice to define a tolerance level below the action level, which serves as a signal in the QA review process that critical parameters may be trending toward the action limit. This tolerance level is different for each clinic based on the available equipment and user expertise. The standard industry method to define a site-specific appropriate tolerance level is statistical process control. Sanghangthum et al.[9] describe how to implement this method for medical physics applications. Further information about statistical process control can be found in Chapter 12.3.

## 3.3 Surface Dosimeters

### PURPOSE AND CALIBRATION

Surface dosimeters are used to measure patient entrance and exit dose, although the latter is rarely done because of the difficulty in placing a detector reliably and comfortably underneath a patient.

TABLE 3.1 ▦ Characteristics of In-Vivo Dosimeters

| Type | Dosimeter | Dose | Energy Dependence | Readout Time | Price | Best Achievable Uncertainty | Handling |
|---|---|---|---|---|---|---|---|
| **Surface Dosimeter** | TLD | 1D | No (MV therapy range) Yes (HDR[3]) | 1-24 hr | $ | 3% | + No cable + Small size |
| | OSLD | 1D | No (MV photons and electrons) Yes[4] (kV range, LET dependent for protons/carbon) | Immediate | $ | 3% | |
| | Diode | 1D | Yes | Immediate | $$ | 2% | |
| | MOSFET | 1D | Yes | Immediate | $$ | 3% | |
| **Implantable Dosimeter** | | 1D | Yes | Immediate | N/A | 3% | |
| **Transmission Dosimeter** | EPID | 2D/3D | | Immediate | Included in linac | | Not ready for clinical practice |
| | PMH technology | 2D | | Immediate | $$$ | | Under development |
| | Others | 2D | | Immediate | $$$ | | |

**TABLE 3.2 ▦ List of Measurements Recommended for Clinically Commissioning an In-Vivo Dosimetry System**

| | | |
|---|---|---|
| Calibration | TLD: Individual or batch calibration factors<br>MOSFET/OSLD: Verification of manufacturer calibration within clinically used dose range | 2-4 hours |
| Correction Factors | Dosimeter-specific correction factors (dose linearity, fading, energy response, dose rate)<br>Beam dependent correction factors (SSD, field size, compensators, angle of incidence) | 4-8 hours |
| Verification | Performed in anthropomorphic phantom<br>1st step: use of standard beam (e.g., 6 MV 10 cm² field at 100 cm SSD)<br>2nd step: use of patient plans | 2-6 hours |

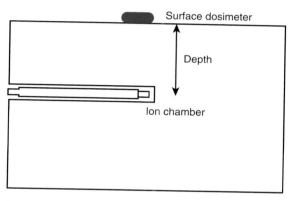

**Figure 3.1** Calibration setup for an in-vivo dosimeter used to infer dose at depth. The in-vivo dosimeter readings are cross-calibrated to the dose measured by a second dosimeter placed at depth in a phantom.

Surface dosimeters for in-vivo DQA can be classified into two purposes: (1) measurement of skin dose and (2) measurement of surface dose to infer dose at depth.

Historically, measurement of surface dose to infer dose at depth for 2D and 3D conformal treatments was the predominant use of in-vivo dosimetry. With modern record & verify (R&V) systems, the advent of multi-leaf collimators (MLCs) for blocking, image-guided setups, the replacement of physical wedges by universal or dynamic wedges, along with more extensive analog and electronic safety systems in place, the routine use of surface dosimeters for depth dose verification has become less common. However, as IAEA Human Health Report No. 8[6] points out, the R&V system only controls the parameters within the software; errors originating from treatment planning or patient setup are not caught.[6,10] Therefore, the IAEA recommends implementing in-vivo dosimetry for every patient.

The measurement of surface dose to infer dose at depth is accepted clinical standard for special procedures and cases such as verifying the correct placement of lead compensators and dose calculation at extended distance in total body irradiation (TBI). In-vivo dosimeters used to infer dose at depth are calibrated in a phantom using a second detector at a predefined depth, usually $d_{max}$. The in-vivo dosimeter readings at the surface are then cross-calibrated to the measured dose at depth (Figure 3.1). To make the detector reading in the high-gradient buildup area more robust, either a buildup cap or small bolus is used. Some diodes have inherent buildup to achieve this purpose.

The use of methods to verify the planned dose to skin is motivated by the large uncertainties of measuring beam data in the buildup region during commissioning and the challenge of modeling the buildup region accurately in treatment planning systems. Skin dose measurement is used to verify dose to surgical scars that need to be irradiated to prevent recurrence from disseminated disease. Dose to the skin in superficial treatments such as total skin electrons (TSET) for mycosis fungoides, melanomas, and tumors invading through the skin are other applications of measuring surface dose. Per ICRU-35,[11] the point of measurement for skin is defined as 0.5 mm below the surface. For very thin surface in-vivo dosimeters, a 0.5 mm buildup such as wax should be used. IAEA Human Health Report No. 8[6] recommends limiting the beam attenuation below the dosimeter to <5% to minimize dose perturbation to the target.

For each detector type, correction factors must be established based on the detector's physical properties. All radiation detectors show nonlinearity of dose response at the low and high ends of the detector range. Therefore, a dose-response curve must be established as part of the in-vivo dosimeter commissioning. Equally, the detector's energy response characteristics must be established through the range of beam energies in which it will be used. Recently, the dose rate of linear accelerators has expanded rapidly. Dose rate response of in-vivo dosimeters through the complete range of clinically available x-ray beams has not been thoroughly studied. Therefore, commissioning of an in-vivo dosimetry system should incorporate careful study of dosimeter response of all available intrinsic beam dose rates, as well as dose rates encountered through the range of SSDs clinically used. The latter is especially important for in-vivo dosimetry of total body irradiation treatments at extended SSDs. Some dosimeters such as TLD and radiochromic film exhibit a change of response as a factor of time to readout. Unless a standardized time interval from measurement to readout can be established, this time-dependent dose response also needs to be characterized.

Two correction factors are dependent on the beam. The first factor is the change of scatter and contaminant electrons reaching the surface dosimeter as beam size or SSD changes. The IAEA recommends assessing the field size and SSD dependence through the clinically expected range of beams; if the correction factors exceed 1%, they should be applied to the clinical measurement. The second factor is the angle-of-incidence correction, which may be needed when measuring steeply sloped incidence angles (e.g., for breast or chest wall treatments). As with the first factor, the IAEA recommends applying this factor only if measurements show that a correction of >1% is needed. Table 3.1 summarizes currently used in-vivo dosimeters and their main characteristics, which are discussed in detail in the following paragraphs.

## THERMOLUMINESCENT DOSIMETERS

There are currently two types of TLD materials used in clinical practice: (LiF:Mg, Ti), which has linear dose response up to 1 Gy and supralinear response >1 Gy, and (LiF:Mg, Cu, P), which has linear dose response up to 10 Gy and sublinear response >10 Gy. During the commissioning process, the dose-linearity curve should be verified within the clinically expected range.

(LiF:Mg, Ti) is less sensitive to thermal treatment than (LiF:Mg, Cu, P), which made it the preferred TLD material choice until programmable ovens to maintain consistent annealing patterns became available. TLDs can be manufactured in many shapes and sizes; powders, cubes, chips, and rods are the most commonly available. Depending on the shape, there may be an angular dependence if the TLD surface is not carefully placed relative to the incident beam angle. Extensive and at times contradictory literature exists on the energy dependence of TLDs. In clinical practice, it is best to measure the dose response for all available beam energies to determine if an energy correction factor may be needed.

The main drawback of TLDs is the decay of lower energy electron traps at room temperature (fading). Three main strategies can be employed clinically to manage the effect of fading on dose measurement accuracy:

1. Reading the TLD within a well-defined time window at a specified time interval after the measurement.
2. Pre-annealing before readout (i.e., heating the TLD using a specified low temperature pattern to force low energy electron trap decay).

3. Reading the TLDs at least 24 hours after measurement, by which time the majority of low energy electrons have decayed.

The readout is performed by subjecting the TLD to a well-defined heating pattern and measuring the luminescence of the resulting glow curves. The low energy glow curves are usually discarded for readout by pre-annealing, fading at room temperature, or electronically subtracting the light output in the low temperature range of the readout curve. To maintain a constant relationship between luminescence and dose, great care must be taken to keep the TLD surface clean and undamaged. TLDs should be handled only with clean tools and/or gloves to avoid surface contamination through oils and cells of the skin. TLDs that are scratched or chipped should also be eliminated from clinical use.

Two calibration methods are used in clinical practice:

1. Each TLD is calibrated individually. Calibration factors are stored in a database and applied at each readout. The advantage is very high accuracy of the dose measurement; the disadvantage is added administrative burden of tracking each individual TLD and the risk of accidentally switching TLDs while handling them.
2. TLDs are calibrated and sorted in batches. For this method, a batch of TLDs is irradiated and divided into smaller batches based on their respective calibration factor. The advantage is easier handling and tracking of batched TLDs; the disadvantage is a slightly larger spread in dose measurement uncertainty, depending on the number of TLDs in the original batch and the spread of dose-response in the sub-batches.

## OPTICALLY STIMULATED LUMINESCENCE DOSIMETERS

Optically stimulated luminescence dosimeters (OSLDs) are made of carbon-doped aluminum oxide ($Al_2O_3$:C) and were first used in personnel dosimetry before being applied in the clinical setting. They are very similar to TLDs in that they are passive dosimeters of small size that can be applied to the range of doses and beam energies encountered in x-ray imaging and therapy. Unlike TLDs, the luminescence for readout of OSLDs does not require heat, only optical stimulation. By carefully setting readout parameters, the depletion of the OSLD signal can be kept to a minimum, thereby enabling near nondestructive, repeat readouts of measured dose. The accuracy and consistency of repeat readouts according to manufacturer's specifications should be verified as part of the OSLD commissioning process. Studies on determining the upper cumulative dose limits are still ongoing and some studies indicate that OSLDs should not be used for repeat irradiation without first photo-bleaching the OSLD in bright light.

## DIODES

AAPM TG-62[1] and Chapter 28 of the 2009 AAPM Summer School[12] provide a summary of silicon diodes used as in-vivo radiation detectors. Diode detectors are small, have a high sensitivity to radiation, and are physically robust, making them very suitable for frequent use in clinical practice.

Change in indirect recombination is the dominant effect that changes diode response, occurring under three conditions: (1) physical or radiation damage of the diode material, (2) increased instantaneous dose rate, and (3) changing temperature. The first is the reason diodes deteriorate with use, leading to a finite lifetime as useful detectors depending on the cumulative radiation dose and energy. The second causes dose rate effects, which may be especially pronounced for linacs with high instantaneous dose rate. Dose rate effects can also be observed in measurements at varying SSDs or with beam attenuators. Indirect recombination is strongly dependent on the detector material. To lower changes in radiation response over the diode lifetime, manufacturers often intentionally introduce defects by doping with metals (e.g., platinum) and/or preirradiating

**TABLE 3.3** ▦ **Recommended Clinical Tests for Diode Material– and Detector Construction–Dependent Characteristics**

| Physical Characteristics | | Clinical Situation | Recommended Test |
|---|---|---|---|
| **Diode Material** | **Dose rate dependence** | SSD dependency | • Measure at commissioning and annually |
| | | Beam modifiers (wedges) | • Measure at commissioning and annually |
| | **Radiation damage** | Decrease in sensitivity | • Vendors should provide estimate for specific beam qualities (AAPM TG-62[1])<br>• Measure at commissioning and annually<br>• Monthly calibration<br>• High energy beams more damaging<br>• P-type diodes generally more resistant than n-type diodes |
| | **Temperature dependence** | Temperature change while diode is in contact with patient | • Measure at commissioning and annually<br>• Typical range 0.1-0.54%/°C (radiation current), 15%/°C (leakage current) (AAPM TG-62[1]) |
| **Detector Construction** | **Directional dependence** | Diode is placed at an angle not normal to the beam CAX | • Vendors should state change in effective sensitivity and conditions (AAPM TG-62[1]) |
| | | Energy dependence | • Use detector designed for energy range and beam quality |
| | | Field size dependence | • Diode at surface has different $S_{c,p}$ compared to $S_{c,p}$ measured at depth<br>• Electron contamination increases with decrease in buildup |
| | | Dose perturbation | • Placement of diode causes dose shadow underneath detector<br>• Photon shadow should not exceed 5-6% in 10 cm × 10 cm field at 5 cm depth (AAPM TG-62[1])<br>• Electron diode shadows ~20% for 6 MeV and 9 MeV |

the diodes. The resulting reduction in diode response is deemed acceptable to gain greater stability in response. Information about a specific diode's behavior is listed in the manufacturer's data sheets and/or published in the scientific literature.

The diode material itself is manufactured into a thin disk called a *die*. The die itself is packaged, often with additional buildup material of varying thickness, depending on the intended beam energy. If diodes are used for in-vivo dosimetry of total body irradiation, the effects of the larger low energy component of the beam at extended SSD must be evaluated. The form factor of the diode itself causes a directional dependence for the diode response, which can be amplified depending on the construction of the buildup. The packaging material can also have an effect on the energy dependence of the diode (Table 3.3).

## MOSFETs

Metal–oxide–semiconductor field-effect transistor (MOSFET) detectors are transistors that can be run in either passive (no voltage applied during measurement) or active (biased) mode. Both modes have been used for in-vivo dosimetry. The advantages of MOSFETs are their small size and real-time readout capabilities similar to diodes. The disadvantage is that MOSFETs do saturate with dose, requiring accurate cumulative dose tracking for multiuse MOSFET systems. Because of this dose saturation, MOSFET detectors are often precalibrated by the manufacturer. Therefore, commissioning measurements are often carefully designed to limit the dose accumulation on the clinical system. Manufacturers also provide upper cumulative dose limits above which the linearity of dose response is not guaranteed. Most MOSFET systems also display temperature dependence, although designs containing dual-bias dual-detector circuits have reduced the temperature effect. The energy and angular dependence of MOSFETs behave very similarly to diodes.

## DIAMOND DETECTORS

Diamond detectors can be manufactured in small sizes and show almost no energy dependence in the energy range encountered in clinical practice. Because of availability and cost, their use has so far been restricted to selected academic centers, and few publications exist reporting on possible applications for in-vivo dosimetry.

# 3.4 Implantable Dosimeters

All in-vivo dosimeters discussed so far provide only one data point either in the entrance or exit surface of the patient. From these, the accuracy of the target dose is inferred. Implantable dosimeters are designed to directly measure dose in the target. For targets surrounding cavities (e.g., esophageal cancer), surface dosimeters in waterproof packaging can be used. A similar technique—implanting and later removing the dosimeters via surgery—has been used for animal research, but this approach is clearly prohibitive in clinical practice for humans. The systems that were on the market have been discontinued and currently, no implantable dosimetry system is commercially available.[13]

# 3.5 Transmission Dosimeters

Transmission dosimeters were developed to give 2D or, with dose reconstruction algorithms, 3D dosimetry information. They can be used for 3D conformal, IMRT and VMAT treatments. Transmission dosimeters fall into two general categories: (1) those mounted on the gantry downstream from the MLC measuring entrance dose to the patient and (2) transmission dosimeters measuring exit dose from the patient.

## PATIENT ENTRANCE FLUENCE

Patient entrance dose transmission dosimeters are mounted using the accessory mounts for electron cones or accessory trays. Because they have to be removed for other accessories, they have to be constructed within a reasonable weight limit for the therapist to lift and also be fairly robust to handling. Entrance dose transmission dosimeters are used to verify dose before entering the patient (i.e., their purpose is for machine QA).

## PATIENT EXIT DOSE: ELECTRONIC PORTAL IMAGING DEVICES

EPIDs are used as patient exit dose transmission dosimeters in addition to their primary purpose for imaging. The electronic components of the EPID are radiation sensitive to direct beam, which limits the maximum permissible field size for EPID dosimetry to the active area of the amorphous silicon detector. The advantage of exit dose in-vivo dosimetry over entrance dose in-vivo dosimetry is the added information on the fluence loss in the patient. However, this also makes it more complicated to distinguish machine delivery errors from uncertainties introduced by patient setup errors and respiratory motion.

**FOR THE PHYSICIAN**

With increasing spotlight on radiation therapy errors in recent years, there has been rising interest in the utilization of in-vivo dosimetry as another step in the QA process. The IAEA Human Health Report No. 8[6] concludes:

> Until recently, the routine clinical implementation of in vivo dosimetry has been quite limited in many radiotherapy centres. However, there is growing interest in establishing in vivo dosimetry programmes. This has been partially triggered by a recent series of radiotherapy accidents in industrialized countries [20] that would have been avoided if such programmes were in place. It is believed that the present publication provides suitable guidance for the preparation and implementation of in vivo dosimetry programmes for stationary techniques in radiotherapy. Once established, in vivo dosimetry constitutes a QA tool that may help to reduce the number of misadministrations of dose to radiotherapy patients. To conclude, in vivo dosimetry is a suitable tool to detect errors in radiotherapy, to assess clinically relevant differences between the prescribed and delivered doses, to document doses received by individual patients, and to fulfil requirements set forth by some national regulations.

In-vivo dosimetry has two main goals: (1) prevent gross misadministration and (2) compare the calculated surface dose to measured surface dose in special clinical scenarios. Examples of special scenarios include match lines for matched electron beams, craniospinal irradiation (CSI) treatments, and surface dose verification for TBI and TSE treatments. In-vivo dosimetry systems such as TLD, OSLD, MOSFETs, or diodes can measure point dose at the surface. Therefore, they are predominantly applied in 3D conformal treatments for safety purposes (to infer dose at depth from surface dose) and in IMRT or electron treatments for point surface dose measurements. Their use adds about 5 to 10 minutes to the patient setup time. Typical clinical tolerances are 5% for routine quality and safety measurements. For clinical surface dose measurements, there is usually no specifically stated tolerance. The physicist will provide the physician with a written physics consult report stating planned dose, measured dose, and estimates of uncertainty of surface dose measurement from the beam commissioning and treatment planning systems. Based on this information, the physician will use clinical judgment on whether the measured dose variance is acceptable or if treatment modifications are indicated.

At least one in-vivo dosimetry system should be available in each radiation therapy department. The selection of the system should be based on recommendations and findings from the IAEA report, as well as applicable AAPM reports such as AAPM TG-62[1] on in-vivo dosimetry using diodes. Physicists, therapists, and physicians should have input on clearly defined policies and procedures on the use of in-vivo dosimetry. The physicist will be in charge of commissioning and maintaining quality assurance for the in-vivo system.

Technical developments are under way to develop in-vivo dosimetry systems that are more automated and can also be applied to IMRT and VMAT deliveries. One approach is to mount a transmission chamber on the accelerator head just below the MLC to measure fluence. This system will be able to catch errors in the MLC pattern or delivered MU/fraction but cannot detect errors in patient setup (SSD, shifts). Another disadvantage is that it needs to be dismounted for treatments requiring external compensators (wedges, blocks) or electron cones. The second approach is to use the EPID to measure exit fluence from the patient. Although this method will put an extra radiation dose on the EPID, which may lead to more rapid aging, it can detect most errors in patient setup and machine delivery. One limit of EPID use is in very large fields, which might irradiate the EPID electronics.

In summary, in-vivo dosimetry is useful for surface measurements in selected clinical situations and as an essential safety feature to prevent errors in clinical practice. As more automated in-vivo dosimetry systems become available, their routine use for every patient and every fraction will add another layer of safety and quality verification to treatment delivery.

## References

1. Yorke E, Alecu R, Ding L, et al. Diode in vivo dosimetry for patients receiving external beam radiation therapy, Report of Task Group 62, Madison, WI: AAPM, 2005.
2. I.E. Commission, Medical electrical equipment—Requirements for the safety of radiotherapy treatment planning systems, Geneva, IEC standard 62083, 2000.
3. Tedgren ÅC, Elia R, Hedtjärn H, et al. Determination of absorbed dose to water around a clinical HDR [192]Ir source using LiF: Mg, Ti TLDs demonstrates an LET dependence of detector response. Med Phys 2012;39:1133–40.
4. Reft CS. The energy dependence and dose response of a commercial optically stimulated luminescent detector for kilovoltage photon, megavoltage photon, and electron, proton, and carbon beams. Med Phys 2009;36:1690–9.
5. ESTRO, Mijnheer B, editors. Guidelines for the verification of IMRT, E-booklet no. 9. 2008. <http://www.estro.org/binaries/content/assets/estro/school/publications/booklet-9—guidelines-for-the-verification-of-imrt.pdf>; ESTRO ISBN 90-804532-9.
6. Development of procedures for in vivo dosimetry in radiotherapy. 2013.
7. ICRU. Report No. 24. Determination of absorbed dose in a patient irradiated by beams of X or gamma rays in radiotherapy procedures. Int Commission on Radiation Units and Measurements, Bethesda, MD (1976).
8. Kutcher GJ, Coia L, Gillin M, et al. Comprehensive QA for Radiation Oncology: Report of AAPM Radiation Therapy Committee Task Group 40. Med Phys 1994;21:581–618.
9. Sanghangthum T, Suriyapee S, Kim G-Y, et al. A method of setting limits for the purpose of quality assurance. Phys Med Biol 2013;58:7025.
10. Ford EC, Gaudette R, Myers L, et al. Evaluation of safety in a Radiation Oncology setting using failure mode and effects analysis. Int J Radiat Oncol Biol Phys 2009;74:852–8.
11. ICRU. Electron beams with energies between 1 and 50 MeV. Bethesda, MD, ICRU Report 35, 1984.
12. Zhu T, Saini A. Diode dosimetry for megavoltage electron and photon beams. In: Clinical Dosimetry Measurements in Radiotherapy. DWO Rogers, JE Cygler (eds.) Medical Physics Publishing, Madison, WI, Medical Physics Monograph No. 34; 2009. p. 913–39.
13. Gardner EA, et al. In vivo dose measurement using TLDs and MOSFET dosimeters for cardiac radio-surgery. J Appl Clin Med Phys 2012;13(3).

# CHAPTER 4

# Quality Assurance and Commissioning of New Radiotherapy Technology

## 4.1 Introduction

Comprehensive acceptance testing and commissioning of new equipment are the foundations for the safe implementation of new technology in a Radiation Oncology department. Once the unit is in clinical use, a routine quality assurance (QA) program must be followed to ensure that the unit continues to perform within acceptable limits. Many of the QA tests will rely on establishing baseline values at the time of commissioning. Beyond verifying the functionality and performance of the equipment, the staff who operate the equipment must be properly trained and evaluated for competence. Clear policy and procedures must be developed prior to clinical use to ensure that all staff members understand the use of the equipment and their role in the clinical process.

The next section discusses precommissioning and equipment purchase considerations. Following that are three sections describing the acceptance testing, commissioning, and QA of different types of equipment: treatment units, imaging units, and ancillary equipment. There is some overlap with treatment planning systems, which is covered in Chapter 5. Section 4.6 is a brief discussion of the QA of data transfer followed by sections on QA program evaluation and future directions in QA.

## 4.2 Precommissioning Considerations and Equipment Purchase

Prior to the equipment purchase, there are important considerations to match the functionality to clinical need. It is helpful to develop a detailed request for proposal (RFP) containing the capabilities desired so that various systems can be compared. Table 4.1 shows a sample list for a linac purchase. It is important to note the request to the vendor for a document of failure mode analysis. The availability of such a document will be helpful in designing procedures and QA processes. This list is in addition to the standard compilation of mechanical and beam parameter specifications. The International Electrotechnical Commission (IEC) has described suggested performance specifications.[1] If specifications different from the manufacturer values are desired, they must be outlined in a contract addendum prior to purchase.

The manufacturer should identify whether each desired feature is currently available or is a work in progress. In addition to the system capabilities, the acceptance procedure from the vendor should be examined to ensure that the vendor specifications match expectations.

The goal of a rigorous presale investigation is to get the system that best matches the clinic needs at the best cost. Each clinic is different and will have different priorities, so a method should be established to weigh the different factors according to local needs. For example, when

TABLE 4.1 ▦ **A Sample Linac Purchase RFP**

| | |
|---|---|
| Vendor | |
| Completed by | |
| Date | |
| Delivery | |
| MLC | Leaf configuration (leaf width/number?)<br>Max overtravel<br>Max IMRT field size without carriage movement<br>Max leaf speed<br>Interdigitation possible<br>Minimum opposed leaf separation<br>Inter-leaf transmission<br>Intra-leaf transmission<br>Position accuracy<br>Reproducibility |
| IMRT | Step and shoot?<br>Sliding window?<br>Dynamic arc?<br>Are you willing to complete 3 test plans submitted by our institution? |
| Treatment modes/energies | |
| Beam modifiers (dynamic/manual) | |
| Photon dose rate | Max in standard treatment mode<br>Max in special mode selectable? If yes, what are the choices? |
| Treatment volume | Max unobstructed treatment volume with imagers deployed<br>Max unobstructed treatment volume with imagers parked<br>Max couch angle G=90, table at max extension<br>Max couch angle G=90, table at min extension<br>Max gantry angle past 180 with couch=90 (vertex field) |
| Remote positioning | Automatic or manual intervention required?<br>Gantry<br>Collimator<br>Table vertical<br>Table lateral<br>Table in/out<br>Table angle |
| Isocenter accuracy | Imaging vs. radiation isocenter (mm)<br>Coincidence of mechanical isocenters (mm) |
| 6D couch top | Yaw/Pitch/Roll limits |
| Table weight limit | |
| Table lowest floor height | |
| Isocenter height | |
| In-room space requirement | |
| Facility requirements (power, HVAC, water chiller) | |
| Record and verify | R&V interface<br>R&V full capabilities (integrated IGRT reporting/conebeam CT storage/fusion)<br>Intermediate software required (software that operates between R&V and the accelerator)? Is the R&V system IHE-RO compliant? |

*Continued*

| TABLE 4.1  ■  **A Sample Linac Purchase RFP—cont'd** | | |
|---|---|---|
| Treament delivery time | | |
| | Prostate IMRT | |
| | Head and neck IMRT | |
| | Whole brain? | |
| | Tangential breast compensated | |
| | VMAT or dynamic arc | |
| Failure mode analysis | | |
| | Is a vendor document available? | |

selecting a linac, features to consider would include delivery speed, delivery accuracy, delivery conformality, imaging resolution, imaging modalities, motion management, ease of use, integration with existing systems, reliability, service, and marketing. To get a reliable cost comparison it is advised to include at least 5 years of service cost.

All members of the Radiation Oncology team should participate in the evaluation and selection process (radiation oncologists, physicists, therapists, and biomedical engineers). It is good practice to contact facilities of a similar size and scope of service that already have the equipment being considered to get feedback on what is working well and what issues there are with the equipment. These facilities should not necessarily be those recommended by the vendor.

Many logistic issues must also be resolved or clarified prior to the purchase. For example, what is the delivery path through the hospital? Will the equipment fit through all hallways and door openings? Will after-hours or weekend delivery be required and will it cost extra? Will the installation staff require clearance from the hospital to be on site? Will modifications to shielding be required? What are the contingencies if there is a construction delay? After the purchase has been completed, regular meetings should be held with the vendor project manager, construction staff, and Radiation Oncology staff to ensure a smooth installation and acceptance testing.

## 4.3 Commissioning and QA of Treatment Units

### LINACS

There are many documents describing the commissioning and QA of linear accelerators used in radiation therapy. This section focuses on the general commissioning and QA of a linear accelerator; the QA of the image-guided radiation therapy (IGRT) components is discussed in Chapter 7. The commissioning tests can be separated into seven categories.

1. Shielding adequacy (see Chapter 10). A preliminary survey should be done immediately after the linac is able to make beam to ensure the safety of the personnel performing the testing and those in surrounding areas. A full shielding and head leakage survey can be done later.
2. Testing of safety interlocks.
3. Testing of mechanical parameters such as gantry, collimator, multi-leaf collimator (MLC), and couch. Each is tested for functionality and performance within specification.
4. Measurement of beam parameters such as energy, flatness, symmetry, penumbra, jaw transmission, MLC leaf transmission, interleaf leakage, wedge transmission, monitor units (MU) linearity, beam stability versus gantry angle, output factors, cone factors, and virtual source distance.
5. Testing of imaging components (see Section 7.4).
6. Measurement of patient plan delivery accuracy.[2,3]
7. Outside audit by an agency such as the Imaging and Radiation Oncology Core (IROC-Houston) (formerly Radiological Physics Center (RPC)). This includes checks of machine output and also irradiation of test phantoms.[4]

It is not the intent of this chapter to describe each test in detail, as they are well covered in the references, but rather to point out some key issues and discuss practical solutions.

## Safety Interlocks

The testing of safety interlocks can vary from a simple test of the door interlock by opening the door to a complex test of the symmetry interlock by steering the beam until the interlock trips and then measuring the symmetry. The more complex tests may not be necessary if a risk analysis is performed showing that the probability of a failure is low. See Chapter 12 for a more detailed discussion of risk-based QA program development.

## Mechanical Checks

Testing of mechanical parameters is fairly straightforward and well described in vendor documents. The sequence of testing, however, is very important as adjustments of one parameter may affect another. A sample sequence could be as follows:

1. Set gantry level for gantry angle of 0. Do this first as all other checks will hinge on it. This can be checked using methods described in the literature.[5-7] Once true zero is established, identify the surface on the collimator face where a level can be placed to reliably confirm zero. A high quality level with 0 and 90 degree indicators is a required tool for a medical physicist. Digital levels can be used but the accuracy must be validated. The accuracy of any level can be checked by placing it on a level surface and then rotating the level 180 degrees to confirm the reading.

2. Confirm gantry angle accuracy at other angles. Use the previously identified surface on the collimator face and the level to check 90, 180, and 270 degrees.

3. Confirm radiation field and light field congruence. Check by marking the light field on film and then exposing the film. Perform for small, medium, and large field sizes for all photon energies. Ensuring a very tight tolerance (<1 mm) at this step will allow for the use of the light field in checks farther down the list. There are commercially available plates with radio-opaque field markings embedded that eliminate the need for manual marking of the light field (Sun Nuclear and Civco). Some of these can be used with EPID devices instead of film.

4. Confirm jaw concentricity and position accuracy. Check by marking the light field on a piece of paper and then rotating the collimator 180 degrees to confirm that the light field still coincides with the marks.

5. Confirm crosshair centering. This can be checked at the same time as Step 3 by marking the crosshair center. Also check that the crosshair center projects along a true vertical line. This can be done by transferring where the crosshair projects at isocenter to the floor using a plumb bob and then confirming that the crosshair projection matches.

6. Confirm mechanical isocenter. This is typically done by using the mechanical front pointer. Place a pointer stick on the treatment couch extending off the superior edge. At gantry angle 0, set the mechanical pointer to 100 cm. Align the pointer on the couch with the front pointer. Rotate the gantry through the full range and confirm that the maximum deviation is within specifications. This also confirms the accuracy of the front pointer. If there is a consistent offset, the front pointer needs to be adjusted. At this point, align the lasers to the mechanical isocenter.

7. Confirm radiation isocenter and radiation/mechanical isocenter congruence. Check with film using the traditional star shot technique. Mark the mechanical isocenter location on the film before exposing. When evaluating the film there are two parameters to measure. First, check that the intersection of the beams from various gantry angles is within specification. Second, check that the mechanical isocenter coincides with the radiation isocenter. If there is a small but acceptable difference, set the lasers to the radiation isocenter.

8. Set lasers to radiation isocenter. Care must be taken to ensure that the lasers are level and orthogonal and that opposing lasers match. The use of a plumb bob can assist in checking level. Another tool that can assist in laser setup is a three-direction, self-leveling construction laser. It can be placed at isocenter and used to project level lines onto the walls, the floor, and the ceiling. The device should be checked for proper calibration before using.

9. Confirm collimator isocenter. This is also measured with film using a star shot technique. Mark the crosshair center on the film before exposing. Check both the concentricity of the beams and the agreement of the center with the crosshair.

10. Confirm collimator angle accuracy. With the gantry at 0, set one of the jaws to 0 in the inplane direction. Open the other jaws all the way. Tape a piece of paper to the couch top and mark the beam center. Rotate the gantry in both directions while observing the light field. The jaw edge will remain on the center mark across the entire field if it is exactly parallel to the gantry motion, indicating a true zero collimator angle. Collimator angles of 90, 180, and 270 degrees can be similarly tested. Intermediate angles can be tested by aligning a protractor to the center and observing the angle indicated by the crosshair.

11. Confirm collimator position accuracy. Vary the collimator jaw/leaf setting and observe the light field compared with a calibrated ruler. MLC position accuracy can also be checked with the electronic portal imaging device (EPID) or film.

12. Confirm couch vertical motion is parallel to the beam. Tape a piece of paper to the couch top and mark the beam center. Set the gantry angle to zero using a level to ensure accuracy. Lower and raise the couch while observing the light field. If the couch is traveling in a true vertical path, the crosshair will remain on the center mark.

13. Confirm couch vertical position accuracy. Raise the couch top so that the lasers are just skimming the top of the couch. Confirm that the couch vertical reads 0. Tape a calibrated ruler to the side of the couch in a vertical direction. Confirm that the couch vertical readout matches the ruler by observing where the laser hits the ruler.

14. Confirm couch isocenter. This is measured with film using a star shot technique. Mark the crosshair center on the film before exposing. Check both the concentricity of the beams and the agreement of the center with the crosshair.

15. Confirm that the couch travels in a straight line when being extended toward the gantry. Tape a piece of paper to the couch top and mark the beam center. Extend the couch top in and out while observing the light field. If the couch is traveling in a straight line the crosshair will remain on the mark throughout the range of travel.

16. Confirm couch angle accuracy. Confirm couch angle 0 using the test in Step 15. Couch angles of 90 and 270 degrees can be similarly tested. Intermediate angles can be tested by aligning a protractor to the center and observing the angle indicated by the crosshair.

17. Confirm couch travel accuracy. Place a calibrated ruler on the couch top and move the couch known distances by observing the crosshairs. Check both direction of travel across the full range of motion. Evenly distributed weight should be added to the couch top to simulate clinical conditions. This can be done with solid water or anthropomorphic phantoms.

18. Confirm couch sag for various table extensions. Tape a ruler to the side of the couch in a vertical direction. Align the laser to a convenient position of, for example, 10 cm on the ruler. Add weight to the couch as described in Step 17, and observe the change in where the laser hits the ruler.

19. Confirm optical distance indicator (ODI) accuracy. Place slabs of precise thickness on top of the couch top. Adjust the table vertical until the lasers just skim the top of the slabs. Confirm that this is 100 cm source-to-surface distance (SSD) using the mechanical front pointer. Confirm that the ODI reads 100 cm within specifications. Remove the slabs one by one and confirm that the SSD reads 100 + total slab thickness removed for each. To check SSD <100 cm, adjust couch vertical so that the couch top is at 100 cm and then add the slabs one at a time while checking the SSD at each step.

This entire process could easily take an entire day, particularly if adjustments need to be made. The commissioning process is the time to make all parameters as accurate as possible. There are uncertainties in the measurements, and the equipment performance will likely degrade in the future. For these reasons, parameters should be adjusted to be well within specification so that adjustments are not needed in the near future. This may take some diplomatic negotiation with the installation engineer to continue adjusting a parameter even if it is barely within specifications. Commercial devices are available that can make some of this testing more efficient.

## Beam Parameters

The measurement of beam parameters must be performed with the highest accuracy because the initial commissioning will be used for beam data modeling and will form the basis of comparison for all future QA measurements. See Chapter 2 for details of how to acquire the necessary data. AAPM TG-106, Accelerator Beam Data Commissioning Equipment and Procedures,[8] includes an excellent description of how to commission photon and electron beams.

As with the mechanical testing, the order of beam data collection is important. A sample sequence could be as follows.

1. Confirm that the beam is perpendicular to level and centered on the collimator rotation axis. After carefully leveling the water tank and the detector motion mechanisms, perform inplane and crossplane profiles at two depths, one at a shallow depth ($d_{max}$) and one at a deeper depth (20 or 30 cm). The centers of the scans should coincide. This process of finding the central axis (CAX) can be automated with some water tank scanning systems. Note that the detector motion is confirmed to be vertical using the crosshairs that were checked in Step 5 above. To check beam centering on the collimator axis, perform scans at collimator angles of 0° and 180°, and confirm that the scans match.
2. Confirm beam energy. Perform depth dose scans and confirm that the relevant parameter is within specification (i.e., percent depth dose at 10 cm for photons and clinical depth (90%) or 50% depth for electrons). This should be checked first because the resulting changes in bending magnet current or radiofrequency (RF) power may affect subsequent steps.
3. Confirm flatness and symmetry. Measure profiles for large fields at $d_{max}$ and 10 cm depth to confirm beam flatness and symmetry. The symmetry should be <1% and flatness within vendor specifications. If beam steering is required, repeat Step 1. Different definitions for flatness exist; make sure the flatness is measured in a consistent manner.
4. Check stability of beam versus gantry angle. This can be done easily with a detector array attached to a special gantry mount.
5. Once these are confirmed, the depth dose, profile, transmission factor, and field size dependence data can be collected. The in-air data can then be collected. Measurement of absolute dose should be done last because adjustments to the other parameters may affect output.

In collecting beam data care must be taken in the choice of detectors. There are numerous considerations, most of which are discussed in AAPM TG-106. For example, large ion chambers will not accurately sample the beam penumbra. Diodes may over-respond out of the field. For electron beams if an ion chamber is used, the percent depth doses (PDDs) must be shifted and converted with depth-dependent stopping power ratios. This is not the case if a diode is used, although care must be taken in choosing electron versus photon diodes for scanning (the difference being in the shielding to low energy scatter photons). See Chapter 2 for more details.

## Ongoing QA

Once the commissioning has been completed, the scope of the ongoing QA should be established according to the reference documents, in particular AAPM TG-142 on QA of Medical Linear Accelerators[9] and other reports.[10-12] These are outlined in Table 4.2. Baseline measurements of

TABLE 4.2 ▓ **Linac Commissioning and QA References**

| Reference | Relevant Topics Included in Reference | Description |
|---|---|---|
| AAPM TG-40, 1994[11] | QA of radiotherapy programs | A document describing a comprehensive QA program in Radiation Oncology. It covers the physical aspects of QA as well as describes the QA team, roles, and responsibilities. It has sections for each type of equipment available at the time. Much of the report has been superseded or augmented by subsequent reports. |
| AAPM TG-45, 1994[10] | Acceptance and commissioning of linear accelerators | Code of practice for radiotherapy accelerators. Describes acceptance testing, commissioning, and QA including special procedures such as TBI, TSET, electron arc, IORT, and SRS. |
| AAPM TG-35, 1993[12] | Safety consideration for linear accelerators | Medical accelerator safety considerations. Describes the classification of potentially hazardous situations, procedures for responding to them, training, and computer control issues. |
| AAPM TG-142, 2009[9] | QA of linear accelerators | The TG accomplished the update to AAPM TG-40, specifying new tests and tolerances, and has added recommendations for not only the new ancillary delivery technologies but also for imaging devices that are part of the linear accelerator. The report also gives recommendations as to action levels for the physicists to implement particular actions, whether they are inspection, scheduled action, or immediate and corrective action. The report is geared to be flexible for the physicist to customize the QA program depending on clinical utility. There are specific tables according to daily, monthly, and annual reviews, along with unique tables for wedge systems, MLC, and imaging checks. The report also gives specific recommendations regarding setup of a QA program by the physicist in regards to building a QA team, establishing procedures, training of personnel, documentation, and end-to-end system checks. |
| AAPM TG-198 | Implementation of AAPM TG-142 | Still in progress as of this writing. Charge (from aapm.org): 1. Provide specific procedural guidelines for performing the tests recommended in AAPM TG-142. 2. Provide estimate of the range of times, appropriate personnel, and qualifications necessary to complete the tests in AAPM TG-142. 3. Provide sample daily/weekly/monthly/annual QA forms. |
| AAPM TG-50, 2001[13] | MLC QA | The aim of this report is to provide basic information and to state fundamental concepts needed to implement the use of a MLC in the conventional clinical setting. The intent of this report is to assist medical physicists, dosimetrists, and radiation oncologists with the acquisition, testing, commissioning, daily use, and QA of MLCs in order to realize increased efficiency of utilization of therapy facilities. It is not the intent of this report to describe research into advanced applications of MLCs in conformal therapy or dynamic treatments. |

## TABLE 4.2 ▪ Linac Commissioning and QA References—cont'd

| Reference | Relevant Topics Included in Reference | Description |
|---|---|---|
| AAPM TG-58, 2001[14] | Commissioning and QA of EPID | Clinical use of electronic portal imaging. Includes sections on commissioning and QA. |
| AAPM TG-106, 2008[8] | Commissioning of linear accelerators | Accelerator beam data commissioning equipment and procedures. Review of the practical aspects and physics of linac commissioning. Provides guidelines on phantom selection, detector selection, scanning of photon and electron beams, and beam data processing. |
| AAPM Report 82[15] | IMRT QA | Guidance document on delivery, treatment planning, and clinical implementation of IMRT. Describes the entire process of implementing IMRT and includes a section on QA specific to IMRT. |
| AAPM TG-210 | Conventional linac acceptance testing | Still in progress as of this writing. **Charge:** 1. Recommendations for (1) technical specifications that should be included in the purchase contract and (2) consideration of technical aspects of purchase contract. 2. To provide definition of performance specifications for major linac subsystems in the acceptance testing procedure (ATP). 3. To make recommendations on the tests to be performed during the ATP, including beam matching and subsequent major repair/upgrades including testing methods that complement vendor-suggested measurements. |
| AAPM TG-148, 2010[16] | QA of helical TomoTherapy | QA of helical TomoTherapy. The specific objectives of this TG are: 1. To discuss QA techniques, frequencies, and tolerances and 2. discuss dosimetric verification techniques applicable to this unit. This report summarizes the findings of the Task Group and aims to provide the practicing clinical medical physicist with the insight into the technology that is necessary to establish an independent and comprehensive QA program for a helical TomoTherapy unit. The emphasis of the report is to describe the rationale for the proposed QA program and to provide example tests that can be performed, drawing from the collective experience of the task group members and the published literature. It is expected that as technology continues to evolve, so will the test procedures that may be used in the future to perform comprehensive QA for helical TomoTherapy units. |

*Continued*

TABLE 4.2 ▨ Linac Commissioning and QA References—cont'd

| Reference | Relevant Topics Included in Reference | Description |
|---|---|---|
| AAPM TG-135, 2011[17] | QA of robotic radiosurgery | QA of robotic radiosurgery. The TG (TG-135) had three main charges: 1. To make recommendations on a code of practice for Robotic Radiosurgery QA; 2. To make recommendations on QA and dosimetric verification techniques, especially in regard to real-time respiratory motion tracking software; 3. To make recommendations on issues that require further research and development. This report provides a general functional overview of the only clinically implemented robotic radiosurgery device, the CyberKnife VR. This report includes sections on device components and their individual component QA recommendations, followed by a section on the QA requirements for integrated systems. Examples of checklists for daily, monthly, annual, and upgrade QA are given as guidance for medical physicists. Areas in which QA procedures are still under development are discussed. |
| AAPM TG-178 | Gamma stereotactic radiosurgery dosimetry and quality | Still in progress as of this writing. **Charge:** Review calibration phantoms versus in-air calibration for gamma stereotactic radiosurgery (GSR) devices Work with Working Group on Dosimetry Calibration Protocol for Beams that are not compliant with AAPM TG-51 (WGDCPB) Suggest a protocol for calibration with ionization chambers calibrated appropriately at an accredited dosimetry calibration laboratory that can be successfully utilized with all GSR devices Update QA protocols for all static GSR devices Create new QA protocols for new GSR devices with rotating or moving sources |
| IAEA | Acceptance testing and commissioning of linear accelerators | Acceptance Tests and Commissioning Measurements. Chapter 10 in *Review of Radiation Oncology Physics: A Handbook for Teachers and Students.* http://www-naweb.iaea.org/nahu/DMRP/documents/Chapter10.pdf |
| IAEA | QA of linear accelerators | QA of external beam radiotherapy. Chapter 12 in *Review of Radiation Oncology Physics: A Handbook for Teachers and Students.* http://www-naweb.iaea.org/nahu/DMRP/documents/Chapter12.pdf |

TABLE 4.3 ■ **Sample QA After Linac Repair**

| Type of Repair | Parameters Affected | QA to Be Done |
|---|---|---|
| Klystron or magnetron | Beam energy | Depth dose and max field size profiles at $d_{max}$ |
| Thyratron | None | None |
| Bend magnet | Beam energy | Full commissioning spot check |
| Field light or mirror replacement | Rad/light field congruence | Rad/light field image |
| MLC motor | MLC position | MLC accuracy |
| Waveguide | Beam energy, flatness, symmetry, spot size | Full commissioning spot check |
| Monitor unit ion chamber | Output, flatness, symmetry | Output, flatness, and symmetry |

daily, monthly, and annual QA should be taken at the time of commissioning to establish a proper baseline. At the time of each annual QA, the daily and monthly QA measurements should also be performed to ensure continued fidelity of these measurements. The description of the test, equipment used, frequency, who performs the test, acceptable ranges, and corrective actions to be taken should be documented for each test.

## QA After Repairs

Another situation requiring QA is after significant equipment repair. The facility should establish a protocol for what measurements should be done after different types of repairs. The vendors can provide guidance documents, but each facility should establish their own policy. A sample is shown in Table 4.3.

Documenting machine problems and their resolution is an important QA activity. The facility should have a log of machine issues, how they were resolved, what QA was done, and authorization for return to service by the physicist. Down time should be documented monthly and repair trends analyzed for any ongoing issues. A log should include at the minimum the date, time, therapist present, who was notified (biomed, physics, manager, service), actions taken to resolve the issue, service call placed if unable to resolve, down time, delay time, number of patients not treated, service hours, follow-up, and physics authorization of return to use for each incident (Table 4.2).

## High Dose Rate Remote Afterloading Units

High dose rate (HDR) remote afterloading systems have been in common use since the 1990s. Typically they use a single $^{192}$Ir source mounted on the end of a long wire that is computer controlled to drive the source to the appropriate distance and then step through a series of dwell positions to deliver the prescribed dose. The units have 5 to 20 channels, allowing for multiple catheter or applicator treatments. Vendors include Elekta (formerly Nucletron) and Varian. A newer unit, BEBIG Multisource, has multiple sources, one $^{192}$Ir and $^{60}$Co.[18]

Acceptance testing and commissioning are described in AAPM TG-41[19] remote afterloading technology and involve completing all of the tests listed in Table 4.4 as well as treatment planning system (TPS) commissioning, which is described in Chapter 5. Further references on commissioning and QA of HDR units is found in Table 4.5. Many of the tests involve the use of film to produce autoradiographs. Recently there have been descriptions of methods using portal imagers[20] and chamber arrays[21] to perform some of the QA tests. In addition, Jursinic has described a methodology to perform many tests without film and with increased efficiency.[22]

There is some discrepancy among the guidelines as to what tests should be performed and the frequency of testing. Without a reference document describing the relative effectiveness of

TABLE 4.4 ▪ HDR QA Guidelines

| QA Test | ESTRO Booklet (2004)[24] | AAPM TG-59 (1998)[25] | AAPM TG-56 (1997)[23] | AAPM TG-40 (1994)[11] |
|---|---|---|---|---|
| Warning lights | daily | daily | daily | daily |
| Room monitor | daily | daily | daily | daily |
| Communication equipment | daily | daily | daily | daily |
| Timer termination | daily | daily | daily | |
| Timer accuracy | | daily | daily | |
| Emergency equipment present | daily | daily | daily | |
| Survey meter functional | daily | daily | daily | |
| Source position | daily and quarterly | daily | daily | weekly |
| Source position multiple channels | | | quarterly | |
| Date, time, and source strength in unit | daily | daily | daily | |
| Output constancy | | daily | daily | |
| Presence of manuals and procedures | | daily | daily | |
| Functioning of dedicated imaging | | daily | daily | |
| Emergency stop | quarterly | | quarterly | |
| Treatment interrupt | quarterly | | quarterly | daily |
| Door interlock | quarterly | daily | daily | daily |
| Power loss | quarterly | daily | quarterly | |
| Obstructed catheter | quarterly | | quarterly | |
| Integrity of transfer tubes | quarterly | | quarterly | |
| Length of transfer tubes | | | quarterly | |
| Handheld monitor | quarterly and annually | | | |
| Source calibration | source exchange | | quarterly | source exchange |
| Facility survey | | | source exchange | |
| Timer accuracy and linearity | annually | | quarterly | source exchange |
| Applicator and catheter attachment | 6 months | | quarterly | source exchange |
| Contamination test | annually | | | |
| Leakage radiation | annually | | quarterly | |
| Practice emergency procedures | annually | | | annually |
| Hand crank function | annually | | | |
| Length of treatment tubes | annually | | quarterly | source exchange |
| Transit time effect | annually | | annually | |
| Source decay accuracy | | | annually | |
| Verification of dummy markers | | | annually | weekly |
| Verify position simulation markers for applicators | | | annually | |
| Review accuracy of standard plans | | | annually | |
| Review QA manual | | | annually | |
| Review compliance with staff training requirements | | | annually | |
| Verify source inventory | | | annually | annually |

TABLE 4.5 ■ **HDR Commissioning and QA References**

| Reference | Description |
|---|---|
| AAPM TG-56, 1997[23] | Code of practice for brachytherapy physics. Describes a complete QA program for brachytherapy including HDR. |
| AAPM TG-41, 1993[19] | Remote afterloading technology. The document reviews the principles of operation, calibration procedures, radiation control procedures, QA procedures, facility design, and dose computation for remote afterloading systems. |
| AAPM TG-59, 1998[25] | HDR treatment delivery. Includes a section on delivery QA. |
| ASTRO white paper, 2014[26] | A review of safety, quality management, and practice guidelines for HDR brachytherapy. |
| ESTRO booklet, 2004[24] | A practical guide to quality control of brachytherapy equipment. Has description of quality procedures for brachytherapy. Although the HDR source calibration procedure is outdated the general description of the quality procedures is current. |

each QA test, failure modes, and hazard analysis it would be prudent to adopt the most frequent testing frequency. Table 4.4 shows a comparison of these guidelines.

In addition to these tests, the AAPM TG-56[23] Code of Practice for Brachytherapy Physics and ESTRO[24] recommend having a tertiary method for verification of source strength. This is usually done with a cylindrical ion chamber in a fixed geometry. A constancy value can be established at the initial commissioning of the system. It is important to reproduce the setup precisely, including the proximity of any scattering material (treatment couch, walls, floors, etc.) to achieve consistent results. See Chapter 1 for details on source calibration. It is useful to have this backup calibration check system in case of malfunction of the well chamber (which is the recommended device for measuring source activity) or to troubleshoot differences between the calibration certificate and the locally measured activity. Another good practice is to calibrate both the old and the new source at the time of source exchange. This provides a check on the well chamber constancy.

## KILOVOLTAGE UNITS

Treatment units with energies in the kilovoltage range can vary from superficial to electronic brachytherapy to orthovoltage. The superficial and orthovoltage units typically treat using fixed applicators with relatively short SSDs. They also use combinations of filters to achieve different penetrating qualities. Electronic brachytherapy units are used either intraoperatively or to treat superficial skin lesions. Electronic brachytherapy is the use of a low energy kV source (typically 50 kV) to deliver radiation inside or adjacent to a tumor similar to brachytherapy methods using radioactive seeds. Instead of a radioactive seed, the kV device target is placed at the desired location. AAPM TG-152, The 2007 AAPM Response to the CRCPD Request for Recommendations for the CRCPD's Model Regulations for Electronic Brachytherapy, contains sections regarding the calibration and QA for these units.[27] The ASTRO Emerging Technology Committee also published a report in 2010 that reviews these technologies.[28] Further references for recommended QA are found in Table 4.6.

Because of the short distances typically used with kV equipment (1 to 30 cm), the setup of any measurement must be very precise, with a much higher requirement for electronic brachytherapy units for treatments in the 1 to 3 cm range. At 1 cm distance a 0.5 mm error in positioning of a measurement device will result in a 10% error. At 30 cm the same error drops to 0.3%.

Because the superficial and orthovoltage units typically use cones and filters, it is important to perform quality control (QC) on all clinically used combinations. The users should be aware of which combinations are released for clinical use to avoid using an uncalibrated combination.

**TABLE 4.6 ▪ kV Unit Commissioning and QA References**

| Reference | Description |
| --- | --- |
| CAPCA, 2005[32] | Standards for Quality Control at Canadian Radiation Treatment Centers: Kilovoltage X-ray Radiotherapy Machines. Describes performance objectives and criteria, system descriptions, acceptance testing and commissioning, QC, and documentation. Table 1 provides a comprehensive list of daily, monthly, and annual tests. |
| AAPM TG-152, 2009[27] | Model regulations for electronic brachytherapy. Discusses treatment unit requirements, physicist support, operating procedures, calibration measurements, routine QA, records, treatment planning, and training. |
| IPEM Report 81, 1999[33] | Physical aspects of quality control in radiotherapy. General book on QC in radiotherapy with a section on kilovoltage units. |

Electronic brachytherapy units pose special challenges because of the short distances involved, as mentioned previously. In addition, the facility may not have an appropriate waterproof chamber for measuring output or depth dose. Because of the low energy, parallel plate chambers are preferred. These are more difficult to waterproof, and thin sheaths may be required. Care should be taken to select an appropriate detector and to apply the appropriate corrections.[29,30] There seems to be consensus that the NACP, Markus, Advanced Markus, and Roos parallel plate chambers can be used to measure depth dose within 3% uncertainty. The application of depth-dependent correction factors may reduce that uncertainty.[31] Cylindrical chambers can be used but cannot measure accurately near the surface because some of the chamber is above the water surface in that range. Beyond 4 to 5 mm depth they can produce accurate results.

# 4.4 Imaging Units

## COMPUTED TOMOGRAPHY

The QA of computed tomography (CT) simulation units is described in AAPM TG-66.[34] Depending on state regulations, the unit may have to comply with some or all of the diagnostic CT requirements. The test descriptions in AAPM TG-66 are well described and do not need elaboration. A brief summary of the recommended tests is shown in Table 4.7.

One issue mentioned in AAPM TG-66 that deserves special consideration is the removal and replacement of the flat couch top insert. If the unit is dedicated to Radiation Oncology this is not an issue because the insert will likely remain in place. This may cause an issue with QA phantom placement as some phantoms are designed to mount using the same mechanism used by the flat table insert. Therefore a new custom mount may need to be designed. Alternatively, the phantom could be placed on top of the insert rather than being suspended from the end of the table. It should be noted that the presence of the couch top will change some of the test values, and baselines different from the manufacturer-specified values will need to be established. If the unit is shared with diagnostic radiology, the removal and replacement may be frequent and the proper alignment should be checked daily. Commercial devices are available that make the testing recommended by AAPM TG-66 more efficient. The Quasar Beam Geometry Phantom (Modus Medical) and CT Sim Check (Integrated Medical Technologies) are examples.

## ULTRASOUND UNITS

Ultrasound (US) use in Radiation Oncology is primarily for the treatment of prostate cancer, either in external beam or interstitial brachytherapy. In addition, US may be used for localization

TABLE 4.7 ▣ **Summary of AAPM TG-66 Recommended Testing for CT Simulators**

| Component | Test |
|---|---|
| Radiation safety | CT dose, shielding |
| Internal lasers | Accuracy of geometrical position |
| Positioning lasers | Accuracy of geometrical position and motion, orthogonality |
| Couch and tabletop | Orthogonality of motion, accuracy of motion, level |
| Gantry | Orthogonality to couch, tilt accuracy |
| Scan localization from scout image | Accuracy of slice indication |
| Collimation | Pre-patient (Radiation Profile Width) and post-patient (Sensitivity Profile Width) collimation measurements |
| X-ray generator | kVp, HVL, mAs linearity, mAs reproducibility, timer accuracy |
| Noise | Standard deviation of CT numbers over region of interest in a uniform density |
| Field uniformity | Consistency of CT numbers at various points in a uniform density. Usually center, 3, 6, 9, and 12 o'clock positions. |
| CT number accuracy | Check CT number for water, air, and various other known densities |
| Spatial integrity | Check distance between objects that are known distance apart and shape of standard objects (i.e., circle, phantoms of known shape) |
| Spatial resolution | Can be determined by calculating modulation transfer function (MTF) from line spread function (LSF) or point spread function (PSF) or by resolving line pairs |
| Contrast resolution | Typically measured using low contrast objects of varying sizes or multiple sets of objects with different contrasts |
| CT simulation software | Image input, contouring, image registration, machine definition, isocenter calculation and movement, image reconstruction, DRRs |

of breast boost treatments or needle placement in interstitial gynecologic treatments. The AAPM has produced a report on QA for each of these, AAPM TG-154, Quality Assurance of US-Guided External Beam Radiotherapy for Prostate Cancer,[35] and AAPM TG-128, Quality Assurance Tests for Prostate Brachytherapy Ultrasound Systems,[36] respectively. Table II in both of these reports lists the recommended tests and frequencies, and a summary is shown in Tables 4.8 and 4.9. Both require the use of a phantom, which may be included with the system or purchased separately. These are usually gel-based phantoms that have a shelf life and need to be replaced periodically. An issue specific to prostate brachytherapy US is the use of a standoff around the transrectal US probe. It has been demonstrated that these may cause image distortion leading to inaccurate volume determination, needle positioning, and dose calculation.[37] The standoff should be carefully tested prior to use.

## POSITRON EMISSION TOMOGRAPHY/CT UNITS

Positron emission tomography (PET)/CT units are also becoming more common in Radiation Oncology departments. The QA of the PET component may be outside the expertise of the Radiation Oncology physicist, and a qualified nuclear medicine physicist should be consulted. The International Atomic Energy Agency (IAEA) has published a document on QA for PET and PET/CT systems,[38] and Xing has published a review of QA for PET/CT in radiation therapy.[39] The IAEA document is very detailed and includes an overview of the technology as well as acceptance testing and routine QA descriptions. The QA performance assessment of the PET component should follow the National Electrical Measurement Association (NEMA)

TABLE 4.8 ▦ Quality Assurance Tests for US-Guided External Beam Radiation Therapy

| Test | Frequency |
| --- | --- |
| Laser alignment | Daily |
| Daily positioning constancy | Daily |
| US unit depth, gain controls | Daily |
| IR (infrared) camera warm-up (IR camera tracks US probe in 3D) | Daily |
| Phantom stability | Quarterly |
| Monthly positioning constancy (includes IR camera calibration) | Monthly |
| Phantom offset test | Monthly |
| Laser offset | Monthly |
| Image quality constancy | Semiannually |
| End-to-end test | Annually or following software upgrade |

TABLE 4.9 ▦ Quality Assurance Tests for Transrectal US Units Used for Brachytherapy

| Test | Frequency |
| --- | --- |
| Grayscale visibility | Annually |
| Depth of penetration | Annually |
| Axial and lateral resolution | Annually |
| Axial distance measurement accuracy | Annually |
| Lateral distance measurement accuracy | Annually |
| Area measurement accuracy | Annually |
| Volume measurement accuracy | Annually |
| Needle template alignment | Annually |
| Accuracy of volume contours in treatment planning system | Acceptance testing |

standard NU2-2001 and the updated version NU2-2007. This standard describes measuring the system sensitivity with line sources and spatial resolution using point sources. The NEMA standard does not address the CT component of a PET/CT, and the reader is referred to the IAEA document. The quantitative use of PET images relies on the standardized uptake value (SUV) calculation. The SUV is the ratio of the image-derived concentration of radioactivity to the injected radioactivity divided by the body weight of the patient. This is done to eliminate differences in values due to different injected activities and different body mass. Because the SUV is important in the determination of malignant areas and their accurate delineation, the consistency of SUV must be checked.

## MAGNETIC RESONANCE UNITS

Magnetic resonance (MR) units dedicated to Radiation Oncology are becoming increasingly common, although still in the minority. In addition, there are now treatment units with MR imaging capability.[40] As MR physics is generally outside the expertise of a Radiation Oncology physicist, the QA of the system should be coordinated with a qualified MR physicist. The recommendations in AAPM Report 100, Acceptance Testing and Quality Assurance Procedures for Magnetic Resonance Imaging Facilities,[41] should be followed. Testing includes vibration measurements, RF shielding testing, magnetic fringe field mapping, mechanical system tests, emergency system tests, patient monitoring equipment tests, static magnetic field subsystem tests, RF subsystem tests, gradient subsystem tests, combined gradient/RF system tests, global system tests, ultrafast imaging tests, and spectroscopy tests. The department should be aware of the pulse sequences used for obtaining different information and optimal target delineation.[42-44]

Of particular concern for treatment units with MR imaging is the functionality of the QA equipment in a high magnetic field environment. Not only must the equipment be nonferrous, but the electronics also must operate in that environment. Further equipment that must be connected to AC power or use cables to connect devices in the treatment room to devices in the control room (i.e., ion chamber to electrometer) may create an antenna effect and distort the MR images. One solution is to place a battery-operated electrometer inside the treatment room and obtain the readings using the monitoring camera. QA devices can be checked for ferrous content using a hand magnet (John Bayouth, personal communication).

If immobilization devices or a flat table insert are to be used, they also must be checked for MR compatibility. Carbon fiber, for instance, may heat up in strong magnetic fields due to the creation of eddy currents. Because of this, flat table inserts and other devices are generally made from fiberglass, which does not exhibit this property.

Finally, staff and patient safety is an important factor in the MR environment. The area should be designed to control and limit access, and clear signage should be present. Staff who enter the high field areas should have regular specialized training on MR safety.

## ON-TREATMENT IMAGING DEVICES

A number of on-treatment imaging devices are available, including cone-beam CT, MV CT, planar radiographs, and nonradiographic localization devices. The technical details and QA concerns of such systems are described in detail in Chapter 7.

## 4.5 Ancillary Equipment

In addition to the complex imaging and treatment delivery equipment there are many ancillary devices in a Radiation Oncology department that require QA. Table 4.10 lists a sample of these devices and how they may be tested.

## 4.6 QA of Data Transfer

Data in many forms are transferred between many systems in a typical department. See the sample data transfer matrix in Chapter 5. A systematic method is needed to validate the accuracy of the data transferred at each step. This can be done by visual inspection of parameter values, qualitative review of images, or more elaborate file comparison methods. AAPM TG-201[46] has described these processes in great detail. A follow-up document with clinical examples is in progress.

## 4.7 QA Program Evaluation

Establishing and maintaining a comprehensive QA program in Radiation Oncology is a complex, time-consuming process. The amount of data accumulated over a year can add up to thousands of discrete results. Much of the data will simply be of a pass/fail nature and the results are simply interpreted. A more complex evaluation of these data can often be achieved using statistical process control methods as discussed in Chapter 12. Regular reporting of these data should be done at monthly QA meetings. Other data should be reviewed on a more global scale. For instance, were any changes made in clinical policy that would require adopting tighter tolerances for some QA tests? Are the results of the imaging QA consistent with PTV margins used

TABLE 4.10 ▨ **Ancillary Equipment QA**

| Device | Test Method |
|---|---|
| Ion chamber | Annual comparison with calibrated chambers or constancy check with long-lived radioisotope in a fixed geometry |
| Electrometer | Annual comparison with calibrated electrometer |
| Barometer | Quarterly comparison with calibrated barometer or comparison with local airport pressure. When comparing to airport pressure, request uncorrected station pressure and account for any difference in elevation. |
| Thermometer | Annual comparison with calibrated thermometer |
| Ruler | Comparison with calibrated ruler prior to use |
| Solid phantom | Check that dimensions are accurate. Perform CT scan of phantom to confirm density, uniformity, and lack of defects. Note some phantoms are near water equivalent at MV energies and not at kV energies. This can have a significant impact on dose calculation if the phantom is used for patient-specific QA. For example, if the phantom has a density of 1.0 at MV energies and 1.08 at kV energies and the phantom is used without a density override in the TPS, the TPS calculation will be 8% low since it is calculating based on a density of 1.08. This can be checked by using an MVCT if available or by transmission measurements if not. |
| Beam Scanning Equipment | See Chapter 2 for details of setup QA. In addition, a rigorous QA should be done as part of acceptance testing.[45] |

clinically? Policies and procedures should also be reviewed on a regular basis to confirm that they meet the latest regulations and recommendations.

These types of reviews can establish whether or not the current tests are within current limits, but they do not address any deficiencies in the program. Internal reviews can be done to address this, but it is better to have independent audits. Practice accreditation is one way to achieve this. In fact, accreditation may become mandatory in the near future. One state in the United States (NY) has already made it a requirement. In the United States, practice accreditation may be performed through the ACR or, as of 2015, through ASTRO's Accreditation Program for Excellence (APEx). Reaccreditation typically occurs on a 3 to 4 year cycle, so there is a question as to the requirements in the intervening years. This is a likely area for internal audits, although external audits would be preferred because an outside opinion is much more likely to identify areas for improvement. This can be done as an informal arrangement with a colleague or a formal contract with a consulting physicist. AAPM TG-103, Peer Review in Clinical Radiation Oncology Physics, describes the components and expectations of an external review.[47]

Routine dosimetry audits are also recommended and are usually required for clinical trial participation. Outside of any required dosimetry audits, every treatment beam should receive outside verification of absolute dose annually. Dosimetry services are available from IROC (formerly RPC), University of Wisconsin, and IAEA.[48-50] Further, it is best practice to perform modality-specific multidimensional audits yearly for those services offered in the clinic. For example, if a facility offers IMRT, SRS, and stereotactic body radiosurgery (SBRT), a dosimetry audit could be done annually on a rotating basis: IMRT in year 1, SRS in year 2, and SBRT in year 3, for example.

In conclusion, as the QA program is multifaceted so must be the evaluation of the program.

## 4.8 Future Directions in QA

The acceptance testing, commissioning, and ongoing QA of radiotherapy equipment are vital to the accurate delivery of radiation. There are many references that describe the technical considerations of these activities. Just as important are having a comprehensive process for testing, identifying risks, training of all involved staff, documenting policy and procedure, developing the QA process, and developing performance metrics. The reference documents and vendor information, along with risk assessment, will guide the testing. Risks can be identified using processes such as failure mode and effect analysis (FMEA) as described in Chapter 12. Training will be guided by the vendor and information gained during the testing process. To implement a new technology safely all staff must have a clear understanding of their roles, which are well described by policy and procedure. The ongoing accuracy and safety of the system must be monitored by a comprehensive QA program. Again, there are many technical references that describe QA programs for most systems, but there is also a growing movement to design QA programs based on risk assessments. Once the system is in clinical use, metrics should be developed to monitor the clinical effectiveness. For instance, if an SBRT program is implemented, the clinical outcomes should be checked after the first group of patients to ensure that the goals of the program have been met and that there are no unexpected acute effects. Two common themes run through these processes: identifying and managing risk and ensuring the competency of the staff. The former is described in the literature while the latter is described by the AAPM document Guidelines for Competency Evaluation for Medical Physicists in Radiation Oncology (currently in review). A more complete discussion of these concepts is found in Chapter 12.

## FOR THE PHYSICIAN

As is shown in the preceding sections, acceptance testing, commissioning, and ongoing QA for modern radiotherapy equipment can be a very complex process. From the relatively simple (US unit) to the very complicated (modern linac with IGRT capabilities), there are numerous professional societies and agencies that have published guidance documents with recommendations for equipment testing to safely implement new technology.

Important issues must be considered before purchasing the equipment. They include:

1. Determine the clinical needs of the department and ensure that the performance specifications of the equipment being considered can meet those needs. This can be done by developing a detailed request for proposal (RFP) that outlines all of the desired functionality.
2. Determine which functions are most important so that proposals from different vendors can be compared and ranked. It is best to include all team members in this evaluation.
3. Review the vendor's acceptance test document and acceptable ranges for performance to ensure that they match your expectations. If a tighter specification of performance is desired, it must be negotiated prior to purchase.
4. A careful site review must be done to ensure that the equipment will fit in the selected space, that the delivery path is clear, and that all electrical and cooling needs can be met.
5. Contact current users of the equipment at facilities similar in scope to find out their experiences.

The actual testing of radiation delivery equipment will focus on many distinct areas. They include:

1. Radiation safety and shielding
2. Safety interlocks
3. Testing of mechanical parameters
4. Testing of radiation delivery parameters
5. Testing of imaging components, if applicable
6. Developing the ongoing QA procedures and procedures for QA after equipment repair or upgrade

The testing of imaging units follows a very similar process. The imaging-specific testing will include radiation dose (if applicable) and image quality.

In addition to the major equipment, the ancillary equipment must be tested. Examples of these are ion chambers, diodes, electrometers, barometers, thermometers, rulers, solid phantoms, and scanning equipment.

Many of the devices in a Radiation Oncology department will be interconnected and will transfer data to and/or receive data from other devices. The accuracy of this data transfer must be verified as this is required for the safe delivery of radiation. The transfer of the MLC leaf sequencing from the treatment planning system to the linac control system is one example.

Once the QA program has been established it must be reviewed on a regular basis to ensure that it continues to meet the safety goals of the department. Technology and treatment protocols are constantly evolving, and the reviews should determine if any changes in technology or clinical parameters require changes to the QA program. For example, if PTV margins are reduced, does the QA program verify the accuracy of the IGRT components to a sufficient level of accuracy? In addition, external audits are extremely valuable in ensuring the quality and safety of the program. These audits can come in the form of remote dosimetry audits, peer reviews, and practice accreditation.

In the future, QA programs will evolve from a performance testing process based on published guidelines to processes that use risk analysis to determine the optimal testing methodologies. These can include process mapping, failure mode effect analysis, fault tree analysis, and statistical process control, which are discussed in more detail in Chapter 12.

## References

1. IEC 60976. Medical electrical equipment—medical electron accelerators—functional performance characteristics. Geneva: International Electrotechnical Commission; 2007.
2. Ezzell GA, Burmeister JW, Dogan N, et al. IMRT commissioning: Multiple institution planning and dosimetry comparisons, a report from AAPM Task Group 119. Med Phys 2009;36(11):5359–73.
3. Low DA, Moran JM, Dempsey JF, et al. Dosimetry tools and techniques for IMRT. Med Phys 2011;38(3):1313–38.
4. Moran JM, Dempsey M, Eisbruch A, et al. Safety considerations for IMRT: Executive summary. Pract Radiat Oncol 2011;1:190–5. Full report available on ASTRO website: <https://www.astro.org/Clinical-Practice/White-Papers/IMRT.aspx>.
5. Beaumont S, Torfeh T, Latreille R, et al. New method to test the gantry, collimator, and table rotation angles of a linear accelerator used in radiation therapy. Proc SPIE 7961. Med Imaging 2011; Physics of Medical Imaging.
6. Chang L, Ho SY, Wu JM, et al. Technical innovation to calibrate the gantry angle indicators of linear accelerators. J Appl Clin Med Phys 2001;2(1):54–8.
7. Rowshanfarzad P, Sabet M, O'Connor DJ, et al. Gantry angle determination during arc IMRT: evaluation of a simple EPID-based technique and two commercial inclinometers. J Appl Clin Med Phys 2012;13(6):203–14.
8. Das IJ, Cheng C-W, Watts RJ, et al. Accelerator beam data commissioning equipment and procedures: Report of the AAPM TG-106 of the Therapy Physics Committee of the AAPM. Med Phys 2008;35(9):4186–215.
9. Klein EE, Hanley J, Bayouth J, et al. Task Group 142 report: Quality assurance of medical accelerators. Med Phys 2009;36(9):4197–212.
10. Nath R, Biggs PJ, Bova FJ, et al. AAPM code of practice for radiotherapy accelerators: Report of AAPM radiation therapy Task Group 45. Med Phys 1994;21(7):1093–121.
11. Kutcher GJ, Coia L, Gillin M, et al. Comprehensive QA for Radiation Oncology: Report of AAPM radiation therapy committee Task Group 40. Med Phys 1994;21(4):581–618.
12. Purdy JA, Biggs PJ, Bowers C, et al. Medical accelerator safety considerations: Report of AAPM Radiation Therapy Committee Task Group No. 35. Med Phys 1993;20(4):1261–75.
13. AAPM Report No. 72, Basic applications of multi-leaf collimators: Report of Task Group 50, American Association of Physicists in Medicine. Madison, WI: Medical Physics Publishing; 2001.
14. Herman MG, Balter JM, Jaffray DA, et al. Clinical use of electronic portal imaging: Report of AAPM Radiation Therapy Committee Task Group 58. Med Phys 2001;28(5):712–37.

15. Ezzell GA, Galvin JM, Low D, et al. Guidance document on delivery, treatment planning, and clinical implementation of IMRT: Report of the IMRT subcommittee of the AAPM Radiation Therapy Committee. Med Phys 2003;30(8):2089–115.
16. Langen KM, Papanikolaou N, Balog J, et al. QA for helical TomoTherapy: Report of the AAPM Task Group 148. Med Phys 2010;37(9):4817–53.
17. Dieterich S, Cavedon C, Chuang CF, et al. Report of AAPM TG-135: Quality assurance for robotic radiosurgery. Med Phys 2011;38(6):2914–36.
18. Palmer A, Mzenda B. Performance assessment of the BEBIG Multisource high dose rate brachytherapy treatment unit. Phys Med Biol 2009;54:7417–34.
19. AAPM Report No. 41, Remote afterloading technology: A report of AAPM Task Group No. 41. New York: American Association of Physicists in Medicine, American Institute of Physics; 1993.
20. Smith RL, Taylor ML, McDermott LN, et al. Source position verification and dosimetry in HDR brachytherapy using an EPID. Med Phys 2013;40(11):111706.
21. Yewondwossen M. Characterization and use of a 2D-array of ion chambers for brachytherapy dosimetric quality assurance. Med Dosim 2012;37(3):250–6.
22. Jursinic P. Quality assurance measurements for high-dose-rate brachytherapy without film. J Appl Clin Med Phys 2014;15(1):4586.
23. Nath R, Anderson LL, Meli JA, et al. Code of practice for brachytherapy physics: Report of the AAPM radiation therapy committee Task Group No. 56. Med Phys 1997;24(10):1557–98.
24. Venselaar J, Perez-Calatayud J, editors. A practical guide to quality control of brachytherapy equipment. In: European guidelines for quality assurance in radiotherapy. ESTRO booklet No. 8. Brussels, Belgium: 2004.
25. Kubo HD, Glasgow GP, Pethel TD, et al. High dose-rate brachytherapy treatment delivery: Report of the AAPM Radiation Therapy Committee Task Group No. 59. Med Phys 1998;25(4):375–403.
26. Thomadsen BR, Erickson BA, Eifel PJ, et al. A review of safety, quality management, and practice guidelines for high-dose-rate brachytherapy: Executive summary. Pract Radiat Oncol 2014;4:65–70. Full report available on ASTRO website: <https://www.astro.org/Clinical-Practice/White-Papers/HDR-White-Paper.aspx>.
27. AAPM Report No. 152, The 2007 AAPM response to the CRCPD request for recommendations for the CRCPD's model regulations for electronic brachytherapy. American Association of Physicists in Medicine; 2009.
28. Park CC, Yom SS, Podgorsak MB, et al. American Society for Therapeutic Radiology and Oncology (Astro) Emerging Technology Committee Report on Electronic Brachytherapy. Int J Radiat Oncol Biol Phys 2010;76:963–72.
29. Hill R, Mo Z, Haque M, et al. An evaluation of ionization chambers for the relative dosimetry of kilovoltage x-ray beams. Med Phys 2009;36(9):3971–81.
30. Li XA, Ma CM, Salhani D. Measurement of percentage depth dose and lateral beam profile for kilovoltage x-ray therapy beams. Phys Med Biol 1997;42(12):2561–8.
31. Ma CM, Li XA, Seuntjens JP. Study of dosimetry consistency for kilovoltage x-ray beams. Med Phys 1998;25(12):2376–84.
32. Standards for quality control at the Canadian radiation treatment centres, Kilovoltage x-ray radiotherapy machines. Canadian Association of Provincial Cancer Agencies; 2005.
33. IPEM Report 81, Physics aspects of quality control in radiotherapy. York, England: The Institue of Physics and Engineering in Medicine; 1999.
34. Mutic S, Palta JR, Butker EK, et al. Quality assurance for computed-tomography simulators and the computed-tomography simulation process: Report of the AAPM Radiation Therapy Committee Task Group No. 66. Med Phys 2003;30(10):2762–92.
35. Molloy JA, Chan G, Markovic A, et al. Quality assurance of U.S.-guided external beam radiotherapy for prostate cancer: Report of AAPM Task Group 154. Med Phys 2011;38(2):857–71.
36. Pfeiffer D, Sutlief S, Feng W, et al. AAPM Task Group 128: Quality assurance tests for prostate brachytherapy ultrasound systems. Med Phys 2008;35(12):5471–89.
37. Diamantopoulos S, Milickovic N, Butt S, et al. Effect of using different U/S probe standoff materials in image geometry for interventional procedures: The example of prostate. J Contemp Brachytherapy 2011;3(4):209–19.
38. IAEA Human Health Series No. 1, Quality assurance for PET and PET/CT systems. Vienna: International Atomic Energy Agency; 2009.

39. Xing L. Quality assurance of PET/CT for radiation therapy. Int J Radiat Oncol Biol Phys 2008;71(1 Suppl.):S38–42.
40. Mutic S, Dempsey JF. The ViewRay system: Magnetic resonance-guided and controlled radiotherapy. Semin Radiat Oncol 2014;24(3):196–9.
41. AAPM report 100, Acceptance testing and quality assurance procedures for magnetic resonance imaging facilities. American Association of Physicists in Medicine; 2010.
42. Bauer S, Wiest R, Molte LP, et al. A survey of MRI-based medical image analysis for brain tumor studies. Phys Med Biol 2013;58:R97–129.
43. Markkola AT, Hannu JA, Lukkarinen S, et al. Multiple-slice spin lock imaging of head and neck tumors at 0.1 tesla: exploring appropriate imaging parameters with reference to T2-weighted spin-echo technique. Invest Radiol 2001;36(9):531–8.
44. Devic S. MRI simulation for radiotherapy treatment planning. Med Phys 2012;39(11):6701–11.
45. Mellenberg DE, Dahl RA, Blackwell CR. Acceptance testing of an automated scanning water phantom. Med Phys 1990;17(2):311–14.
46. Siochi RA, Balter P, Bloch CD, et al. A rapid communication from the AAPM Task Group 201: Recommendations for the QA of external beam radiotherapy data transfer. J Appl Clin Med Phys 2010;12(1):3479.
47. Halvorsen PH, Das IJ, Fraser M, et al. AAPM Task Group 103 report on peer review in clinical Radiation Oncology physics. J Appl Clin Med Phys 2005;6(4):50–64.
48. <http://www.mdanderson.org/education-and-research/resources-for-professionals/scientific-resources/core-facilities-and-services/radiation-dosimetry-services/index.html>.
49. <http://www-naweb.iaea.org/nahu/DMRP/tld.html>.
50. <http://uwmrrc.wisc.edu/index.php?option=com_content&task=view&id=33&Itemid=59>.

# CHAPTER 5

# Quality Assurance of Radiotherapy Dose Calculations

## 5.1 Introduction

In modern radiotherapy the vast majority of dose calculations are performed by computerized systems. There may be minor exceptions such as radiopharmaceuticals used in nuclear medicine. The system may calculate all or some of the following: point doses, 2D isodoses, 3D isodoses, and doses to volumes. In addition, a whole host of nondosimetric information may be used to inform clinicians as to the quality of the treatment plan. This includes imaging information (computed tomography (CT), magnetic resonance (MR), positron emission tomography (PET), ultrasound (US) etc.), derived imaging information (beam's-eye view (BEV), digitally reconstructed radiographs (DRRs)) and beam apertures (both static and dynamic). The radiation source could be either electrically produced (linac, orthovoltage, cyclotron, etc.) or from a radioactive material ($^{60}$Co, $^{137}$Cs, $^{192}$Ir, $^{125}$I, $^{103}$Pd, $^{223}$Ra, etc.). The general term for these kinds of systems is treatment planning system (TPS). An overview of the commissioning and quality assurance (QA) testing methodologies that can be employed for these systems is given below and then each is discussed in greater detail in the following sections.

It is imperative that the dose calculations are accurate to within acceptable limits. ICRU report 62 recommends that the overall uncertainty in the dose delivered to a patient not exceed 5%.[1] To meet this goal, a comprehensive QA program must be implemented for every clinically used TPS. This includes QA prior to treating patients (acceptance and commissioning) and ongoing QA afterward (routine and patient specific and after every upgrade). The backbone of any dose calculation QA is the comparison of calculated doses to doses measured in the clinic. In addition, comparisons can be made with peer-reviewed reference data and calculations from other systems or Monte Carlo calculations.

In addition to the dosimetric QA, the nondosimetric components mentioned above must have a QA program. This is generally accomplished with the use of geometric phantoms and the comparison of imported/exported data.

A comprehensive test of all components is called an end-to-end (E2E) test. This type of test involves using phantoms to test the complete clinical process from beginning to end, just as an actual patient would be treated. It is important to involve the clinical staff that would perform the duties on actual patients to ensure that the proper workflow is employed and that errors are not missed due to missed steps or improper sequencing.

There are recommendations for TPS QA from various entities as well as many sources of reference data. One standard reference is AAPM TG-53 on QA for Clinical Radiotherapy Treatment Planning,[2] which discusses many of the issues noted here at a general level. In the following sections, the appropriate sources will be described and summarized for each category of radiotherapy. A sample checklist for TPS commissioning is shown in this chapter's Appendix 1.

This chapter is closely related to the previous chapter on commissioning and QA of technical systems. While some of the content in this chapter discusses beam measurements that are part of equipment commissioning, the majority of these data are intended for the characterization of the radiation source and the validation of the dose calculations and are therefore covered in this chapter.

# 5.2 Treatment Planning System Commissioning

## DOSIMETRIC TESTING

Dosimetric data can be in the form of point doses, 2D isodoses, 3D isodoses, dose/volume information, or activity. To test the accuracy of the calculations from a system, three strategies can be employed:

1. Comparison of calculated doses to measurements
2. Comparison of calculated doses to benchmark data
3. Comparison of calculated doses from one system to another system that has already been validated

A full commissioning of a system will usually involve using at least two of these strategies.

Another factor that must be evaluated is the dose calculation grid resolution. A system may give clinically different results for a 4 mm grid spacing compared to a 2 mm grid. It is very important to recognize when to use smaller or larger grids. For example, some studies recommend a 2.5 mm or smaller grids for intensity-modulated radiation therapy (IMRT) calculations,[3] and the grid spacing should be proportional to the multi-leaf collimator (MLC) leaf width, meaning that a micro-MLC will need 2 mm or smaller grid spacing.[4] Other special considerations include the use of Monte Carlo–based treatment planning to account for tissue inhomogeneities, the dose effects of couch tops, and biological models.

The user must be aware of how the TPS reports dose to heterogeneities. The system may calculate dose to the medium or convert to dose to water by using stopping power ratios. These two methods will lead to different results. The relative merits have been discussed in the literature but no standard has yet emerged.[5-9] This issue is of particular concern for MC algorithms. See AAPM TG-105, Issues Associated with Clinical Implementation of Monte Carlo–Based Photon and Electron External Beam Treatment Planning, for details.[5] Monte Carlo calculations have long been used to accurately calculate doses, particularly in heterogeneous tissues where electron transport issues are not properly handled by model-based calculations. The long calculation times for Monte Carlo algorithms have prevented their general use in the clinic. With the advent of faster computing hardware and optimized codes, they are now entering the mainstream. The issues of statistical uncertainty, the ability to account for the exact geometry of the accelerator treatment head, and other features are unique to Monte Carlo algorithms and must be well understood for accurate implementation. For example, because of the statistical uncertainty of the dose to any voxel, normalization to point doses can lead to unexpected results. This is especially relevant for electron Monte Carlo, where treatment dose is often prescribed to $d_{max}$. For dose prescriptions to an isodose line, a Monte Carlo calculation uncertainty of 2% at prescription isodose has evolved as a clinical standard. It should be noted, though, that uncertainties of dose calculation are higher for organs at risks (OARs) receiving lower doses than the prescription dose. A Monte Carlo treatment planning system should be able to display the uncertainty of dose calculation on the treatment planning scan to allow the clinicians to thoroughly assess the dose distribution.

AAPM TG-176, Dosimetric Effects Caused by Couch Tops and Immobilization Devices,[10] discusses how the treatment couch and immobilization devices can cause increased skin dose, reduced tumor dose, and a change in the dose distribution if not properly addressed. In particular, beam entrance through high density components should be avoided. Attenuation through carbon fiber couch tops can range from 2% for normally incident beams to 6% for highly oblique beams at low energies. In addition, denser sections can have up to 17% attenuation. The attenuation will increase if the couch top is paired with other immobilization devices. The skin dose can reach 100% of the maximum dose. Simple attenuation corrections can lead to inaccurate dose calculation, and the explicit inclusion of the devices by the TPS is recommended.

AAPM TG-166, The Use and QA of Biologically Related Models for Treatment Planning,[11] discusses four issues with biological models:

1. Strategies, limitations, conditions, and cautions for using biological models
2. The practical use of the most commonly used biological models: equivalent uniform dose (EUD), normal tissue complication probability (NTCP), tumor control probability (TCP), and probability of complication free tumor control ($P_+$)
3. Desirable features and future directions of biological models
4. General guidelines and methodology for acceptance testing, commissioning, and ongoing QA of biological models

Because the use of biological models represents a paradigm shift, they must be implemented carefully to avoid a dangerous misapplication of the models. The use of biological models can have advantages in both optimization and plan evaluation. This is because if the model is accurate the results are directly correlated with outcomes and can more reliably rank plans for a given patient. More detail on biological models is given in Chapter 14.

## COMPARISON OF CALCULATED DOSES TO MEASUREMENTS

A forthcoming Medical Physics Practice Guideline (MPPG) #5 from AAPM on Commissioning and QA of TPS in external beam therapy will have a summary of the minimum requirements for dosimetric testing (AAPM TG-244). Nondosimetric testing is not part of the scope of the planned document.

When commissioning a TPS there are two types of measurements taken: beam data needed to characterize the beam model and data needed to validate the model. For linear accelerators, this is the subject of AAPM TG-106 on accelerator beam data commissioning equipment and procedure.[12] The characterization set varies by vendor but includes items such as output factors, wedge transmission factors, depth dose curves, and profiles. These are typically measured in a water phantom. Specifics related to these measurements can be found in Chapter 2. The user must be careful to perform the measurements under the conditions described by the vendor. Particular attention must be paid to the definition of the normalization condition and the definition of wedge transmission. For instance, some systems normalize to 90 cm source-to-surface distance (SSD) and 10 cm depth while others require 100 cm SSD. In addition, some systems require wedge transmission relative to a 10 × 10 cm field while others require a ratio of wedge to open field for each field size.

As discussed in Chapter 2, the measurement of surface dose must be done using the appropriate detector (extrapolation or parallel plate chamber). This is typically an area of weakness for many dose calculation algorithms and should be carefully evaluated. If the system cannot accurately calculate surface dose, more frequent patient-specific measurements may be required to confirm the skin dose.

Out-of-field doses are important for characterizing the risk for situations such as a pregnant patient and patients with implanted electronic devices. AAPM TG-158, Measurements and Calculations of Doses Outside the Treatment Volume from External Beam Radiation Therapy, is developing recommendations in this area. The accuracy of out-of-field dose measurements should be checked using an anthropomorphic phantom. In recent years, a few clinical studies have emerged emphasizing the importance of assessing integral dose and dose to distant organs to avoid late secondary cancers.[13-14] Studies have shown that some systems may have difficulty in calculating these doses accurately.[15-16] At distances close to the irradiated volume, internal scatter is the largest component of the dose, whereas at larger distances machine scatter and leakage dominate.[17] For 3D conformal systems internal scatter contributes up to 70% of the dose and dominates up to 25 cm from the irradiated volume. For IMRT, internal scatter dominates only up to 10 cm from the irradiated volume, with collimator scatter dominating for the next 10 cm and head leakage beyond 20 cm.[18]

The validation set is a more extensive set of measurements encompassing the range of clinical situations expected to be used at that facility. This will include depth dose and profile data at multiple SSDs, oblique angle data, the effect of inhomogeneity, and complex field shaping. Appendix 2 in this chapter shows suggested validation test measurements compiled from various sources including Appendix 3 of AAPM TG-53[2] and in International Atomic Energy Agency (IAEA) TRS-430, Commissioning and Quality Assurance of Computerized Planning Systems for Radiation Treatment of Cancer.[19] Two other IAEA documents, TECDOC-1540 and TECDOC-1583, expand on TRS-430 and provide practical examples.[20-21] The European Society of Therapeutic Radiation Oncology (ESTRO) and the Netherlands Commission on Radiation Dosimetry have also produced documents showing practical examples.[22,23]

When performing these measurements many methods can be used. The most basic is the use of the appropriate detectors in a water phantom. Again, the details are described in Chapter 2. The water phantom can acquire 1D and point dose data. Similarly, solid phantoms can be used in combination with point dosimeters. The point dosimeter is in actuality a (very small) volume dosimeter, so the user must ensure that the dosimeter is appropriate for the gradients and field sizes used.

By using a combination of water equivalent and non-water slabs, inhomogeneity effects can be analyzed. Because of the changes in beam spectra and scattering properties within or near non-water materials, corrections may need to be made to the dosimeter readings. For film embedded in non-water material the measured dose is the dose to the film, not dose to the inhomogeneity.[24] The comparison can be made by using the dose to water for the calculation or applying the appropriate correction to the measurement using stopping power ratios. Ion chamber measurements will need similar corrections.[25]

Film and detector arrays can be used to measure 2D data. Film has the advantage of much greater spatial resolution but can be problematic when trying to measure larger fields. Most radiotherapy departments no longer have film processors, so radiochromic film is used. The scanners used to analyze radiochromic films suffer from a lack of uniformity of response over larger areas, which limits the accuracy of the results. Detector arrays have a good uniformity of response over larger areas but suffer from poor spatial resolution. The detectors are situated 5 to 10 mm apart depending on the exact model used. There can also be directional response differences. Again these detectors can be used to evaluate inhomogeneity effects but are limited to transmission data since their design does not allow them to measure inside or proximal to an inhomogeneity.

## TISSUE HETEROGENEITY IN THE CONTEXT OF TPS DOSE CALCULATIONS

Some systems will use a CT number to density correction curve created using physical density while others use electron density. Not all dose calculation algorithms perform equally in and around tissue inhomogeneities, and the user should be aware of the algorithm uncertainties and limitations.[26] AAPM TG-65, Tissue Inhomogeneity Corrections for Megavoltage Photon

Beams, presents a detailed evaluation of inhomogeneity corrections.[27] It describes the performance of different algorithms in various conditions and present recommendations. A summary of
the recommendations is as follows:

1. Heterogeneity corrections should be applied to dose calculations and prescriptions. Even if
   there are inaccuracies in the algorithm, it will be closer to reality than if no correction is
   applied.
2. For head and neck, larynx, and lung treatments, even simple algorithms will calculate
   adequately in areas away from bone and air interfaces. Near these interfaces convolution
   and Monte Carlo algorithms will perform better. For high electron density materials, refer to
   AAPM TG-63, Dosimetric Considerations for Patients with Hip Prostheses Undergoing
   Pelvic Irradiation, for details.[28]
3. For lung treatments energies of 12 MV or less are recommended.
4. For breast treatments, the doses near the chest wall/lung interface are more accurately calculated with convolution or Monte Carlo methods.
5. For gastrointestinal treatments, barium contrast areas should be contoured and the density
   should be overridden.
6. For prostate and pelvis treatments, the main concern is with high electron density hip prostheses. Again, see AAPM TG-63.

The calculation of dose to non-water structures is performed by using the CT numbers
of the planning scan to account for differences in density. Typically a TPS will use a stored table
to convert CT number to density. This table is established by scanning phantom materials of
known density and correlating with the measured CT numbers. This CT–density relationship
depends on the kVp of the scan and can be different from scanner to scanner even for the
same kVp. The stability of this relationship must be verified over time and when the CT tube is
replaced.

How would the tolerance levels be established for this QA measure? One way to approach
this is to look at the typical clinical applications. Most tissue is near water equivalent, so to
establish a clinically relevant range you could change the density of a water phantom and note
when the calculated dose at 20 cm depth changes by more than 1%. For lower densities such as
lung, a typical thickness is about 15 cm. Tolerance levels can be calculated by placing a calculation
point distal to the lung volume and again changing the density until the dose changes by 1%.
High density regions would not be expected to exceed 4 cm in thickness. Using this methodology
yields ranges of +/–20 in CT number for low density to water and +/–100 for high density
values. By comparison, AAPM TG-66, Quality Assurance for Computed-Tomography Simulators
and the Computed-Tomography Simulation Process, recommends a generic +/–5 over the entire
range of CT numbers.[29]

Another issue with CT number to density conversions is the number of bits used to store the
CT data, i.e., grayscale values. Using a traditional 12 bit storage will truncate the data at a CT
number of approximately 3000, while 16 bit storage will allow much higher values. This will
provide more accurate dosimetry and improved visualization.[30]

## COMPARISON OF CALCULATED DOSES TO BENCHMARK DATA

There are many sources of benchmark data in the peer-reviewed literature. These detail either a
specific parameter such as output factors, a compilation of data, or test plans. Table 5.1 summarizes some of the literature. In addition, AAPM TG-23, Radiation Treatment Planning
Dosimetry, has dosimetry data for characterization and validation,[31] but it is somewhat old and
may not have adequate data for some modern systems. It also does not have MLC data. IAEA
TECDOC-1540[20] also has a set of benchmark data. Both data sets are available for download

TABLE 5.1 ▦ **Summary of Benchmark Data**

| Vendor(s) | Type of Data | Publication |
|---|---|---|
| Any | IMRT commissioning sample plans | Ezzell et al., IMRT commissioning: Multiple institution planning and dosimetry comparisons, a report from AAPM Task Group 119. Med Phys 2009;36(11):5359-5373. Sample plans available for download on AAPM website. |
| Any | Measurement of collimator scatter factor | AAPM TG-74, Zhu et al., In-air output ratio Sc for megavoltage photon beams, Med Phys 2009;36(11):5261-5291. |
| Varian 4 MV, Siemens 15 MV | Lung transmission dose data | Rice et al., Benchmark measurements for lung dose corrections for x-ray beams, IJROBP 1988;15:399-409. |
| Any | Phantom scatter | Stochi et al., A table of phantom scatter factors of photon beams as a function of the quality index and field size, PMB 1996;41:563-571. |
| Elekta, Siemens, Varian | Small field photon OF | Followill et al., The Radiological Physics Center's standard dataset for small field size output factors, JACMP 2012;13(5):3962. |
| Elekta (Philips), Siemens, Varian | WF | Followill et al., Standard wedge transmission values for Varian, Siemens, Philips, and AECL accelerators, Med Phys 1997;24:1076. Kennedy and Hanson, A review of high-energy photon beam characteristics measured by the Radiological Physics Center, Med Phys 1992;19:838. |
| Elekta, Siemens, Varian | Electron cone ratios | Tailor et al., Predictability of electron cone ratios with respect to linac make and model, JACMP 2003;4:172. |
|  | Electron PDD, electron cone ratios | Davis et al., Electron percent depth dose and cone ratios from various machines, Med Phys 1994;22:1007. |
| CyberKnife | Output factors | Bassinet et al., Small fields output factors measurements and correction factors determination for several detectors for a CyberKnife and linear accelerators equipped with microMLC and circular cones, Med Phys 2013;40(11):117201. |
| CyberKnife | OF, PDD, OAR | Deng et al., Commissioning 6MV photon beams of a stereotactic radiosurgery system for Monte Carlo treatment planning, Med Phys 2003;30(12):3124-3134. |
| CyberKnife | OF, OAR | Francescon et al., Monte Carlo simulated correction factors for machine specific reference field dose calibration and output factor measurement using fixed and iris collimators on the CyberKnife system, Phys Med Bio 2012;57:3741-3758. |
| Elekta | Agility MLC data and some sample data for MLC shapes | Bedford et al., Beam modeling and VMAT performance with the Agility 160-leaf multi-leaf collimator, JACMP 2013;14(2):172-185. |
| Elekta | Penumbra, OAR, OF | Cranmer-Sargison et al., Small field dosimetric characterization of a new 160-leaf MLC, Phys Med Bio 2013;58:7343-7354. |

TABLE 5.1 ▒ **Summary of Benchmark Data—cont'd**

| Vendor(s) | Type of Data | Publication |
|---|---|---|
| Elekta | PDD, OF | Paynter et al., Beam characteristics of energy-matched flattening filter free beams, Med Phys 2014;41(5):052103. |
| Siemens | OAR, PDD, OF | Cho and Ibbott, Reference photon dosimetry data: A preliminary study of in-air off-axis factor, percent depth dose, and output factor of the Siemens Primus linear accelerator, JACMP 2003;4(4):300-306. |
| TomoTherapy | OAR, OF | Balog et al., Clinical helical TomoTherapy commissioning dosimetry, Med Phys 2003;30:3097-3106. |
| Varian | PDD, OAR, OF | Beyer, Commissioning measurements for photon beam data on three TrueBeam linear accelerators, and comparison with Trilogy and Clinac 2100 linear accelerators, JACMP 2013;14:273. |
| Varian | PDD, OF, OAR, penumbra, WF, MLC leakage, electron effective SSD, electron cone ratios, electron PDD | Chang et al., Commissioning and dosimetric characteristics of TrueBeam system: Composite data of three TrueBeam machines, Med Phys 2012;39(11):6981-7018. |
| Varian | PDD, OAR, OF, MLC transmission, electron PDD, electron cone ratios; includes staff time estimates | Glide-Hurst et al., Commissioning of the Varian TrueBeam linear accelerator: A multi-institutional study, Med Phys 2013;40(3):031719. |
| Varian | PDD, OF, Sc, WF, OAR, electron cone ratios, electron depth dose, electron effective source distance | Watts, Comparative measurements made on a series of accelerators by the same vendor, Med Phys 1999;26(12):2581-2585. |
| Brachy sources | Benchmark data, AAPM TG-43 parameters | The Imaging and Radiation Oncology Core (formerly Radiological Physics Center) has extensive data on their website: http://rpc.mdanderson.org. |

on the AAPM website, http://www.aapm.org/pubs/reports/. Another older source of data is BJR Supplement No. 25,[32] which contains depth dose data for various beam qualities. The data contain averages of many beams from different vendors, so care should be used when comparing to these data and a greater level of disagreement should be expected (2% to 5%). The Imaging and Radiation Oncology Core in Houston (IROC-H), formerly known as the Radiological Physics Center (RPC), has documentation on standard data for various linear accelerator models for both photon and electron beams.[33-34] Their website also has many useful references (http://rpc.mdanderson.org/RPC/home.htm). AAPM TG-67, Benchmark Datasets for Photon Beams, produced a report describing the contents of a photon beam benchmark data set. Based on this report an Small Business Innovation Research (SBIR) grant was awarded to measure the data sets. Sun Nuclear Corporation was awarded this grant and maintains the data. The vendor may also supply benchmark data. This should be used for comparison only and is not a substitute for local measurements. The use of vendor data as clinical data should only be done after validating the accuracy to within 1% to 2%.

Brachytherapy sources benchmark data are available for vendor-specific sources. The general calculation methodology is described in AAPM TG-43, Dosimetry of Interstitial Brachytherapy Sources, and Its Supplements.[35-37]

## COMPARISON OF CALCULATED DOSES FROM ONE SYSTEM TO ANOTHER SYSTEM THAT HAS ALREADY BEEN VALIDATED

This is a relatively simple process with several caveats. First, the limitations of the previous system must be known. For instance, differences would be expected when comparing a convolution model to a pencil beam model, and the comparison would not be valid for inhomogeneity calculations. In that case a comparison could be made for simple water calculations but measurements would have to be made for the more complex situations. Second, the capabilities of the two systems may not match. For example, the newer system may have volumetric arc therapy (VMAT) while the older does not. In the end, this type of comparison is of limited use for dosimetric commissioning. However, it is a valuable process to review with the clinical team any differences among the systems so that the results can be correlated with past experience. As mentioned previously, differences in inhomogeneity calculations should be understood as well as how penumbra differences may affect field size selection.

One of the most common examples of this is the verification of TPS MU calculation. AAPM TG-114, Verification of Monitor Unit Calculations for Non-IMRT Clinical Radiotherapy, describes this in detail.[38] Typically the treatment plan data are transferred to the independent system using the Digital Imaging and Communications in Medicine (DICOM) protocol (http://dicom.nema.org/). Depending on the system, the plan file, image files, and structure sets may be transferred. Some systems only calculate the MU based on an effective depth to the reference point and the treatment field fluence pattern. Other systems will perform a complete recalculation including dose-volume histograms (DVHs) for comparison. It is typical for second check systems to use the same input beam data as the commissioned TPS. This will speed up the implementation process; however, a rigorous QA of the second check system still needs to be performed.

### END-TO-END TESTS

End-to-end tests are a valuable QA activity that closes the loop on the entire planning process. The basic concept is to treat a phantom just like you would a patient. Ideally the phantom would contain a target that is visible using the desired imaging modality (CT, MR, PET, US). The phantom would be immobilized and imaged as per clinical policy. Next a treatment plan is performed according to clinical protocol. If it is a treatment modality that requires patient-specific QA, that should be performed according to department policy. The phantom is then reimmobilized on the treatment couch, imaged according to department policy, and then treated as per the treatment plan. Finally, the measured dose is compared to the calculated dose to check the agreement. It is important for the phantom to have the ability to embed film and point detectors to get both an accurate absolute dose measurement as well as 2D verification of the positional accuracy in at least 2 orthogonal planes. For small targets like those encountered in stereotactic radiosurgery (SRS) this may require separate deliveries for the film and point dosimeters as there may not be enough space to accommodate both at the same time. As mentioned above, it is critical that the team members who would perform a task for a patient also perform the task during the end-to-end test so that the real clinical process is tested.

### DOSE–VOLUME TESTING

The dose–volume information in a plan is often used by clinicians to evaluate the quality of a plan and therefore must be accurate. For external beam systems, utilizing a beam that is as flat as possible will enable a simple evaluation. By using a single beam and structures that are within the flat portion of the beam, the dose–volume relationship will follow the depth dose curve. For example, if the proximal surface of the structure is at the 80% depth and the distal surface is at the 50% depth, and 1000 cGy is given to $d_{max}$ depth, the minimum dose to the structure will be

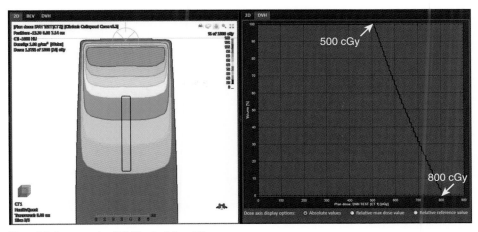

**Figure 5.1** An example of DVH calculation QA.

500 cGy and the maximum dose 800 cGy. The volume receiving between 500 and 800 cGy will follow the depth dose curve as shown in Figure 5.1.

For brachytherapy systems this validation can be simple. By placing a point source at the center of a spherical structure a very predictable dose–volume relationship can be determined. Again, the importance of dose grid size must be evaluated. This can be done by looking at the dose–volume changes by grid size for structures of various volumes. This is true for any type of system, not just brachytherapy. If small volumes are to be evaluated, smaller grid sizes may be needed. This will depend on the system's interpolation algorithms and the method by which voxels are assigned to structures.

The example in Figure 5.2 shows differences in effect based on the size and location of the structure. The smaller structure near the beam edge (high gradient) has the most dramatic change when the dose grid is changed from 4 mm to 1 mm. Clinical examples of this could be the optic chiasm or the penile bulb.

## NONDOSIMETRIC TESTING

AAPM TG-53 and IAEA TRS-430 describe in detail the nondosimetric testing that is recommended. In addition, AAPM TG-201, Quality Assurance of External Beam Treatment Data Transfer, describes data transfer testing.[39] To complete all of the tasks described would take many hours of dedicated time. A comprehensive plan must be developed that can be accomplished with the resources at hand. A list of areas to check would include patient anatomic representation, contouring, autocontouring, volume determination, density determination, image display, dose display, coordinate systems, machine description, machine capabilities, machine parameters, readout conventions (i.e., International Electrotechnical Commission (IEC)), aperture display, automatic field shaping, beam geometry display, SSD, and data import/export. A sample set of tests is shown in Appendix 3 in this chapter.

Testing of autocontouring can be done using different density materials of a known size and shape. For example, an acrylic sphere inside a container of water could be imaged by CT and then contoured on the TPS. The same test can be used to determine the accuracy of the density and volume reported by the TPS. A more elaborate test would involve the use of different density plastics approaching water density to test the minimum contrast difference the algorithm can detect.

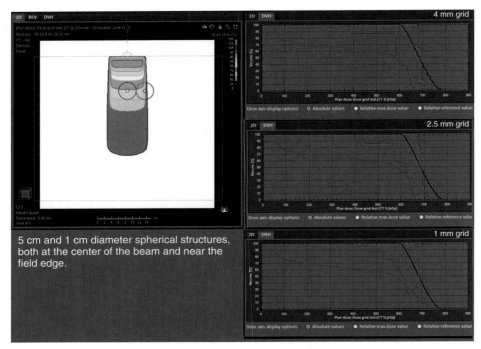

5 cm and 1 cm diameter spherical structures, both at the center of the beam and near the field edge.

**Figure 5.2** The effect of grid size on DVH calculation.

Image display can be done by testing objects of known size and shape. A bowling ball is an example of a test object that can be used to test BEV, DRR, and SSD accuracy. By design, bowling balls need to be perfectly spherical and are ideal for these purposes. Obtain a CT scan of the ball and import it into the TPS. Place many beams at the center of the ball with a field size equal to the diameter of the ball using different combinations of gantry, collimator, and couch angles. Since the ball is spherical, the BEV, DRR, and SSD should be identical for every beam. The MU should also be identical and can be used as part of the dosimetric testing. Slab phantoms can similarly be used. More elaborate phantoms are available as well, such as the Quasar phantoms from Modus Medical, the Baltas phantom from Pi Medical Research, and the ISIS phantom from Radiation Products Design.

The accuracy of the coordinate systems and patient orientation is extremely important. These can be checked by placing markers on slab phantoms at known locations (i.e., left anterior) and then scanning and importing into the TPS to confirm that the location of the markers is correct. The DOVe phantom from Integrated Medical Technologies is engraved with text and objects that make the determination of the image orientation obvious for any orientation. In addition, there are holes at known coordinates to confirm the accuracy of the coordinate system. A sample image of the phantom is shown in Figure 5.3.

Connectivity testing is important to ensure the accuracy of information at all steps in the process. Image data may come from within the department, a Picture Archiving and Communication system (PACS), or media from outside facilities. The data may be transferred directly to the TPS or to a contouring system first. From the TPS data may be sent to the Record & Verify (R&V) system and a second check system. A data transfer matrix can be created as shown in Table 5.2. The matrix lists the sources and destinations of information, and a description of the types of data is shown in each cell in the matrix. Cells are only populated for transfers that are used, so many may be blank. This will help guide what is to be tested. For example, in

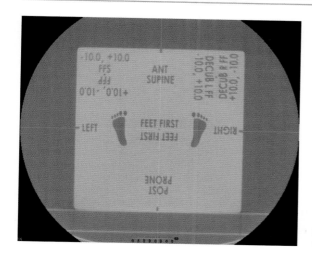

**Figure 5.3** Sample phantom for the verification of patient orientation.

a CT-to-TPS transfer the geometric accuracy, density information, and orientation must be checked. For a TPS-to-R&V transfer, the beam parameters, leaf sequence information, and dose information must be checked. For all transfers the patient identification information must be checked.

Different machine capabilities must be checked such as maximum MLC leaf over-travel, maximum and minimum gantry speeds, or minimum MU for dynamic wedges. It is important to check these settings so that plans are not created that are undeliverable. One area that many TPS systems can improve is in collision detection. More systems are now allowing the placement of the treatment couch onto the image data set, which helps in determining where collisions may occur. A cylindrical structure can be created that has a diameter equal to the effective "bore" size of the linac to visualize the safe zone. This can be augmented by creating a table of allowable beam angles based on couch height and rotation.

## TIME ESTIMATES AND RESOURCES FOR COMMISSIONING AND QA PROGRAM DEVELOPMENT

The commissioning of a TPS can be part of opening a new center, part of a new program (i.e., new linac or HDR system), or as a replacement TPS. The amount of time required is substantial. Beam or source data must be collected and input into the system. The beam or source is then modeled. Then output is verified by measurements and/or benchmark data. In addition, the full functionality of the system must be validated including the nondosimetric features mentioned above. After commissioning a new TPS, it is recommended to perform an outside audit to confirm the accuracy of the system. This can be done using remote dosimetry services. These services will either mail an anthropomorphic phantom to be used in an end-to-end test with point and film dosimeters embedded or will mail radiochromic film to the institution to be returned for evaluation after irradiation in the institution's phantom. Once the system is commissioned, an ongoing QA program must be developed.

As mentioned throughout this chapter, extensive testing is required to fully ensure the performance of treatment planning dose calculations. Completing this testing is a significant investment. How much time should you allocate and what strategies can you employ to speed up the process? AAPM TG-106[12] discussed the time for linac commissioning and reported 4 to 6 weeks for testing a modern linac with electrons. Their estimate does not include nonscanned data measurements, baseline QA readings, benchmarking, and validation of the TPS. Nonscanned

**TABLE 5.2 ■ Data Transfer Matrix**

| Source | Destination | | | | | | | | | |
| --- | --- | --- | --- | --- | --- | --- | --- | --- | --- | --- |
| | CT Sim Lasers | CT Sim Software | TPS | R&V | Contouring Station | MU Second Check | HDR Console | Linac Console | Linac 4DTC | Data Archive |
| CT | | Images (DICOM) | Images (DICOM) | | Images (DICOM) | | | | | |
| CT Sim Lasers | | | | | | | | | | |
| CT Sim software | Isocenter, coordinates (FTP) | | Images, structures, fields, isocenter (DICOM) | | | | | | | |
| Gating System | | Respiratory cycle (FTP) | | | | | | | | |
| PACS | | | Images (DICOM) | | Images (DICOM) | | | | | |
| CD | | | Images (DICOM) | | Images (DICOM) | | | | | |
| TPS | | | | Field data (DICOM), PDF (FTP), isocenter | | RT Plan | Delivery file (FTP) | | | Archive data (may be semi-automated) |
| R&V | | | | | | | | Field data | Field data | |
| Contouring Station | | | | PDF (FTP) | | Images, structures (DICOM) | Images, structures (DICOM) | | | |
| MU Second Check | | | | | | | | | | |
| Linac Console | | | | | | | | Treatment complete, MU | | |
| Linac 4DTC | | | | | | | | Treatment complete, MU | | |
| Linac CBCT | | | | | | | | Images, shift data (DICOM) | | |
| Data Archive | | | Restored patients | | | | | | | |

TABLE 5.3 ■ **Time Estimates for TPS Commissioning**

| Task | Time Estimate (days) |
|---|---|
| Photon scanning (3 energies, depth doses, profiles) | 7 |
| Point data collection (OF, Sc, WF) | 5 |
| Electrons (5 energies, scans, cone factors, VSD) | 5-10 |
| Verification | 5 |
| Nonscanned data (MLC transmission, jaw transmission, head leakage) | 2-3 |
| Baseline QA measurements | 1-2 |
| Benchmarking | 1 |
| TPS validation | 4 |
| Analysis and report generation | 5-10 |
| Total | 35-47 |

data typically take 2 to 3 days for a modern linac with electrons. Daily and monthly QA baselines could be acquired in 8 to 12 hours spread over several days so as to confirm the reliability of the tests and the consistency of the linac. Benchmarking involves comparison of the measured data to published values. This can be done for PDD, OF, Sc, WF, and electron cone ratios, for example. This process could take an entire day. A list of reference documents is shown in Table 5.1. IAEA TECDOC-1583[21] provides an estimate of 2 working days for TPS validation, excluding IMRT tests. Adding IMRT testing could easily double this estimate. Adding all of this up results in approximately 35 to 47 working days as shown in Table 5.3.

The time estimates shown are based on an 8-hour workday. Clearly a solo physicist in a busy clinic cannot realistically commission the TPS and cover the clinical work without extending the work over 6 to 9 months or working 12-hour days and weekends. One common strategy is to contract for temporary physics support. Extra physics support staff could either perform the routine clinical work so that the staff physicist(s) can concentrate on the new system or the opposite. Having the staff physicist perform the commissioning has the advantage of allowing him or her to become expert with the system and have full knowledge of its strengths and weaknesses. It has a disadvantage in that the temporary staff will not be familiar with clinical process at the facility and will need time to be trained. A combination of the two strategies may be more practical. For example, the scanning data and point measurements could be done by a contractor. Contractors typically work in teams and have done the measurements many times and are therefore very efficient in acquiring the data. This could reduce a 17 to 20 day process to 5 to 7 days. The on-site physicist could concentrate on benchmarking and TPS validation testing to confirm the quality of the contractor's work. Another way to speed up the time to clinical release is to release one beam energy at a time. Releasing a system over a period of time has the advantage of being able to use the system earlier, but it must be done very carefully and may result in repeating some work. Releasing 3D before IMRT may cause reworking the beam model to fine tune the MLC penumbra, for example, and would not be advised. A more reasonable approach would be to release one beam energy for clinical use while modeling the others. A sample sequence might be 6 MV photons (with IMRT), electrons, and then higher energy photons.

## BRACHYTHERAPY-SPECIFIC TESTING

For brachytherapy dose calculation most systems use the AAPM TG-43 formalism. The systems calculate based on unit density and do not account for tissue inhomogeneity. Validating the input parameters can be done using the references listed on the IROC website as shown in Table 5.1. The references also show dose values at various points around a 1 U source strength, which can be used to validate the dose calculation. AAPM TG-138, A Dosimetric Uncertainty Analysis for Photon-Emitting Brachytherapy Sources,[40] discusses the uncertainties in the measurement of the source strength and the AAPM TG-43 parameters. They recommend using consensus values for the AAPM TG-43 parameters because using other values or multiple investigators will increase the uncertainty of the calculated doses. Since the seed orientation may not be known precisely in a prostate seed implant, calculations for seeds are generally done using a point source model except if otherwise specified in a clinical trial protocol. Therefore the anisotropy factor (average value) is used rather than an anisotropy function that describes the change in dose rate versus angle relative to the seed axis. For HDR brachytherapy the orientation is known because the catheter(s) path is input into the system for accurate dose calculation. In either case, the proper implementation must be verified by checking the dose rate at various distances and angles relative to the seed axis. Once the dose distribution is verified for a single source the accuracy for multiple sources should be evaluated. Some areas of recent development in brachytherapy dose calculation are the use of Monte Carlo algorithms (for both calculating AAPM TG-43 parameters and direct calculation),[41-42] incorporating inhomogeneity corrections,[43-44] and accounting for transit time.[45] AAPM TG-186, On Model-Based Calculations in Brachytherapy, has recommended transitioning from the AAPM TG-43 formalism to model-based dose calculation algorithms (MBDCA).[46] Since this is a new development, they recommend continued use of AAPM TG-43 for dose specification and reporting MBDCA information along with AAPM TG-43 dose information to allow for a systematic transition. They further recommend a unified methodology for assigning particular tissues to particular densities so that there will be consistency from institution to institution. A recommended commissioning process for MBDCAs is also discussed in the document.

## 5.3 Ongoing QA

After commissioning the TPS, routine QA must be established to ensure the continued accuracy of the system. Both the functionality of the system and the integrity of the beam model must be checked. Typically the beam model integrity is checked using a checksum function on the data files. AAPM TG-53 recommends that at least once every 12 months or after a software upgrade a subset of the dosimetric and nondosimetric testing must be performed.[2] A sample list is shown in Table 5.4. If performing QA after an upgrade it is best to review the release notes and design specific tests for any changes in functionality.

## 5.4 Patient-Specific QA

Patient-specific QA falls into two categories. First, the MU calculation of the TPS must be verified by an independent method as recommended by ACR-ASTRO Practice Guidelines.[47-48]

TABLE 5.4 ▓ **Sample Ongoing TPS QA**

| TPS QA Test | Description | Frequency |
|---|---|---|
| Beam data integrity | Checksum | Monthly |
| Dosimetric | Recalculation of 3D test plans. Use all beams and modifiers. Recalculation of IMRT plan. Compare results of dose matrix, point doses, and DVH to commissioning baseline. Investigate any differences. | Annually or upgrade |
| Connectivity | Test DICOM import and export of images and plans. | Annually or upgrade |
| Nondosimetric | Compare BEV/DRR to baseline for test case. | Annually or upgrade |
| New features | Test and compare to expected functionality. | On upgrade |

TABLE 5.5 ▪ **Action Levels for MU Verification as Recommended by AAPM TG-114**

| Primary calculation geometry | Similar Calculation Algorithms | | Different Calculation Algorithms | |
|---|---|---|---|---|
| | Same patient geometry (%) | Approximate patient geometry (%) | Same patient geometry (%) | Approximate patient geometry (%) |
| Large field | 2 | 3 | 2.5 | 3.5 |
| Wedged fields, off-axis fields | 2 | 3 | 3.5 | 4.5 |
| Small fields and/or low density heterogeneity | 3 | 3.5 | 4 | 5 |

This is typically done by comparing to the calculation of another system and is described in section 5.3.4 of AAPM TG-114.[38] Table 5.5 shows the AAPM TG-114 suggested action levels for disagreement between the verification and primary calculations including inhomogeneity.

AAPM TG-71, Monitor Unit Calculations for External Photon and Electron Beams,[49] and ESTRO booklet 6, Monitor Unit Calculation for High Energy Photon Beams: Practical Examples,[50] are also good references on MU verification. If the MU verification is done by a manual calculation, AAPM TG-71 gives a detailed description of the methodology. Factors included in the calculation are reference dose rate, collimator scatter, phantom scatter, depth, beam modifiers, off-axis ratios, and distance. Selecting an appropriate calculation point is important. Points that are shielded, within approximately 2 cm of the field edge, or within 1 cm of an inhomogeneity interface should be avoided, for example. It may not be possible to use the same point for all fields with a plan.[49]

The second category is the validation of IMRT dose distributions.[51-52] Originally this involved the use of an ion chamber to verify absolute dose and film to verify the spatial accuracy. Subsequently, detector arrays became the most widely adopted tool for this verification. In either method the patient fluence is recalculated on a phantom in which the measurement devices are placed. The recalculated phantom doses are then compared to the phantom measurements. There is currently some controversy in the field as to whether patient-specific measurements need be performed in every case. However, it is worth noting that in the United States, at the time of writing, CPT code #77301, which controls reimbursements, specifically calls for measurement in a phantom.

The most common evaluation method is the gamma index originally described by Low and Dempsey.[53] This method uses both dose difference and distance to agreement criteria to evaluate the difference between planned and measured doses on a point-by-point basis. This is to allow for different criteria to be used in different areas of the dose distribution based on the gradient in that area. Dose difference is used for the low gradient areas, and distance to agreement is used in high gradient areas. Results are generally reported as the percentage of points passing a combination of the two criteria (i.e., 95% of points passing with 2%/2 mm criterion). There is some controversy regarding how the beams should be measured (fixed gantry versus clinical angles, field by field versus composite) and what criteria to use.[54-55] If clinical gantry angles or arcs are being measured, the measurement device angular dependence must be carefully characterized.[56-59] If using the standard gamma index method many institutions use a 3%/3 mm criterion or even 5%/5 mm; however, it has been shown that this may not detect significant errors. With the absence of a standard, each institution must determine its own criteria based on the known weaknesses in the institution's system. AAPM TG-119 suggests that these limits should be set based on a determination of statistical variability in clinical practice.[47] The 3%/3 mm criterion would be a reasonable upper limit, with 2%/2 mm as an alternative. AAPM TG-120 on dosimetry tools and techniques for IMRT gives a description of the dosimeters, phantoms, and analysis

TABLE 5.6 ■ Commonly Used Detector Arrays for Patient-Specific QA

| Device (Manufacturer) | Description |
| --- | --- |
| MapCHECK (Sun Nuclear Corporation) | 2D diode array with nonuniform spacing |
| MapCHECK 2 (Sun Nuclear Corporation) | 2D diode array with uniform 7 mm spacing. 32 × 26 cm max field size |
| ArcCHECK (Sun Nuclear Corporation) | 3D diode array with 1 cm spacing in cylindrical configuration. 21 cm max field length |
| Octavius 729 (PTW Corporation) | 2D ion chamber array (729 detectors) with 1 cm spacing. 27 × 27 cm max field size |
| Octavius 1500 (PTW Corporation) | 2D ion chamber array (1500 detectors) with 7 mm spacing. 27 × 27 cm max field size |
| MatriXX (IBA Dosimetry) | 2D ion chamber array (1020 detectors) with 7.6 mm spacing. 24.4 × 24.4 cm max field size |
| Delta4 (Scandidos) | Two orthogonal 2D diode arrays (1069 detectors) with 5 mm spacing in the central 6 × 6 cm area and 1 cm spacing outside that area. 20 × 20 cm max field size |

techniques in use.[48] Other devices are also starting to be used, including portal imager dosimetry and 3D detector arrays. Table 5.6 shows some detector arrays commonly used for patient-specific QA. In addition, other methodologies that omit any measurement have been proposed and used at some centers. These involve recalculation of the dose based on the MLC leaf sequencing. While this does confirm the dose calculation, it removes the QA of the actual delivery hardware. In this case the institution must have a rigorous MLC QA program.

## FOR THE PHYSICIAN

Accurate dose calculation during treatment planning is critical to achieving the goals of treatment. The first step involves characterizing the radiation source in the treatment planning system (linac or brachytherapy), either by verifying the consensus parameters that describe the source or measuring the appropriate source parameters to accurately model the source. Once this is done, further measurements and/or calculations must be made to validate the calculation model. The comparisons can be done using another independent calculation methodology such as Monte Carlo or by using published benchmark data for the same source. An important step in the validation process is a comprehensive test of the entire clinical process called an end-to-end test. This involves the use of patient phantoms with embedded dosimeters that are subjected to the same process as a real patient, with each task being performed by the staff member who would perform it on a patient. In this manner the entire process can be evaluated for dose accuracy and geometrical accuracy.

Some issues that must be addressed in the dosimetric testing are:

1. Calculation in standard conditions (square or rectangular fields at different SSDs for a homogeneous phantom)
2. Calculation in clinical scenarios (oblique beams, inhomogeneous materials, surface irregularity, flash, lack of scatter equilibrium, beam modulation)
3. Dose volume calculations. Many clinical judgments are based on the dose volume information and it is critical that they are accurate.
4. Patient-specific QA. This involves the verification of the beam MU or treatment time and the validation of the absolute dose and geometrical accuracy of modulated beams (IMRT).

In addition to the dosimetric accuracy of a TPS, the nondosimetric components of the system must be evaluated for accuracy. These include:

1. Patient anatomic representation
2. Contouring, manual and automatic
3. Volume determination
4. Density determination
5. Image display
6. Dose display
7. Aperture display
8. Beam geometry display
9. Coordinate systems
10. Machine description (capabilities, parameters)
11. Readout conventions (i.e., IEC)
12. SSD
13. Data import/export

All of this testing takes a considerable amount of time, and this must be factored in to the implementation of a new system. Typically this can take 6 to 8 weeks of standard 8-hour workdays. In smaller clinics with limited resources, alternative strategies may need to be employed for a smooth implementation without disrupting the clinical work flow. This could involve the use of temporary contracted physics staff or a staggered release of equipment capabilities, one beam energy at a time, for example.

Once the system has been commissioned, the continued accuracy must be ensured by establishing an ongoing QA process. This will involve the calculation of dose and display of information for benchmark cases for which baselines were established during commissioning. A subset of tests should also be performed after software upgrades.

The ICRU has recommended that the calculation of absorbed dose be accurate to within 5% uncertainty. As more data are accumulated regarding dose response, it is imperative that the calculated doses are as accurate as possible so that meaningful relationships can be determined. The accurate commissioning and QA of the TPS are key to achieving that goal.

## References

1. Prescribing, recording and reporting photon beam therapy (Report 62). Bethesda, MD: International Commission on Radiation Units & Measurements, ICRU; 1999.
2. Fraass B, Doppke K, Hunt M, et al. American Association of Physicists in Medicine Radiation Therapy Committee Task Group 53: Quality assurance for clinical radiotherapy treatment planning. Med Phys 1998;25(10):1773–829.
3. Dempsey JF, Romeijn HE, Li JG, et al. A Fourier analysis of the dose grid resolution required for accurate IMRT fluence map optimization. Med Phys 2005;32(2):380–8.
4. Bortfeld T, Oelfke U, Nill S. What is the optimum leaf width of a multi-leaf collimator? Med Phys 2000;27(11):2494–502.
5. Chetty IJ, Curran B, Cygler JE, et al. Report of the AAPM Task Group No. 105: Issues associated with clinical implementation of Monte Carlo-based photon and electron external beam treatment planning. Med Phys 2007;34(12):4818–47.
6. Han T, Mikell JK, Salehpour M, et al. Dosimetric comparison of Acuros XB deterministic radiation transport method with Monte Carlo and model-based convolution methods in heterogeneous media. Med Phys 2011;38(5):2651–64.
7. Siebers JV, Keall PJ, Nahum AE, et al. Converting absorbed dose to medium to absorbed dose to water for Monte Carlo based photon beam dose calculations. Phys Med Biol 2000;45(4):983–95.
8. Walters BRB, Kramer R, Kawrakow I. Dose to medium vs dose to water as an estimator of dose to sensitive skeletal tissue. Phys Med Biol 2010;55(16):4535–46.
9. Ma CM, Li J. Dose specification for radiation therapy: dose to water or dose to medium? Phys Med Biol 2011;56(10):3073–89.
10. Olch AJ, Gerig L, Li H, et al. Dosimetric effects caused by couch tops and immobilization devices: Report of AAPM Task Group 176. Med Phys 2014;41(6):061501-1-30.

11. Li A, Alber M, Deasy JO, et al. The use and QA of biologically related models for treatment planning: Short report of the AAPM TG-166 of the therapy physics committee of the AAPM. Med Phys 2012;39(3):1386–409.
12. Das IJ, Cheng CW, Watts RJ, et al. Accelerator beam data commissioning equipment and procedures: Report of the AAPM TG-106 of the Therapy Physics Committee of the AAPM. Med Phys 2008;35(9): 4186–215.
13. Tubiana M, Diallo I, Chavaudra J, et al. Can we reduce the incidence of second primary malignancies occurring after radiotherapy? A critical review. Radiother Oncol 2009;91(1):4–15.
14. Diallo I, Haddy N, Adjadj E, et al. Frequency distribution of second solid cancer locations in relation to the irradiated volume among 115 patients treated for childhood cancer. Int J Radiat Oncol Biol Phys 2009;74(3):876–83.
15. Huang JY, Followill DS, Wang XA, et al. Accuracy and sources of error of out-of-field dose calculations by a commercial treatment planning system for intensity-modulated radiation therapy treatments. J Appl Clin Med Phys 2013;14(2):4139.
16. Howell RM, Scarboro SB, Kry SF, et al. Accuracy of out-of-field dose calculations by a commercial treatment planning system. Phys Med Biol 2010;55(23):6999–7008.
17. Kase KR, Svensson GK, Wolbarst AB, et al. Measurements of dose from secondary radiation outside a treatment field. Int J Radiat Oncol Biol Phys 1983;9(8):1177–83.
18. Ruben JD, Lancaster CM, Jones P, et al. A comparison of out-of-field dose and its constituent components for intensity-modulated radiation therapy versus conformal radiation therapy: Implications for carcinogenesis. Int J Radiat Oncol Biol Phys 2011;81(5):1458–64.
19. IAEA TRS-430, Commissioning and quality assurance of computerized planning systems for radiation treatment of cancer. Vienna: International Atomic Energy Agency; 2004.
20. IAEA TECDOC-1540, Specification and acceptance testing of radiotherapy treatment planning systems. Vienna: International Atomic Energy Agency; 2007.
21. IAEA TECDOC-1583, Commissioning of radiotherapy treatment planning systems: Testing for typical external beam techniques. Vienna: International Atomic Energy Agency; 2008.
22. Quality assurance of treatment planning systems practical examples for non-IMRT photon beams. Brussels: European Society for Therapeutic Radiology and Oncology; 2004.
23. Quality assurance of 3-D treatment planning systems for external photon and electron beams. Netherlands Commission on Radiation Dosimetry report; 2005. http://radiationdosimetry.org/files/documents/0000016/69-ncs-rapport-15-qa-3-d-tps-external-photon-and-electron-beams.pdf.
24. Wilcox EE, Daskalov GM, Lincoln H, et al. Accuracy of dose measurements and calculations within and beyond heterogeneous tissues for 6 MV photon fields smaller than 4 cm produced by CyberKnife. Med Phys 2008;35(6):2259–66.
25. El-Khatib E, Connors S. Conversion of ionization measurements to radiation absorbed dose in non-water density material. Phys Med Biol 1992;37(11):2083–94.
26. Kry SF, Alvarez P, Molineu A, et al. Algorithms used in heterogeneous dose calculations show systematic differences as measured with the radiological physics center's anthropomorphic thorax phantom used for RTOG credentialing. Int J Radiat Oncol Biol Phys 2013;85(1):e95–100.
27. AAPM Report No. 85, Tissue inhomogeneity corrections for megavoltage photon beams: Report of Task Group No. 65 of the Radiation Therapy Committee of the AAPM. Madison, WI: American Association of Physicists in Medicine, Medical Physics Publishing; 2004.
28. Reft C, Alecu R, Das IJ, et al. Dosimetric considerations for patients with HIP prostheses undergoing pelvic irradiation. Report of the AAPM Radiation Therapy Committee Task Group 63. Med Phys 2003;30(6):1162–82.
29. Mutic S, Palta JR, Butker EK, et al. Quality assurance for computed-tomography simulators and the computed-tomography simulation process: Report of the AAPM Radiation Therapy Committee Task Group No. 66. Med Phys 2003;30(10):2762–92.
30. Glide-Hurst C, Chen D, Zhong H, et al. Changes realized from extended bit-depth and metal artifact reduction in CT. Med Phys 2013;40(6):061711.
31. AAPM TG-23 Report 55, Radiation treatment planning dosimetry verification. Available for download on the AAPM website: <http://www.aapm.org/pubs/reports/>.
32. BJR Supplement 25, Central axis depth dose data for use in radiotherapy. Br J Radiol 1996; London.
33. Followill DS, Kry SF, Qin L, et al. The Radiological Physics Center's standard dataset for small field size output factors. J Appl Clin Med Phys 2012;13(5):3962.

34. Followill DS, Davis DS, Ibbott GS. Comparison of electron beam characteristics from multiple accelerators. Int J Radiat Oncol Biol Phys 2004;59(3):905–10.
35. Nath R, Anderson LL, Luxton G, et al. Dosimetry of interstitial brachytherapy sources: Recommendations of the AAPM Radiation Therapy Committee Task Group No. 43. Med Phys 1995;22:209–34.
36. Rivard MJ, Coursey BM, DeWerd LA, et al. Update of AAPM task group No. 43 Report: A revised AAPM protocol for brachytherapy dose calculations. Med Phys 2004;31(3):633–74.
37. Rivard MJ, Butler WM, DeWerd LA, et al. Supplement to the 2004 update of the AAPM Task Group No. 43 report. Med Phys 2007;34(6):2187–205.
38. Stern RL, Heaton R, Fraser MW, et al. Verification of monitor unit calculations for non-IMRT clinical radiotherapy: Report of AAPM Task Group 114. Med Phys 2011;38(1):504–30.
39. Siochi RA, Balter P, Bloch CD, et al. A rapid communication from the AAPM Task Group 201: Recommendations for the QA of external beam radiotherapy data transfer. J Appl Clin Med Phys 2010;12(1):3479.
40. DeWerd LA, Ibbott GS, Meigooni AS, et al. A dosimetric uncertainty analysis for photon-emitting brachytherapy sources: Report of AAPM Task Group No. 138 and GEC-ESTRO. Med Phys 2011;38(2):782–801.
41. Aryal P, Molloy JA, Rivard MJ. A modern Monte Carlo investigation of the AAPM TG-43 dosimetry parameters for an [125]I seed already having AAPM consensus data. Med Phys 2014;41(2):021702.
42. Zhang M, Zou W, Chen T, et al. Parameterization of brachytherapy source phase space file for Monte Carlo-based clinical brachytherapy dose calculation. Phys Med Biol 2014;59(2):455–64.
43. Mason J, Al-Qaisieh B, Bownes P, et al. Investigation of interseed attenuation and tissue composition effects in [125]I seed implant prostate brachytherapy. Brachytherapy 2014;6:S1538–4721.
44. Gaudreault M, Reniers B, Landry G, et al. Dose perturbation due to catheter materials in high-dose-rate interstitial [192]Ir brachytherapy. Brachytherapy 2014;Jun 10:epub.
45. Fonseca GP, Landry G, Reniers B, et al. The contribution from transit dose for [192]Ir HDR brachytherapy treatments. Phys Med Biol 2014;59(7):1831–44.
46. Beaulieu L, Carlsson Tedgren A, Carrier JF, et al. Report of the Task Group 186 on model-based dose calculation methods in brachytherapy beyond the AAPM TG-43 formalism: Current status and recommendations for clinical implementation. Med Phys 2012;39(10):6208–36.
47. ACR Technical Standard for the Performance of Radiation Oncology Physics for External Beam Therapy.
48. http://www.acr.org/~/media/7B19A9CEF68F4D6D8F0CF25F21155D73.pdf.
49. Gibbons JP, Antolak JA, Followill DS, et al. Monitor unit calculations for external photon and electron beams: Report of the AAPM Therapy Physics Committee Task Group No. 71. Med Phys 2014; 41(3):031501-1-34.
50. Mijnheer B, Bridier A, Garibaldi C, et al. Monitor unit calculation for high energy photon beams—Practical examples, Physics for clinical radiotherapy booklet No. 6. Brussels: European Society for Therapeutic Radiology and Oncology; 2001.
51. Ezzell GA, Burmeister JW, Dogan N, et al. IMRT commissioning: Multiple institution planning and dosimetry comparisons, a report from AAPM Task Group 119. Med Phys 2009;36(11):5359–73.
52. Low DA, Moran JM, Dempsey JF, et al. Dosimetry tools and techniques for IMRT. Med Phys 2011;38(3):1313–38.
53. Low DA, Dempsey JF. Evaluation of the gamma dose distribution comparison method. Med Phys 2003;30:2455–64.
54. Nelms BE, Zhen H, Tomee WA. Per-beam, planar IMRT QA passing rates do not predict clinically relevant dose errors. Med Phys 2011;38(2):1037–44.
55. Nelms BE, Chan MF, Jarry G, et al. Evaluating IMRT and VMAT dose accuracy: Practical examples of failure to detect systematic errors when applying a commonly used metric and action levels. Med Phys 2013;40(11):111722.
56. Boggula R, Birkner M, Lohr F, et al. Evaluation of a 2D detector array for patient-specific VMAT QA with different setups. Phys Med Biol 2011;56(22):7163–77.
57. O'Daniel J, Das S, Wu QJ, et al. Volumetric-modulated arc therapy: Effective and efficient end-to-end patient-specific quality assurance. Int J Radiat Oncol Biol Phys 2012;82(5):1567–74.
58. Zhu J, Chen L, Jin G, et al. A comparison of VMAT dosimetric verifications between fixed and rotating gantry positions. Phys Med Biol 2013;58(5):1315–22.
59. Jin H, Keeling VP, Johnson DA, et al. Interplay effect of angular dependence and calibration field size of MapCHECK 2 on Rapid Arc quality assurance. J Appl Clin Med Phys 2014;15(3):4638.

APPENDIX **1**

# A Sample Checklist for TPS Commissioning

1. NONDOSIMETRIC AND GEOMETRIC COMMISSIONING
   1.1 Patient Anatomic Representation
      1.1.1 Acquisition of patient information
         CT scan process
         Contour acquisition
      1.1.2 Entry or transfer of input anatomic data
         Contour acquisition
      1.1.3 Anatomic model
         Contouring
         3D objects
         3D density description
         Points and lines
         Image display and use
         Coordinate systems
   1.2 External Beam Plans: Machine Capabilities and Beams
         Machine description and capabilities
         Machine parameters
         Machine readout conventions and scales
         Limitations
         Field size and shaping
         Collimator jaw setting
         Asymmetric jaws
         Blocks (and trays)
         MLC shape
         Automated field shaping
         Beam setup (SSD–SAD)
         Beam location (x, y, z)
         Gantry, collimator, and table angle
         Arcs
         Accessories
         Beam display
         BEV
         Multiple beam tools
   1.3 Plan Evaluation Tools
      1.3.1 Dose display
         Plan normalization
         Isodose lines and surfaces
         Cold and hot spots
         Relevant points

　　　1.3.2　Dose–volume histograms
　　　　　　DVH type
　　　　　　Plan normalization
　　　　　　Relative and absolute dose
　　　　　　Volume determination
　　　　　　Histogram dose bin size
　　　　　　Compound structures
　　　　　　Consistency and dose display
　　　　　　Calculation of grid size and points distribution
　　　　　　DVH comparison guidelines
　　　　　　Dose statistics
2.　DOSIMETRIC TESTING
　　2.1　1D Scans (Depth Doses)
　　2.2　2D Scans (Combinations of Depths, SSD, Open and Wedge Fields, About 55 Total)
　　2.3　Inhomogeneity (Plastic Water, Al, Lung Equivalent, ICCR Case)
　　2.4　IMRT Plans (Real Clinical Cases, SMLC, DMLC, VMAT, 6 Patients Used)
　　2.5　MU Validation (Compared to Independent System, Test Plans From 2.2, 2.3, 2.4, and Real Patient Plans)
3.　RECORD AND VERIFY (EMR EXPORT, VERIFIED EACH DCM PLAN PARAMETER)
4.　NETWORKING (TO AND FROM ALL CTS, OTHER PLANNING SYSTEMS, ETC.)

# A Sample Compilation of Dosimetric Testing from AAPM TG-53 and IAEA TRS-430

## Photon Beam Calculation Testing

### REFERENCES:

1. AAPM TG-53
2. AAPM TG-67
3. IAEA TRS-430

### TESTS:

1. Depth Dose, Profiles, and 2D Data Multiple SSDs
2. Output Factors and MU Calculation
3. Patient Shape Effects
4. Density Corrections
5. IMRT

**Depth Dose, Profiles, and 2D Data**

| Description | AAPM TG-53 | IAEA TRS-430 | Sample Institution Tests | Example Measurement Device |
|---|---|---|---|---|
| Square fields | 3, 5, 10, 20, 30, 40 cm fields @ 100 cm SSD; 5, 10, 20, 30 cm fields @ 90 cm and 110 cm SSD | 3, 5, 10, 40 cm fields @ 100 cm SSD; $d_{max}$, 10 cm, 20 cm for 2D profiles (photon test 1) | 3, 5, 10, 20, 30, 40 @ 100 cm SSD; 5, 10, 20, 30 @ 90 cm and 110 cm SSD depth doses. 10 and 20 cm fields at 10 cm depth 80, 90, 100, 110 SSD for 2D. | 0.6 cc ion chamber water tank for 90 and 110 SSD depth dose and profiles. Chamber array for 2D. |
| Rectangular fields | No specific fields recommended | 5 × 30, 30 × 5 @ 100 cm SSD; $d_{max}$, 10 cm, 20 cm for 2D (photon test 1) | 5 × 25, 25 × 5 @ 100 cm SSD depth doses; $d_{max}$, 10 cm, 20 cm for 2D | 0.6 cc ion chamber in water tank for depth dose and profiles. Chamber array for 2D. |

| Description | AAPM TG-53 | IAEA TRS-430 | Sample Institution Tests | Example Measurement Device |
|---|---|---|---|---|
| Asymmetric fields | Table A3-9 @ 100 cm SSD | 10 × 10 offset X, Y, and X & Y; max over travel; with max hard and dynamic wedges; with MLC and wedge (photon test 2) | 10 × 10 offset X, Y, and X & Y; max over travel; with max hard and dynamic wedges; with MLC and wedge. 90 cm SSD. 10 cm depth for 2D. | 0.6 cc ion chamber in 1D tank for depth dose. Chamber array for 2D. |
| MLC fields | Table A3-8 | Central block, corner blocks, asymmetric oval, C shape (photon test 3) | Central block, corner blocks, asymmetric oval, C shape 90 SSD. 10 cm depth for 2D. | 0.6 cc ion chamber in 1D tank for depth dose. Chamber array for 2D. |
| Physical wedges | 5, 10, 20 @ 100 cm SSD; 10, 20 @ 80 cm and 110 cm SSD | 5, 10, max @ 90 cm SSD; 20 or max @ 80 cm SSD (photon test 7) | 5, 10, max @ 90 cm SSD; 20 or max @ 80 cm SSD | 0.6 cc ion chamber in 1D tank for depth dose. Chamber array for 2D. |
| Dynamic wedges | | 5, 10, max @ 90 cm SSD; 20 or max @ 80 cm SSD (photon test 9) | 5, 10, max @ 90 cm SSD; 20 or max @ 80 cm SSD | Chamber array |

## Output Factors and MU Calculation

| Description | AAPM TG-53 | IAEA TRS-430 | Sample Institution Tests | Measurement Device |
|---|---|---|---|---|
| Square fields | 3, 5, 10, 20, 30, 40 cm fields @ 100 cm SSD; 5, 10, 20, 30 cm fields @ 90 cm and 110 cm SSD | Same as above section | 5, 10, 20, 30 @ 90 cm and 110 cm SSD 10 cm depth; 10 and 20 cm fields at 10 cm depth 80, 90, 100, 110 SSD | 0.6 cc ion chamber in 1D tank |
| Rectangular fields | | Same as above section | | |
| Asymmetric fields | | Same as above section | | |
| MLC fields | | Same as above section | | |
| Physical wedges | 5, 10, 20, max @ 10 cm depth, 90 cm SSD | Same as above section | | |
| Dynamic wedges | | Same as above section | | |

## Patient Shape Effects

| Description | AAPM TG-53 | IAEA TRS-430 | Sample Institution Tests | Measurement Device |
|---|---|---|---|---|
| Oblique beam | 30 × 30 at 30 degrees or 10 × 10 at 40 degrees | 10 × 10 at 30 degrees (photon test 10) | 10 × 10 at 30 degrees | Chamber array |
| Surface irregularity | Step phantom | | Step phantom | Chamber array |
| Tangential geometry | 10 × 20 tangent beam on square phantom | | 10 × 20 tangent beam on square phantom | 0.6 cc ion chamber in solid phantom and film |
| Square phantom | Beam centered and beam flashing | 20 × 20 beam on square phantom with differing amounts of flash (photon test 11) | 20 × 20 beam on square phantom with differing amounts of flash | 0.6 cc ion chamber in solid phantom |
| Thin phantom | Not mentioned | Not mentioned | Thin phantom, 2 cm thick, 30 × 30 placed on top of styrofoam, lateral beam | 0.6 cc ion chamber in solid phantom |

## Density Corrections

| Description | AAPM TG-53 | IAEA TRS-430 | Sample Institution Tests | Measurement Device |
|---|---|---|---|---|
| Lateral equilibrium | No specific fields recommended | Profiles in various densities (photon test 13) | Profiles in various densities. 5 and 10 cm fields in plastic water, lung equivalent, and aluminum | Film |
| Attenuation | Compare to Rice et al | 5 × 5 and 20 × 20 fields with slab geometry (photon test 13) | 5 × 5 and 20 × 20 fields with slab geometry | 0.6 cc ion chamber in solid phantom |
| ICCR test case (ref) | Not mentioned | Not mentioned | ICCR test case | 0.6 cc ion chamber and film in solid phantom |

## IMRT

| Description | AAPM TG-53 | IAEA TRS-430 | Sample Institution Tests | Measurement Device |
|---|---|---|---|---|
| Optimize dose to plane | Not mentioned | Calculate leaf sequence to optimize dose to a plane with beam at 30 degrees | Calculate leaf sequence to optimize dose to a plane with beam at 30 degrees | Chamber array |
| Inverse planned IMRT | Not mentioned | Detailed checks of the dynamic MLC or other delivery device must be conducted, for example, for leaf position calibration, interleaf effects, small field output factors, linearity of dose per MU and the relationship of jaws to MLC leaves. Leaf sequences must be exported to the linear accelerator and delivered to appropriate phantoms.<br>The absolute dose and spatial distribution of the dose are then measured using ionization chambers, film, thermoluminescent dosimeters, or gel dosimeters and are compared with the predicted dose. | Planning of 3 prostate, 3 H&N, and 3 "other" IMRT. Use both static fields and VMAT | Chamber array |

# Sample Nondosimetric Testing

| Test | Method |
|------|--------|
| Export Field TPS-R&V: prescription | Test what exports for POI and all ROI methods |
| Export Field TPS-R&V: dicom coordinates | Confirm export to existing site setup. Confirm xyz for all pt orientations |
| Export Field TPS-R&V: dose | RT dose populating field for 100% IDL or other IDL? Confirm dose sum |
| Export Field TPS-R&V: field name | Confirm field ID (number of characters, text). Confirm spacing for field name (5 spaces) |
| Export Field TPS-R&V: machine name | Test for all machines, include STPS machine |
| Export Field TPS-R&V: tolerance tables | Confirm nothing exports |
| Export Field TPS-R&V: field type | Investigate setup fields |
| Export Field TPS-R&V: modality | CT, kV, x-rays |
| Export Field TPS-R&V: MU | Investigate rounding |
| Export Field TPS-R&V: time | Confirm × 1.2. EDW? |
| Export Field TPS-R&V: dose rate | Confirm 400 default |
| Export Field TPS-R&V: arc mode | Direction, MU/deg, start/stop angles |
| Export Field TPS-R&V: wedges | Test all wedges, all orientation on one machine |
| Export Field TPS-R&V: bolus | Does this export? What format? |
| Export Field TPS-R&V: gantry angle | Investigate rounding, number of decimal points |
| Export Field TPS-R&V: collimator angle | Investigate rounding, number of decimal points |
| Export Field TPS-R&V: field size | Investigate rounding, number of decimal points |
| Export Field TPS-R&V: couch parameter | If any |
| Export Field TPS-R&V: MLC shape import, static and dynamic segments | |
| Export Field TPS-R&V: SSD | To skin? To bolus? |
| Export Field TPS-R&V: field setup notes | If any |
| Export Field TPS-R&V: DRTPS | Export, mag, overlying structures, graticule, FS, |
| Export Field TPS-R&V: planning CT and structure set | Export, 4d/OBI function all the way to image acquisition/registration |
| Export Field TPS-R&V: | |
| Export Field TPS-R&V: | |
| Export Field TPS-R&V: | |
| Export Field TPS-R&V: | |
| Documentation: Tx plan report | Investigate pdf and paTPSing erroTPS. Customization? Compile how dosimetry will put the plan together |
| Documentation: physician tx plan approval | Showing on reports |
| Documentation: time/date stamps | Last approved |
| Documentation: editing approved plans | What can get changed after approval |

# CHAPTER 6

# Immobilization Techniques in Radiotherapy

## 6.1 Introduction

Proper immobilization techniques accomplish a variety of clinical goals including the following:

- **Reduce patient motion and improve day-to-day reproducibility of setup.** External beam treatments typically require several tens of minutes to complete, and during this time the operator is essentially blind to any motion of the patient or tissue with notable exceptions (e.g., orthogonal fluoroscopic imaging, 3D surface mapping, or combination magnetic resonance (MR) therapy devices). Although delivery techniques such as volumetric arc therapy (VMAT) can reduce treatment times, the addition of other technologies such as Image-guided radiation therapy (IGRT) increase the overall time of a treatment session. Movement during treatment is particularly important for stereotactic treatments, especially "frameless" stereotactic radiosurgery,[1] since these are long treatments delivering high doses. Effective immobilization is crucial for minimizing motion during treatment.
- **Improve patient comfort.** This is not only an end in itself but also is also a key factor in reducing motion. An uncomfortable patient will tend to move to try to find a more comfortable position; therefore, ensuring that the patient is as comfortable as possible will reduce motion. In addition to reducing motion, immobilization devices also help ensure that the patient anatomy is aligned reproducibly from day to day. Patient comfort also plays into reproducibility in that patients will settle into a comfortable position. Though this may be thought to be less important in the era of IGRT, the reality is that most patients do not receive IGRT on every day of treatment and some sites still provide challenges even with IGRT. An example is the head and neck. Because of neck flexion or extension it may only be possible to accurately align one anatomical region (see Chapter 18).
- **Accommodate the requirements of physical devices.** Immobilization devices and patients must fit not only through the bore of the computed tomography (CT) simulator (or magnetic resonance imaging (MRI) or positron emission tomography (PET) unit) but must also fit within the envelope of devices used during treatment (e.g., a lung patient with a lateralized lesion whose arms collide with the IGRT imaging panel on treatment).
- **Avoidance of normal tissue.** The thoughtful use of immobilization technologies can result in better avoidance of normal tissue, a classic example being the "belly board," whereby a patient undergoing abdominal treatment is placed prone in order to pull the bowel out of the high dose region.

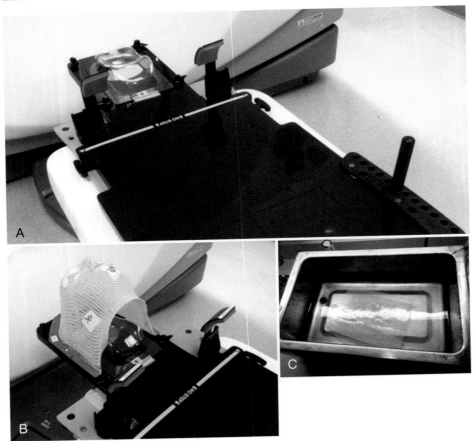

**Figure 6.1** Head and neck immobilization with a thermoplastic mask. **A,** Carbon fiber table top with head rest, shoulder bars and hand grips. **B,** Thermoplastic mask for head immobilization. **C,** High temperature water bath used to soften thermoplastic material.

## 6.2 Immobilization Devices and Techniques

### CRANIAL IMMOBILIZATION

Head frames using pins represent what is arguably the most accurate (and most invasive) methods of cranial immobilization and also allow localization using the Brown-Roberts-Wells (BRW) stereotaxy system. Examples include the Leksell G frame (Elekta Inc.) or the Talon system (Best Nomos Inc.), the latter of which allows multiple fraction treatments with two self-tapping titanium screws anchored in bone. A relocatable head frame was introduced in the early 1990s, the Gill-Thomas-Cosman (GTC) frame, which employs a dental appliance on the maxillary bone to anchor the cranium.[2] One version uses a vacuum to maintain the position of the dental appliance combined with a patient-controlled release mechanism, an example of which is the HeadFix system (Elekta Inc.) available since the late 1990s.[3] For further information see AAPM TG-68 on intracranial stereotactic systems.[4]

A widely used noninvasive cranial immobilization option relies on a thermoplastic mask (Figure 6.1B). These perforated plastics are typically 1/16″ to 1/8″ thick and soften when heated in a water bath at approximately 150° to 165° F (Figure 6.1C). Some masks are designed to soften in a convection oven. Some newer formulations include Kevlar for rigidity or may have reinforced areas to increase rigidity. Others have large holes around the eyes to increase patient comfort. Vendor recommendations should be followed to minimize mask shrinkage after formation. Numerous studies have examined the reproducibility of patient positioning with these devices[5] and have noted small intrafraction motion.

## HEAD AND NECK IMMOBILIZATION

Thermoplastic masks are also commonly used for immobilization of head and neck cancer patients (Figure 6.1). As with cranial masks, a head holder is used that sets the head extension (Figure 6.1A). Various standard reusable head holder devices are available: Timo foam (polyurethane foam with a plastic coating), Silverman (clear radiologically thin plastic shell), or PosiFix (low density polyethylene foam, Civco Medical Solutions, Inc.). Alternatively, a custom device can be made such as the MoldCare cushion (Alcare Co. Inc.), which is a formulation of polystyrene beads coated in a moisture-curing resin in a fabric bag. The custom devices provide more support in the neck area and may be more reproducible. For head and neck treatments it is important to control the position of the shoulders, especially if supraclavicular nodal regions are to be included in the treatment. This can be accomplished with shoulder bars (Figure 6.1A) or with a thermoplastic mask that extends down over the shoulders, though there appears to be no clear advantage of one over the other.[6] Hand grips set at known positions also aid with arm and shoulder position (Figure 6.1A). Thermoplastic mask arrangements are available that support prone treatments as required, for example, in craniospinal irradiation.

One problem with thermoplastic devices is that they hold a rigid shape formed at the time of simulation. If a patient loses weight or the tumor volume resolves, the thermoplastic device may become loose. An example is shown in Figure 6.2 for a head and neck patient; the mask initially fits snugly (Figure 6.2A) but becomes loose by day 20 of treatment (Figure 6.2B). Similarly, a patient on steroids may develop swelling, which causes a mask to fit too tightly. In either case, resimulation and planning may be required. The use of a mask makes it difficult to measure the true source-to-surface distance (SSD). A simple depth gauge can be used to monitor the distance between the mask and skin.

## THORACIC, ABDOMINAL, AND PELVIC IMMOBILIZATION

A major consideration in the thorax is the position of the patient's arms. Arms down at the sides is the most comfortable position for most patients but can present a challenge for three-point setup and precludes the use of some beam angles. Treating through the arms introduces dosimetric uncertainty (due to daily differences in arm position) and can also cause skin toxicity in the folds. A commonly used device is the wingboard (Figure 6.3B). Patients rest their heads on the headrest in the center and grip the two posts on the top with their hands. The arm position is set reproducibly by controlling the position of the grips.

Body-forming immobilization devices are in common use, either on their own or in combination with other devices like the wingboard shown in Figure 6.3. One type is based on expandable polyurethane foam, such as AlphaCradle (Smithers Medical Products Inc.) or RediFoam (CIVCO Inc.), which consists of a two-part solution poured into a plastic bag that hardens after a few minutes into a rigid foam. Care must be taken because some foaming agents are toxic to the skin. It has been reported that KY jelly mixed into the foam can clean it from skin. One feature of the foam cradle system is that areas can be cut out once the cradle is formed. A section that prevents reading of an SSD can be removed, for instance. A downside is that if the foam cradle is not acceptable, it must be discarded and the process started over from the beginning. An alternative is the vacuum cushion system, which consists of polystrene beads in a plastic bag that is made rigid by evacuating the bag down to a pressure of approximately 650 mbar and then sealing it. One such device is shown in Figure 6.4—the BlugBag (Medical Intelligence Inc.)—which shows the vacuum-sealed immobilization bag under the patient (blue) and the optional

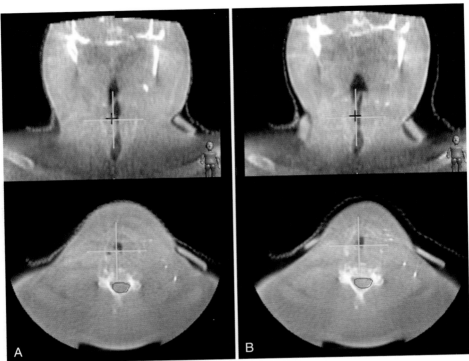

**Figure 6.2** Cone-beam CT scans of a head and neck patient on day 1 of treatment (**A**) and day 20 of treatment (**B**) showing the fit of the thermoplastic mask.

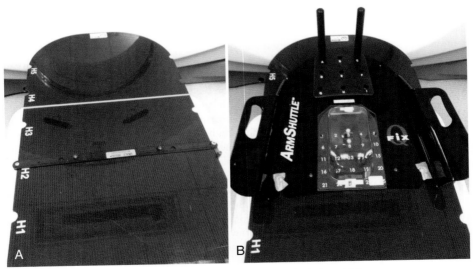

**Figure 6.3** Carbon fiber table top with indexing bar (**A**) and indexed wingboard (**B**).

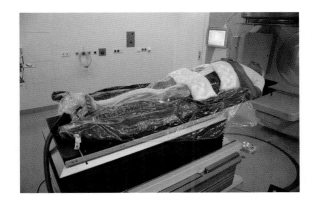

**Figure  6.4** Vacuum  bag  for  pelvic immobilization.

cover sheet that also vacuum seals over the top of the patient. Similar products are available from other vendors (e.g., Vac-Lok, CIVCO Medical Solutions Inc.). Care must be taken in handling and storing these vacuum bags since a rupture of the seal will inflate the device, which may necessitate resimulation and replanning. Vendor recommendations should be followed regarding periodic reapplication of the vacuum to maintain the proper rigidity.

A third immobilization option, particularly useful for the pelvis, is a thermoplastic mold that stretches over the patient (e.g., HipFix, CIVCO Medical Solutions, Inc.). These are similar to the thermoplastic head mask but are constructed of thicker plastic. For the pelvis and abdomen special consideration must be given to the legs and feet because their large lever arm can affect the position of the hips. Leg and knee positions can be set with a vacuum bag (Figure 6.4) or a separate indexable knee roll and foot holder, which are commercially available. In addition, a "saddle" can be formed in the vacuum cushion to assist with accurate superior/inferior positioning.

## INDEXING OF IMMOBILIZATION DEVICES

Figure 6.3A and B illustrate an important principle common to almost all modern immobilization devices: indexing. With indexing, the immobilization devices are clamped to labeled positional notches in the table (e.g., "H2" in Figure 6.3A). This ensures that the device and patient will be at the same position on the table for each day of treatment. Indexing enables an important safety feature—namely, an interlock for the position of the treatment table. Since the table is expected to be in the same place each day, the treatment delivery system can read its position and determine whether it is at its intended location to within a predetermined tolerance. This can help prevent inadvertent treatment of the wrong location.

Immobilization equipment must sometimes be used in combination with other devices. An example is an abdominal compression plate that might fit on a bridge over the patient or an array of stereo-camera markers that may also be fixed on a bridge over the patient. Such devices must be accommodated within the constraints of the immobilization devices.

## BREAST IMMOBILIZATION AND SETUP

Immobilization for breast treatments presents some unique challenges. If a supine setup is used, elevation on an adjustable incline board is often helpful to increase comfort and to provide a more reproducible fall of the breast. It is important to reduce rotations and to provide a reproducible position for the arm, particularly when matching supraclavicular or axilla fields to the breast tangent fields. Commercial devices are available for positioning the ipsilateral arm. Supine setups on an incline board are also subject to problems with clearance with the treatment devices or CT simulator bore. Alternatively, prone setups can be used, which have the advantage of pulling the breast tissue away from the lung and heart and may have a particular advantage for larger women. Special care must be taken, however, to reduce rotation for these setups. It is also important to position the breast at the proper place relative to the opening in the prone board and to avoid having the breast touch the table top as this may cause excess skin dose. Some prone breast devices are attached as a table extension to eliminate this effect. Bolus presents a special challenge for breast treatments because the bolus should conform to the skin as much as possible, which may be difficult with typical tissue equivalent bolus material. Alternatives include a brass metal mesh,[7] a beam spoiler, or even a thick coating of Vaseline.

## IMMOBILIZATION FOR EXTREMITIES

Extremities represent a special challenge for immobilization and setup. If a single leg or arm is to be treated, it is necessary to avoid the contralateral limb with the creative use of immobilization devices, elevating and holding one of the legs in place with a vacuum cushion, for example. For treatments of the hand or foot, the hand or foot can sometimes be clamped down with a thermoplastic head mask. If bolus is required for the foot or hand it can sometimes be treated in a water bath.

# 6.3 Dosimetric Effects of Table Tops and Immobilization Devices

Immobilization devices and table tops disturb radiation beams that pass through them, a topic that is considered in detail in AAPM TG-176[8] with reference to roughly 20 studies that have been published on the topic. Two issues are considered: 1) increased skin dose due to the blousing effect of devices and 2) attenuation of the beam by devices.

## INCREASED SKIN DOSE

A standard reference for dose-related skin toxicities is Archambeau et al.[9] (the topic is not considered in the QUANTEC study, which is more focused on late effects). For a patient receiving standard 2 Gy fraction treatment, skin erythema starts at approximately 20 Gy, dry desquamation at 45 Gy, and moist desquamation above that. Most damage heals within 4 weeks of the completion of therapy, and late skin necrosis is a rare phenomenon in modern practice. The two skin layers relevant to acute and late effects are the epidermal layer (approximately 0.1 mm deep), which is home to proliferating cells, and the dermal layer (1 to 3 mm deep), which supplies the vasculature.[9]

AAPM TG-176[8] notes that thermoplastic devices can increase surface does by 30% to 70%, depending on the final thickness of plastic and the beam parameters. Vacuum bags and foam cradles have also been observed to increase skin dose by roughly the same amount. It is important to note that solid carbon fiber table tops also have a skin bolusing effect. These tables (e.g., Figure 6.3A) are now in wide use, especially for IGRT, and can substantially increase skin dose. For low energy posterior beams this increase can be a factor of two or more, to the point that most skin sparing may be lost.

## BEAM ATTENUATION

Carbon fiber tables also attenuate the transmitted beam with dose reductions of 3% to 6% depending on the energy, angle, and field sizes. The table top support rails present on some units may severely attenuate the beam, and treatment through these should be avoided. AAPM TG-176[8] recommends that attenuation and bolusing effects of table tops be explicitly included in the treatment plan. Some treatment planning system vendors provide an automatic means of accomplishing this, while others require users to develop their own method using CT scans of these devices.

## 6.4 Emerging Questions

Clinical requirements for patient immobilization continue to evolve. One important question in the near future will be the compatibility of the devices with MRI. This is important for two reasons. First, to facilitate the image fusion of diagnostic MRI for sites outside the cranium, it is highly desirable to scan the patient in a pose that mimics treatment. In this sense, large bore MRI units are valuable, such as the MAGNETOM Espree (Siemens Inc.), a 1.5 T MRI unit with a bore that is 70 cm diameter wide and 120 cm long. Whenever possible the patient should be scanned on a flat surface with the immobilization devices used for treatment. Second, the emerging use of MRI-guided radiation therapy (MRgRT) necessitates the use of MR-compatible immobilization devices. Many modern devices are designed to be MR compatible, a notable exception being the carbon fiber table top, which can exhibit large eddy currents that can distort images or even harm the patient.

---

**FOR THE PHYSICIAN**

Immobilization is one of the first technical steps taken in providing radiation treatment. The subsequent quality of treatment depends crucially on this step. Good immobilization acts not only to reduce motion during treatment, but also to provide reproducible patient setup from day to day. This is important even in the era of image guidance, because some alignment issues cannot be corrected by imaging alone (e.g., variability in flexion of the neck, which means only one region can be aligned with the intended position). Immobilization can also be used to increase normal tissue sparing, the classic example being the prone "belly board" that moves bowel away from the high dose region.

A variety of immobilization technologies exist, including thermoplastic masks, bite blocks, wing boards to assist in arm positioning, and inclined boards for breast cancer patients. Though most modern devices, including table support assemblies, are made to be radiologically thin, care must be taken to avoid excess skin toxicity since some immobilization devices and couch tops can increase skin dose by a factor of two or more. The recently published AAPM Task Group 176 report[8] offers a wealth of information on this topic.

Most modern immobilization devices provide indexing, which offers a means of locking the device into the treatment support table at exactly the same place each day. Because the device is in the same place each day relative to the table, this means that the table X, Y, and Z coordinates should also be the same each day. These table coordinates can be checked by the treatment delivery computer. Indexing therefore provides an important double-check safety mechanism to prevent the treatment of the patient in the wrong location.

---

### References

1. Bova FJ, Buatti JM, Friedman WA, et al. The University of Florida frameless high-precision stereotactic radiotherapy system. Int J Radiat Oncol Biol Phys 1997;38:875–82.
2. Gill SS, Thomas DG, Warrington AP, et al. Relocatable frame for stereotactic external beam radiotherapy. Int J Radiat Oncol Biol Phys 1991;20:599–603.
3. Olch AJ, Lavey RS. Reproducibility and treatment planning advantages of a carbon fiber relocatable head fixation system. Radiother Oncol 2002;65:165–8.

4. Lightstone AW, Benedict SH, Bova FJ, et al. Intracranial stereotactic positioning systems: Report of the American Association of Physicists in Medicine Radiation Therapy Committee Task Group no. 68. Med Phys 2005;32:2380–98.
5. Tryggestad E, Christian M, Ford E, et al. Inter- and intrafraction patient positioning uncertainties for intracranial radiotherapy: A study of four frameless, thermoplastic mask-based immobilization strategies using daily cone-beam CT. Int J Radiat Oncol Biol Phys 2011;80:281–90.
6. Sharp L, Lewin F, Johansson H, et al. Randomized trial on two types of thermoplastic masks for patient immobilization during radiation therapy for head-and-neck cancer. Int J Radiat Oncol Biol Phys 2005;61:250–6.
7. Healy E, Anderson S, Cui J, et al. Skin dose effects of postmastectomy chest wall radiation therapy using brass mesh as an alternative to tissue equivalent bolus. Pract Radiat Oncol 2013;3:e45–53.
8. Olch AJea. Dosimetric effects of immobilization Devices: Report of AAPM Task Group 176. Med Phys 2014;41(6), 061501-1 to 061501-30.
9. Archambeau JO, Pezner R, Wasserman T. Pathophysiology of irradiated skin and breast. Int J Radiat Oncol Biol Phys 1995;31:1171–85.

# CHAPTER 7

# Image Guidance and Localization Technologies for Radiotherapy

## 7.1 Introduction

A key component of safe and effective modern radiotherapy is the ability to align a patient with respect to the radiation beam during treatment. Current means of accomplishing this include 3D visualization of soft tissue structures (via computed tomography (CT) or ultrasound and soon magnetic resonance imaging (MRI)), 2D or 3D localization of bony landmarks or fiducials (planar kV/MV images or implanted marker tracking), and alignment of surrogates such as a bite block or reflective markers. The most extensive use of these techniques is for image-guided radiotherapy (IGRT), which uses imaging on a regular (sometimes daily) basis, typically with a volumetric modality. This chapter focuses on the technical aspects of these on-treatment localization approaches. Clinical motivations and considerations are considered further in Chapter 18, which includes a comparison of the various advantages/disadvantages of various image guidance systems.

This chapter includes 1) an overview of technologies for imaging and localizing patients during treatment, 2) basic concepts underlying image quality, and 3) principles and practice of commissioning and quality assurance. While the primary literature on imaging and localization technologies is vast, this chapter draws from consensus documents including AAPM Task Groups, standards from the Canadian Association of Provincial Cancer Agencies (CAPCA), and other sources.[1-12] A resource reference list appears in Table 7.1 in shorthand form. Appendix I has more complete details for each reference.

## 7.2 Overview of Clinical Imaging Systems

The technology and use of on-treatment imaging systems continue to evolve at a fast pace. A literature search reveals 236 papers published in the Radiation Oncology literature with the phrase "cone-beam" in 2013 alone. Several of the consensus reports attempt to provide overviews, of which AAPM TG-104,[7] The Role of In-Room kV X-Ray Imaging for Patient Setup and Target Localization is notable for its historical perspective dating back to the use of kV sources coupled to $^{60}$Co treatment units in the late 1950s. Currently the most commonly used technologies include the following (see lists in AAPM TG-104/AAPM TG-179[2]):

- Kilovoltage cone-beam CT (kV-CBCT), e.g., On-Board Imaging (OBI) system (Varian Inc., Palo Alto, CA); Synergy X-ray Volume Imager (XVI) system (Elekta, Inc., Crawley, UK). Flat panel imaging device in fluoroscopic mode; 2 projection images per degree with 200° to 360° gantry rotation range; 1 to 2 minute acquisition. These units are also capable of radiographs and fluoroscopy. **Reference document: AAPM TG-104[7] (Sec. II.C).**
- Megavoltage planar images (portal images) used in gantry-based systems. **Reference documents: AAPM TG-58[8] (circa 2001) and CAPC QC Standards for EPIDs.** Efforts are now in development to utilize MV imaging to verify delivery of dose either just before treatment or during treatment itself, an approach referred to as *in-vivo EPID dosimetry*.

TABLE 7.1  ▤  Resource Documents for On-Treatment Imaging and Localization
(See Appendix I for Full Citations)

| Report # | Date | Description |
|---|---|---|
| AAPM TG-132 | Pending | Image registration and data fusion algorithms and techniques |
| AAPM TG-226 | 2014 | Medical physics practice guideline (MPPG), QA of x-ray-based IGRT systems |
| AAPM TG-179 | 2012 | QA of CT-based IGRT |
| AAPM TG-174 | 2012 | QA of non-radiographic localization systems |
| AAPM TG-154 | 2011 | Ultrasound for external beam radiation therapy (EBRT) prostate |
| AAPM TG-135 | 2011 | QA for CyberKnife |
| AAPM TG-148 | 2010 | QA for TomoTherapy |
| AAPM TG-104 | 2009 | In-room kV imaging |
| AAPM TG-75 | 2007 | Dose in IGRT |
| CAPCA QC: EPID | 2005 | Canadian Quality Control Standards for EPID |
| AAPM TG-58 | 2001 1999 | EPID imaging IPEM document, Report 81 (IPEM, 1999); EPIDs |
| ACR/ASTRO | 2009 | ACR-ASTRO practice guidelines on IGRT |
| ASTRO IGRT Safety | 2013 | Safety considerations for IGRT |

- Fan-beam MV-CT (TomoTherapy/Accuray, Madison, WI). CT using the 3.5 MeV beam, 4 mm collimated beam with pitch 1 to 3. **Reference document: AAPM TG-148.[6]**
- In-room CT on rails. Less widely used than the above technologies, although diagnostic-quality images are available. **Reference document: AAPM TG-104[7] (Sec. II.A).**
- Planar stereoscopic kV-imaging. CyberKnife system (Accuray Inc., Sunnyvale, CA) and Novalis ExacTrac system (BrainLab AG, Feldkirchen, Germany) use paired x-ray tube/flat panel imagers mounted in the floor and ceiling to determine shifts relative to DRRs. Dual-energy kV systems are now becoming commercially available, which enable subtraction imaging to enhance soft tissue visualization.[13] **Reference documents: See AAPM TG-104,[7] AAPM TG-135.[5]**
- "Combined systems" (i.e., stereoscopic planar plus kV-CBCT). NovalisTx platform (Varian Inc., Palo Alto, CA). Vero (Mitsubishi Heavy Industries, Ltd. & Brainlab AG), using the MHI-TM2000 accelerator and a pair of x-ray tubes/flat panel imagers mounted in a pivoting O-ring assembly. **Reference document: AAPM TG-104.[7]**
- Digital tomosynthesis. Lying somewhere between planar imaging and CT, this technique renders a "thick plane" perpendicular to the beam by acquiring images over a small range of angles (<40 degrees). **Reference document: AAPM TG-104[7] and references therein.**

In addition to the above systems, various "add-on" technologies are available for on-treatment localization. Ultrasound has been used to localize the prostate and surgical cavity in breast during treatment. A camera system establishes the geometric relationship between the ultrasound transducer probe and the treatment isocenter. Commercial products include SonArray (Varian Medical Systems, Palo Alto, CA) and Clarity (Resonent Medical, Montreal, Canada) marketed as "I-beam" (Elekta Inc., Crawley, UK). Challenges include interuser variability (and the associated importance of user training), abdominal pressure (displacements of 5 mm have been noted), and intrafraction motion (one study noted 5 mm displacements 3% of the time). **Reference documents: AAPM TG-154[4] for external beam and AAPM TG-128[14] for ultrasound (US) in brachytherapy.**

Several localization systems are available that rely on imaging the surface of the patient and/or superficial markers (i.e., nonradiographic localization systems). **Reference document: AAPM**

TG-147,[3] cf. Table 1, list of systems. One class of systems uses two or more stereoscopic cameras to image infrared reflective markers. These include the FreeTrack system (Varian Medical Systems, Palo Alto, CA), which aligns a bite block for intracranial treatments; ExacTrac (BrainLab AG, Feldkirchen, Germany); DynaTrac (Elekta Inc., Crawley, UK); and CyberKnife (Accuray Inc., Sunnyvale, CA), all of which use reflective markers in some modes of operation. Other systems rely on the projection of structured light patterns onto the surface of the patient (e.g., AlignRT, VisionRT Ltd., London, UK) or projected lasers (Sentinel, C-Rad, Uppsala, Sweden). One fundamental limitation of all such systems is their reliance on features on the surface of a patient, which may not correlate with the position of internal anatomy of interest.

A final class of nonradiographic localization relies on implanted electromagnetic transponders whose location can be determined through a source/receiver coil at or near the surface of the patient. One system, Calypso (marketed by Varian Medical Systems, Palo Alto, CA) uses 8 × 2 mm implanted transponder devices. It is currently FDA approved for prostate radiotherapy and its use in lung is under investigation. In the prostate, three beacons are typically implanted from which gland rotation/translation can be determined.

Other on-treatment imaging systems are under development but are not yet the subject of society-level reports. These include the MR-$^{60}$Co treatment unit (ViewRay Inc., Bedford, OH)[15] and MR-coupled linear accelerators.[16] This is an area of active research on the image guidance aspects and also the effect of the magnetic field on radiation transport (e.g., electron-return effect[17]). Proton radiotherapy centers also employ on-treatment image guidance, which is briefly described in AAPM TG-104.[7] Almost all proton radiotherapy centers currently rely on kV planar radiography and do not utilize on-treatment CT.[18]

There are few studies that directly compare the IGRT technologies mentioned above and almost none that does this in a prospective manner. This may be an area of future investigation. An example study for prostate cancer is found in Mayyas et al.,[19] who evaluated ultrasound, kV planar images, CBCT, and implanted electromagnetic beacons in 27 patients prospectively. A benefit was shown to IGRT (relative to standard three-point setup) in terms of possible margin reduction. Though similar overall, some modality-dependent differences were noted in the different dimensions.

## 7.3 Concepts in Radiographic Imaging: Image Quality and Dose

The image quality performance of radiographic systems is commonly characterized by five parameters: geometric accuracy, spatial resolution, low contrast resolution, noise, and uniformity. A particularly useful discussion about contrast and noise in planar imaging can be found in AAPM TG-58,[8] while many reports discuss CT imaging (e.g., AAPM TG-66,[20] AAPM TG-104,[7] and AAPM TG-179[2]). Recently it has been proposed that a system might be developed to predict the optimal imaging technique for visualizing feature detection during IGRT.[21]

For on-treatment CT systems, AAPM TG-179 quotes the following typical performance: geometric accuracy <1 mm, a spatial resolution of 6 to 9 line pairs/cm (kV-CBCT) or 1.6 mm high contrast object (MV-CT), and a contrast resolution of 1% for a 7 mm object (kV-CBCT) or 2% for a 13 mm object (MV-CT). It must be noted, though, that image quality is highly dependent on technique.

CT image quality is also affected by patient-related factors. Metallic implants cause streaking on CT due to beam hardening, which can obscure the visualization of tissue and impact dosimetric calculations if not handled properly. Examples of such implants are orthopedic hardware (spinal support, rods in the humerus or femur, hip prostheses, and the like), dental fillings, and implanted fiducial markers. Artifacts are more prominent on kV-CT (versus MV-CT) because kV imaging is more affected by the photoelectric interaction, which has a high absorption coefficient in high atomic number materials. Intravenous or oral contrast is sometimes used to visualize vessels or esophagus/bowel. This can result in artifacts as well and can also affect dose calculations. Another patient-related artifact is noise due to photon starvation and beam hardening. This can be especially pronounced in large patients, though noise can be reduced in such cases by increasing the kVp of the x-ray tube. If any of the patient anatomy lies outside the CT reconstruction region, edge effects can appear (i.e., bright "rings" at the outer edge of the CT image).

Image quality in kV-CBCT deserves special consideration. The cone-beam geometry produces more scatter than a fan beam, resulting in increased noise, reduced contrast, and reduced uniformity (in particular, "cupping" artifact). When patient sizes are different from those used for calibration incorrect CT numbers may be returned (AAPM TG-179 Section IV.D). This is an important consideration if CBCT scans are used for dose calculation. Similarly, imaging effects must be considered when using MV TomoTherapy images for planning.[22] kV-CBCT is also subject to other image artifacts, including blurring due to patient motion, streaks due to gas bubble motion, ring artifacts from underresponding pixels in the image detector, and streak artifacts due to an incomplete number of projection images. Examples of image artifacts can be found in AAPM TG-104 Figure III-B-1.

## DOSE CONSIDERATIONS

AAPM TG-75[9] provides a comprehensive consideration of dose from on-treatment radiographic imaging. AAPM TG-75 and other reports quote approximate values for imaging dose. These are listed in Table 7.2. In considering these numbers, it must be recognized that imaging dose is strongly dependent on the devices, techniques, and the site being imaged.

Most of the values in Table 7.2 may seem small, but it must be remembered that the patient receives dose to the whole volume being imaged. Also as further context, the imaging dose may exceed the linear accelerator (linac) leakage dose by an order of magnitude, as pointed out in AAPM TG-75. Furthermore, the dose to bone may be approximately three times higher than

TABLE 7.2 ■ Estimated Typical Doses for On-Treatment Imaging Studies

| Modality | Typical Dose | Reference |
|---|---|---|
| kV-CBCT | 10-30 mGy/scan<br>Sometimes 80 mGy/scan | AAPM TG-75 (AAPM TG-179) |
| MV-CT | 10-30 mGy/scan<br>7-40 mGy/scan | AAPM TG-75, AAPM TG-148<br>AAPM TG-179 |
| MV portal images | 0.1 mSv/MU (neck)[1]<br>2.6 mSv/MU (chest)[1] | AAPM TG-75 |
| kV planar images | <1 mGy/image | 27,28 |
| CyberKnife | 0.1-2 mGy/image<br>0.1-0.7 mGy/image[2]<br>Cranium Tx: 7.5 mGy[3]<br>Sacrum Tx: 200 mGy[3] | AAPM TG-75<br>AAPM TG-135<br>AAPM TG-75<br>AAPM TG-75 |

[1]AAPM TG-75 Table X. This estimate assumes an 18 × 16 cm field and is based on the work of Waddington and McKensie.[29] AAPM TG-75 notes that "direct target dose [from portal imaging] should be included in the planned therapeutic dose."
[2]AAPM TG-135 estimates were based on the literature and unpublished reports. Estimates may be lower than AAPM TG-75 because newer image analysis methods have allowed for a significant reduction in image dose.
[3]Estimated total entrance dose based on repeated planar imaging (≈30 image pairs per treatment depending on the site).

the doses listed in Table 7.2 due to the photoelectric effect (see AAPM TG-104 and references therein). Imaging dose is therefore worth considering. It is recommended that the dose be discussed with the radiation oncologist from a clinical cost/benefit perspective (AAPM TG-179). This is especially true for pediatric patients, who are at high risk of secondary malignancy.

AAPM TG-75 discusses ways to limit effective dose, in particular, restricting the superior/inferior extent of the scan to the minimum needed. AAPM TG-75 recommends that imaging dose should be included in the planned therapeutic dose at least in the context of MV portal imaging. Tracking imaging dose during therapy may be a future requirement, just as some states now require that dose from diagnostic CT scans be tracked.

There are some technical aspects to measuring and reporting CT dose that must be considered. AAPM TG-75 and other reports advocate the reporting of CT dose in units of CT dose index (CTDI), a quantity also referred to in United States Code of Federal regulations under 21 CFR 1020.33 though with a slightly different definition. AAPM TG-66 Appendix II provides concise definitions of this and related quantities (c.f. also AAPM TG-75 Section II.C.1, which presents similar material but with some errors in definitions). Important parameters are:

- $CTDI_{100}$, the measured dose in one scan rotation over a longitudinal length of 100 mm
- $CTDI_w$, the weighted average of $CTDI_{100}$ measurements at two locations in a specified phantom (one central and one peripheral)
- $CTDI_{vol}$, the "volume CTDI," which includes the effect of scan pitch and is defined as $CTDI_w$/pitch. Typical values for $CTDI_{vol}$ and DLP in fan-beam kV CT scans circa 2000 are given in AAPM TG-75 Table VII, assembled from extensive data from European centers (10 to 80 mGy)
- Dose length product (DLP), defined as $CTDI_{vol}$ multiplied by scan length

There are challenges with using $CTDI_{100}$ in a cone-beam geometry that is wider than 100 mm because the full dose is not measured (see the discussion in International Atomic Energy Agency (IAEA) Human Health Report #5 on dosimetry in CBCT). Finally, in terms of impact to patients, the most relevant quantity is not absorbed dose but effective dose (organ weighted). There are, however, many challenges in estimating effective dose for on-treatment CT. Section IV of AAPM TG-75 describes the methodology for effective dose calculations and the related challenges. Reports of measured dose from on-treatment systems are often simply quoted in units of mGy (e.g., AAPM TG-75).

## 7.4 Quality Assurance for Imaging Systems

Acceptance testing and commissioning are first steps in QA and largely consist of gathering baseline performance data against which future QA tests will be benchmarked. During acceptance testing and commissioning the key features of the system need to be evaluated including functionality, safety features, calibration, and system integration, including connectivity with the treatment planning system (e.g., transfer of reference images and contours to the image guidance system). Further tests include geometric calibration, position/reposition test, and image quality tests, all of which are described further in the following sections. All modes of operations and settings should be considered during acceptance testing and commissioning. Several reports from ASTRO and ACR specifically recommend the use of end-to-end localization tests at the time of commissioning or upgrades.[12,23]

### ONGOING QUALITY ASSURANCE

A variety of ongoing QA tests are needed to ensure safe, high quality operation. Table 7.3 provides an overview of the standard QA tests. One immediately obvious feature in Table 7.3 is

**TABLE 7.3** ■ Quality Assurance Recommendations for Image-Based Alignment Systems

| QA Test | Planar kV/MV Daily | Planar kV/MV Monthly | Planar kV/MV Annually | CBCT Daily | CBCT Monthly | CBCT Annually | MV-CT Daily | MV-CT Monthly | MV-CT Annually |
|---|---|---|---|---|---|---|---|---|---|
| Safety: collision, interlocks, warning lights | AAPM TG-142, AAPM TG-135, AAPM TG-226, CAPCA | | | AAPM TG-142, AAPM TG-179, AAPM TG-226 | | | AAPM TG-179, AAPM TG-226 | | |
| Positioning/registration with offset phantom | AAPM TG-142, AAPM TG-226[b] | | | AAPM TG-142, AAPM TG-179[a], AAPM TG-226[b] | | | AAPM TG-179[a], AAPM TG-148, AAPM TG-226[b] | | |
| Image and Tx coordinate coincidence | AAPM TG-142, AAPM TG-135[c], AAPM TG-226[b] | CAPCA[d] | | AAPM TG-142, AAPM TG-179[a], AAPM TG-226[b] | | | AAPM TG-179[a], AAPM TG-148, AAPM TG-226[b] | | |
| Image and Tx coordinate coincidence (4 gantry angles) | | AAPM TG-142 | | | AAPM TG-142, AAPM TG-179[e] | | | AAPM TG-179[e] | |
| Isocentric end-to-end test (orthogonal films) | | AAPM TG-135 | | | | | | | |
| Geometric dimensions | | AAPM TG-142, CAPCA[f] | AAPM TG-226[SA] | | AAPM TG-142 | AAPM TG-179[SA], AAPM TG-226[SA] | | AAPM TG-148 | AAPM TG-179[SA], AAPM TG-226[SA] |
| Spatial resolution | | AAPM TG-142, AAPM TG-135 | AAPM TG-226, CAPCA[SA] | | AAPM TG-142 | AAPM TG-226, AAPM TG-179[SA] | | AAPM TG-148 | AAPM TG-226, AAPM TG-179[SA] |
| Contrast | | AAPM TG-142, AAPM TG-135 | AAPM TG-226 | | AAPM TG-142 | AAPM TG-226, AAPM TG-179[SA] | | AAPM TG-148 | AAPM TG-226, AAPM TG-179[SA] |
| Noise | | AAPM TG-142, AAPM TG-135 | CAPCA[SA] | | AAPM TG-142 | AAPM TG-179[SA] | | AAPM TG-148 | AAPM TG-179[SA] |

| | | | | | | |
|---|---|---|---|---|---|---|
| Uniformity | AAPM TG-142 | | AAPM TG-142 | AAPM TG-226, AAPM TG-179[SA] | AAPM TG-148 | AAPM TG-226, AAPM TG-179[SA] |
| CT number (if used for dose calculation) | | | AAPM TG-142 | AAPM TG-179[SA] | AAPM TG-148 | AAPM TG-179[SA] |
| Imaging dose | | AAPM TG-142, AAPM TG-226 | AAPM TG-142, AAPM TG-179, AAPM TG-226 | AAPM TG-142, AAPM TG-179, AAPM TG-226 | AAPM TG-148, AAPM TG-179, AAPM TG-226 | AAPM TG-148, AAPM TG-179, AAPM TG-226 |
| Beam quality | | AAPM TG-142, AAPM TG-135[g] (kV) | | AAPM TG-179[g] | | AAPM TG-179[g] |
| Other image quality tests | | AAPM TG-135[h] | | | | |
| Orientation | | | | AAPM TG-179 | AAPM TG-148 | AAPM TG-179 |
| Resource planning (manpower, IT, etc.) | | | | AAPM TG-179 | | AAPM TG-179 |
| End-to-end phantom test | | | | ACR & ASTRO[C&U] | | AAPM TG-148 |

Frequencies are listed as: Daily (D), Monthly (M), Annually (A). Some reports also call for QA semiannually (SA) or upon Commissioning & Upgrade (C&U) as noted. Superscripts are used in cases where the recommended frequency differs from that in the column heading. The semiannual tests in AAPM TG-179 are suggested after "stability has been demonstrated, 6-12 months after commissioning." "CAPCA" refers to the Canadian report "CAPCA Quality Control Standards: EPID,"[*10] "ACR" refers to reference [11]. "ASTRO" refers to reference [12].

[a] For daily tests AAPM TG-179 recommends that EITHER positioning or coordinate coincidence needs to be tested on a daily basis but not both.

[b] AAPM TG-226 MPPG suggests that the frequency for this test should be weekly for conventional treatments and daily only for SRS/SBRT applications.

[c] AAPM TG-135 for CyberKnife describes the "AQA" test for this purpose (section III.C.1), i.e., a hidden-target test consisting of localization and films of a tungsten ball embedded in a plastic cube.

[d*] CAPCA Quality Control Standards: EPID" calls for monthly tests of positioning in the image plane and perpendicular to the image plane. The report also calls for a daily check of EPID image quality.

[e] In place of this geometric test, AAPM TG-179 recommends "Geometric calibration maps OR kV=MV=laser alignment," usually performed with an aligned BB phantom aligned to the radiation isocenter. In addition, AAPM TG-179 calls for monthly "Couch shifts: accuracy of motions."

[f] For monthly QA "CAPCA Quality Control Standards: EPID" calls for image quality, artifacts, spatial distortion, positioning in the image plane, and perpendicular to the image plane.

[g] AAPM TG-179 recommends somewhat more extensive tests of "tube potential, mA, ms accuracy, and linearity;" and AAPM TG-135 for kV planar imaging in CyberKnife recommends QA of "kVp accuracy, mA station exposure linearity, exposure reproducibility, focal spot size."

[h] AAPM TG-135 for CyberKnife (Table IV.D) also recommends annual tests for "signal to noise ratio, contrast-to-noise ratio, relative modulation transfer function, imager sensitivity stability, bad pixel count and pattern, uniformity corrected images, detector centering, and imager gain statistics."

the disagreement among reports as to frequency and tolerance of tests, an issue that we discuss further below. One aspect of QA that is not explicitly noted in Table 7.3 is the need for QA after major upgrades, repairs, or maintenance. Most reports call for such QA. For example, AAPM TG-226 recommends that the medical physicist should verify or reestablish QA baselines after upgrade, repair, or service. Table 7.3 presents the most important specific recommendations but does not list all QA-related resources. Other documents include the ACR-ASTRO report on IGRT[11] and the ASTRO safety white paper on IGRT.[12] Although these documents offer general guidance on the management of IGRT programs they do not provide specific QA test recommendations, deferring instead to the AAPM task group reports listed here. Another imaging-related resource is AAPM TG-104. However, this report is from the early days of IGRT and only provides a sample QA test battery (from Princess Margaret Hospital, Toronto, Ontario, Canada).

## GEOMETRIC QA

Table 7.3 lists several varieties of geometric QA tests. One test is for geometric scaling and typically employs an object of known size to assess the geometric dimensions generated by the imaging system. This should test all three dimensions, and the recommended frequency is monthly (or semiannually, depending on the report). Some reports suggest an annual test for geometric orientation of CT systems to ensure that the correct image orientation is returned in the three cardinal dimensions. This is typically accomplished using a phantom with multiple markers. A final geometric test assesses the alignment of the imaging and treatment isocenters. This is particularly important in systems in which a different mechanical system is employed for imaging versus treatment, such as any of the current kV-based imaging systems. Figure 7.1 shows one example device for geometric imaging alignment tests on linac-based systems. The plastic cube contains cavities and/or radio-opaque markers that can be visualized on CBCT as well as kV and MV planar imaging. This provides a quick daily test of the imaging and treatment coordinate coincidence (see Table 7.3). Similar recommendations can be found in AAPM TG-148 for TomoTherapy. Daily positioning/repositioning tests can also be accomplished with a device like that shown in Figure 7.1. The plastic cube is aligned to the set of markers at the upper left. A CT scan is then performed and the embedded fiducials are aligned to a reference image. The linac table is shifted by the measured alignment offset. If the imaging and alignment are correct then the set of marks at the center of the cube (the "bull's-eye") will be aligned with the lasers at isocenter. AAPM TG-142 and AAPM TG-226 call for such a test daily while AAPM TG-179 calls for monthly "couch shifts: accuracy of motions." AAPM TG-179 suggests that offset shifts be <2 cm and unequal in all axes to uncover possible errors.

On a monthly basis more extensive "geometric alignment tests" are indicated in some reports (e.g., AAPM TG-179 but not AAPM TG-226). Descriptions of this test for CBCT can be found in some detail in AAPM TG-104 (Section II.B.4), in overview in AAPM TG-179 (Section IV.A), and in the reference.[24] Briefly, it consists of aligning a "ball bearing (BB)" with the MV isocenter by acquiring portal images at four cardinal gantry angles (opposed collimator angles are also acquired to eliminate the effect of possible jaw asymmetry). The step precisely aligns the BB with the radiation isocenter and decouples it from any possible misalignment with the lasers. This step of aligning the BB to the radiation isocenter is similar to that used in a Winston-Lutz test.[25] Once the BB is aligned, it can then be used to acquire "flexmaps" if the CT system needs to be recalibrated. According to AAPM TG-179, geometric recalibration should be performed as recommended by the manufacturer after major hardware or software upgrades or after service that could impact the CT system. If recalibration is not needed a CT can be acquired and the geometric alignment can be measured as the distance from the center of the BB to the center of the reconstructed CT volume. AAPM TG-148 recommends that the alignment between the treatment and imaging coordinate systems be tested on an annual basis

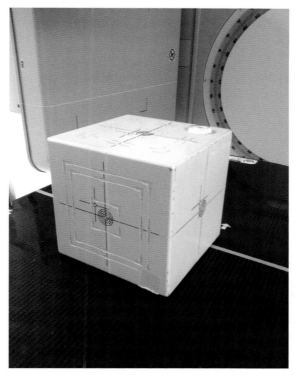

**Figure 7.1** An example device for QA of imaging alignment on a linac-based system. Markers embedded at the bull's-eye position are imaged with CBCT and then aligned. The measured table shifts for alignment should match the distance between the two crosshairs.

using an end-to-end phantom with embedded film, diode arrays, or other means of measuring the delivered dose distribution.

## IMAGE QUALITY QA

Table 7.3 provides an overview of recommended tests of image quality. Numerous commercial devices are available for image quality tests. For QA of MV planar imaging quality the vendors of linear accelerators typically supply the Las Vegas phantom. This phantom is insufficient, however, for accomplishing the tests of resolution and geometry outlined in Table 7.3. Figure 7.2 shows an alternative device (QC-3 Phantom, Standard Imaging, Middleton, WI) for QA of MV planar imaging. Spatial resolution is measured with the line-pair objects embedded in the middle row while contrast is measured with the squares and numbers along either edge. A similar device exists for the QA of kV planar image quality. Vendors often supply the Leeds TRO18FG phantom for this purpose.

For routine QA, the performance of the imaging system is not usually measured in an absolute sense but rather against performance at the time of commissioning. AAPM TG-179 and AAPM TG-142 refer to tolerances as "baseline" or "reproducibility." Further recommendations for the QA of planar imaging quality (both kV and MV) can be found in AAPM TG-142 and in the CAPCA QC Standards for EPIDs.

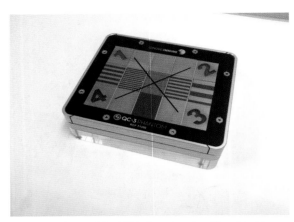

**Figure 7.2** An example device for image QA of MV planar imaging. The object has embedded features for spatial resolution (line pair etchings) and contrast (squares of varying thickness).

Similar test devices exist for the QA of CT scans. Most clinics use the CatPhan (Phantom Laboratories, Salem, NY), which consists of various modules arranged into transverse slices, each of which can be evaluated for a different imaging endpoint including resolution, uniformity, and contrast. The CatPhan 503 (supplied with Elekta accelerators) has three modules and the CatPhan 504 (supplied with Varian accelerators) has four modules, the extra module being one for low contrast resolution at 1%, 0.5%, and 0.3% levels. Other devices are available as well, including the AAPM CT performance phantom (CIRS Inc., Norfolk, VA). If CT numbers are used for dose calculations in a kV-CBCT system, AAPM TG-179 recommends they be tested annually.

## QA OF IMAGE REGISTRATION

One important aspect of the imaging chain is image registration (e.g., registration of a pretreatment MRI to the simulation CT to assist in planning). The topic of quality assurance for image registration is the subject of the forthcoming AAPM TG-132, Use of Image Registration and Data Fusion Algorithms and Techniques in Radiotherapy Treatment Planning. QA is especially important when automatic algorithms are employed.

## IMAGE DOSE

As can be seen in Table 7.3, most consensus reports recommend that dose be measured on an annual basis for on-treatment CT and planar imaging (kV or MV). It is therefore necessary for the clinical medical physicist to know how to make these measurements. AAPM TG-66 (Appendix II.2) provides guidance on measuring CT dose, and other references are AAPM TG-2 (Report 39) from 1993 and AAPM TG-8 (skin dose from radiographic procedures). AAPM TG-75 provides little support, other than to refer the reader to a study of Islam et al. for kV CBCT.[26] The measurement of dose from kV planar images is described in AAPM TG-2 (Report 39). Description of the principles of measured absorbed dose can be found in AAPM TG-7 on mammography. Some centers have found it beneficial to work with a diagnostic imaging physicist to measure dose and evaluate imaging protocols on an annual basis.

## QA OF OTHER LOCALIZATION SYSTEMS

The QA of nonradiographic localization systems is discussed in AAPM TG-147 (see Table 2). AAPM TG-154 focuses specifically on ultrasound systems for external beam (see Table 2 for QA information). AAPM TG-154 recommends daily alignment tests, monthly phantom and laser offset tests, as well as quarterly QA of the ultrasound phantoms themselves, which are subject to desiccation. QA of image quality is recommended on a semiannual basis (AAPM TG-154) and should include spatial resolution, contrast, and sensitivity (i.e., constant penetration depth and freedom from artifacts). Many nonradiographic systems use infrared cameras for localization of patients, markers, or devices. The accuracy of these systems must be tested, as they are subject to possible movement and warm-up effects (AAPM TG-154).

## RECOMMENDATIONS ON TESTS, FREQUENCIES, AND TOLERANCES

Table 7.3 offers a guide as to the frequency with which QA tests should be performed. These recommendations are based on a notion of what errors would be detectable with each test. For example, AAPM TG-179 specifies daily QA tests that are designed to "identify any sudden performance changes or gross errors that could result from collisions, upgrades, or afterhours service." It must be noted, however, that the various task group reports and consensus documents do not agree on which tests should be performed or on the frequency of such tests.

To take an example from Table 7.3, the recommended frequency for testing the spatial resolution of a CBCT system varies from monthly (AAPM TG-142) to semiannually (AAPM TG-179) to annually (AAPM TG-226). Another example is beam quality tests for CBCT. This is recommended on an annual basis in AAPM TG-179 but has no specific recommendation in AAPM TG-142 or AAPM TG-226. Some reports even appear inconsistent within themselves. For example, AAPM TG-142 recommends an annual test of beam quality for kV planar imaging systems but offers no such recommendation for CBCT systems (though a test of CT number constancy may serve as a surrogate). Recommended tolerance levels also differ between reports and some reports advocate different tolerances for some specialized techniques (e.g., stereotactic radiosurgery (SRS)/stereotactic body radiation therapy (SBRT)).

Partially in an attempt to rectify these disagreements, the AAPM has recently developed a Medical Physics Practice Guideline (MPPG) document, AAPM TG-226, Commissioning and Quality Assurance of X-Ray Based Image-Guided Radiotherapy Systems.[1] AAPM TG-226 is designed to provide recommendations that are practicable in a small, resource-limited environment. As such they are *minimum* practice guidelines. As can be seen Table 7.3, some of the recommendations in AAPM TG-226 differ substantially from other TG reports.

## QA MANAGEMENT AND DOCUMENTATION

As outlined above, there is a wealth of information as to which QA tests should be performed and how often. There is relatively little practical information, however, as to how to structure a quality management program. Most reports[1,11,12] state that a qualified medical physicist is responsible for "implementing and managing a QA program," though the physicist may not actually perform every QA test. In addition, the ASTRO safety white paper on IGRT recommends that "reporting and results should be transparent to RTTs, RadOncs and administrators." The reports of the Canadian Association of Provincial Cancer Agencies (CAPCA) offer some additional guidance. They provide suggestions as to the information that should appear on QA forms (e.g., name of institution, equipment, dates, and signatures) and suggestions for annual "independent quality control review" and other review recommendations.[10]

## FOR THE PHYSICIAN

A wide variety of systems are commercially available that enable on-treatment image guidance and localization. These rely on radiographic imaging (e.g., MV images, kV images, kV CBCT, and MV CT), nonradiographic imaging (e.g., in-room US), imaging the surface of the patient (e.g., reflective surface markers), and tracking the location of implanted markers or electromagnetic beacons. Key to the effective use of these IGRT systems is an understanding and control of system performance. Relevant parameters include geometric accuracy, spatial resolution, contrast, noise, and uniformity. A structured QA program is necessary to assess these properties on a daily, monthly, and annual basis. The basic QA tests are well understood, though there is some disagreement in society-level reports as to the type of test and frequency. A qualified medical physicist should oversee the QA, and the reporting and results should be transparent to the staff, physicians, and administrators. A final issue to consider is the dose received from radiographic imaging. Although the doses are much lower than therapeutic doses (e.g., 1 to 3 cGy for a CBCT scan), society-level reports suggest that the imaging dose should be considered from the cost/benefit perspective and minimized to the extent possible. The technical aspects of IGRT considered in this chapter are supplemented by Chapter 18, which considers the clinical aspects of image guidance and localization.

## *References*

1. Fontenot JD, Alkhatib H, Garrett JA, et al. Commissioning and quality assurance of x-ray based image-guided radiotherapy systems: AAPM TG-226 MPPG therapy #1. J Appl Clin Med Phys 2014;15(1):3–13. http://www.jacmp.org/index.php/jacmp/article/view/4528/html_1.
2. Bissonnette JP, Balter PA, Dong L, et al. Quality assurance for image-guided radiation therapy utilizing CT-based technologies: A report of the AAPM TG-179. Med Phys 2012;39(4):1946–63.
3. Willoughby T, Lehmann J, Bencomo JA, et al. Quality assurance for nonradiographic radiotherapy localization and positioning systems: Report of Task Group 147. Med Phys 2012;39(4):1728–47.
4. Molloy JA, Chan G, Markovic A, et al. Quality assurance of US-guided external beam radiotherapy for prostate cancer: Report of AAPM Task Group 154. Med Phys 2011;38(2):857–71.
5. Dieterich S, Cavedon C, Chuang CF, et al. Report of AAPM TG-135: Quality assurance for robotic radiosurgery. Med Phys 2011;38(6):2914–36.
6. Langen KM, Papanikolaou N, Balog J, et al. QA for helical TomoTherapy: Report of the AAPM Task Group 148. Med Phys 2010;37(9):4817–53.
7. Yin F, Wong J. The role of in-room kV x-ray imaging for patient setup and target localization: Report of Task Group 104. College Park, MD: AAPM; 2009.
8. Herman MG, Balter JM, Jaffray DA, et al. Clinical use of electronic portal imaging: Report of AAPM Radiation Therapy Committee Task Group 58. Med Phys 2001;28(5):712–37.
9. Murphy MJ, Balter J, Balter S, et al. The management of imaging dose during image-guided radiotherapy: Report of the AAPM Task Group 75. Med Phys 2007;34(10):4041–63.
10. Arsenault C, et al. Standards for quality control at Canadian radiation treatment centres: Electronic portal imaging devices, in Standards for Quality Control at Canadian Radiation Treatment Centres. 2005. https://www.medphys.ca/content.php?doc=58.
11. Potters L, Gaspar LE, Kavanagh B, et al. American Society for Therapeutic Radiology and Oncology (ASTRO) and American College of Radiology (ACR) practice guidelines for image-guided radiation therapy (IGRT). Int J Radiation Oncol Biol Phys 2010;76(2):319–25.
12. Jaffray D, Langen KM, Mageras G, et al. Safety considerations for IGRT: Executive summary. Pract Radiat Oncol 2013;3(3):167–70.
13. Hoggarth MA, Luce J, Syeda F, et al. Dual energy imaging using a clinical on-board imaging system. Phys Med Biol 2013;58(12):4331–40.
14. Pfeiffer D, Sutlief S, Feng W, et al. AAPM Task Group 128: Quality assurance tests for prostate brachytherapy ultrasound systems. Med Phys 2008;35(12):5471–89.
15. Dempsey JF, Dionne B, Fitzsimmons J, et al. A real-time MRI guided external beam radiotherapy delivery system. Med Phys 2006;33:2254.

16. Raaymakers BW, Lagendijk JJW, Overweg J, et al. Integrating a 1.5 T MRI scanner with a 6 MV accelerator: Proof of concept. Phys Med Biol 2009;54(12):N229–37.
17. Oborn BM, Metcalfe PE, Butson MJ, et al. Electron contamination modeling and skin dose in 6 MV longitudinal field MRIgRT: Impact of the MRI and MRI fringe field. Med Phys 2012;39(2):874–90.
18. Bortfeld T, Paganetti H, Kooy H. Proton beam radiotherapy—The state of the art. Med Phys 2005;32:2048.
19. Mayyas E, Chetty IJ, Chetvertkov M, et al. Evaluation of multiple image-based modalities for image-guided radiation therapy (IGRT) of prostate carcinoma: A prospective study. Med Phys 2013;40(4):041707.
20. Mutic S, Palta JR, Butker EK, et al. Quality assurance for computed-tomography simulators and the computed-tomography-simulation process: Report of the AAPM Radiation Therapy Committee Task Group No. 66. Med Phys 2003;30(10):2762–92.
21. Thapa BB, Molloy JA. Feasibility of an image planning system for kilovoltage image-guided radiation therapy. Med Phys 2013;40(6):061703.
22. Yadav P, Tolakanahalli R, Rong Y, et al. The effect and stability of MVCT images on adaptive TomoTherapy. J Appl Clin Med Phys 2010;11(4):3229.
23. ACR–ASTRO practice guidelines for image-guided radiation therapy (IGRT). Reston, VA: American College of Radiology; 2009.
24. Sharpe MB, Moseley DJ, Purdie TG, et al. The stability of mechanical calibration for a kV cone beam computed tomography system integrated with linear accelerator. Med Phys 2006;33(1):136–44.
25. Lutz W, Ken RW, Nasser M. A system for stereotactic radiosurgery with a linear accelerator. Int J Radiat Oncol Biol Phys 1988;14(2):373–81.
26. Islam MK, Purdie TG, Norrlinger BD, et al. Patient dose from kilovoltage cone beam computed tomography imaging in radiation therapy. Med Phys 2006;33(6):1573–82.
27. Walter C, Boda-Heggemann J, Wertz H, et al. Phantom and in-vivo measurements of dose exposure by image-guided radiotherapy (IGRT): MV portal images vs. kV portal images vs. cone-beam CT. Radiother Oncol 2007;85(3):418–23.
28. Steiner E, Kostresevic B, Ableitinger A, et al. Imaging dose assessment for IGRT in particle beam therapy. Radiother Oncol 2013;109(3):409–13.
29. Waddington SP, McKenzie AL. Assessment of effective dose from concomitant exposures required in verification of the target volume in radiotherapy. Br J Radiol 2004;77(919):557–61.

# CHAPTER 8

# Brachytherapy

## 8.1 Introduction

Brachytherapy is defined as the temporary or permanent application of small, sealed radioactive sources in close proximity to or within the target volume. The treatment dose distribution is characterized by localized high dose and a steep dose drop-off. Soon after radium was first chemically isolated by Marie and Pierre Curie, the effects of radiation damage on skin were observed and led to the earliest application of radioactive material for the treatment of superficial tumors. A few decades later, radium needles were used in low–dose rate interstitial implants. Implant patterns and dose calculations were performed using the Patterson-Parker or Quimby implant systems. Although those dose calculation methods have been retired with the implementation of computer-based treatment planning systems, the basic implant geometry from these systems is still used today.

Currently, the predominant treatment sites for brachytherapy are cancers of the prostate, uterine cervix, endometrium, and partial breast irradiation. It is also used intraoperatively in partial breast irradiation and some abdominal/pelvic applications. Interstitial brachytherapy is also sometimes performed for soft tissue sarcomas. With the implementation of intensity-modulated radiation therapy (IMRT), use of brachytherapy in head-and-neck cancers or bronchial lesions has been decreasing. Similarly, easier access to proton therapy has diminished the use of brachytherapy for ocular melanomas. Medicated stents have replaced intravascular brachytherapy treatments (IVBT), although more recently IVBT is being reconsidered as salvage therapy for medical stent failures. On the other hand, new developments in surface applicators have sparked renewed interest in using brachytherapy for the treatment of superficial tumors. Several groups are also working to develop novel brachytherapy applicators for anal and rectal cancer, but these have not yet emerged from the research and development (R&D) stage. Figure 8.1 shows the classification scheme for brachytherapy treatments with a reference to the respective clinical chapters covering individual treatment techniques.

An excellent historical review of brachytherapy was published by Williamson in 2006.[1] This review discusses the evolution of brachytherapy and provides a description of future developments that remains relevant today. Another review was published in 2008 by Thomadsen et al.[2] The role of AAPM in the development of brachytherapy dosimetry is described in a paper by Ibbott et al.[3] Another excellent source of information is AAPM TG-56, Code of Practice for Brachytherapy Physics.[4] The reference dosimetry of brachytherapy sources is discussed in Chapter 1 of this book, commissioning and quality assurance (QA) of high dose rate (HDR) afterloaders in Chapter 4, and computerized dose calculation QA in Chapter 5. Specific applications of brachytherapy are described in other chapters as shown in Figure 8.1. This chapter describes the basics of brachytherapy, including the brachytherapy process, description of sources, and description of common applicators. The description of the brachytherapy process will include a general workflow, QA of the process, personnel requirements and qualifications, source handling, source transport, source storage, source assay, imaging, and treatment planning.

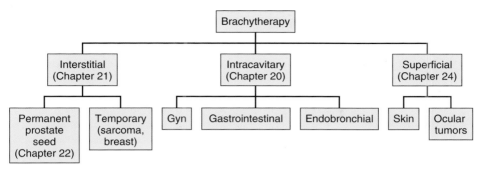

**Figure 8.1** Classification scheme for brachytherapy treatments.

## 8.2 Radioisotopes for Brachytherapy

The original sources used for brachytherapy were radium and radon, which were naturally occurring isotopes. With the advent of artificially produced isotopes many options became available. These isotopes are produced by particle bombardment in a reactor (neutron-rich isotopes) or a cyclotron (proton-rich istotopes) (Table 8.1).

## 8.3 Brachytherapy Applicators

There are many types of brachytherapy applicators. Chapters 20 and 21 have more details, but a brief summary is shown in Table 8.2.

## 8.4 The Brachytherapy Process

Brachytherapy can be performed in many ways. It can be differentiated by the dose rate, the type of implant, and whether or not it is a permanent implant. Low dose rate (LDR) is defined by International Commission on Radiation Units and Measurements (ICRU)-38[5] and US Nuclear Regulatory Commission (NRC) Code of Federal Regulations 10 CFR 35 as implants delivering less than or equal to 2 Gy/hour at the prescription point. Similarly, these references define HDR as greater than or equal to 12 Gy/hour at the prescription point, though the dose rate is often much higher. The type of implant can be intracavitary, interstitial, or surface. Finally, the implant can be permanent or temporary. Permanent implants initially have a dose rate in the range of 8 to 32 cGy/hour, which decays exponentially according to the half-life of the radionuclide. Table 8.3 shows typical applications of brachytherapy.

HDR brachytherapy is delivered using remote afterloaders. These systems have a high activity source at the end of a long wire. When not in use, the source is housed in a heavily shielded enclosure. Typically the source is $^{192}$Ir (10 to 12 Ci at install) although $^{60}$Co sources are available as well. Because of the short half-life for $^{192}$Ir, the HDR source is typically replaced every 3 months. The applicator is connected to the HDR unit using what is called a transfer tube. For multiple channel implants some units have the ability to key the transfer tube to a particular channel, allowing treatment only when it is connected to the correct channel. The source wire is driven out of the shielded enclosure and stepped through the various applicators or catheters to deliver the treatment. The position where the source stops is called a dwell position. The amount of time spent at each dwell position is called the dwell time. Both LDR and HDR treatments require shielded rooms. See Chapter 10 for details.

Temporary implants can also be performed with LDR sources (typically $^{137}$Cs). Historically this was accomplished by manually loading sources into the applicators or catheters, though LDR

TABLE 8.1 ▦ **Isotopes for Brachytherapy**

| Source | Energy | Half-Life | HVL | Comments |
|---|---|---|---|---|
| $^{228}$Ra | γ 0.047-2.45 MeV<br>Average 0.83 MeV | 1626 years | 12 mm Pb | Sealed cells to prevent radon gas leakage<br>Activity in mg Ra<br>Filtration in mm Pt<br>Oldest source; not in use |
| $^{222}$Rn | γ 0.047-2.45 MeV | 3.83 days | 12 mm Pb | |
| $^{192}$Ir | γ 0.136-1.06 MeV<br>Average 0.38 MeV | 73.8 days | 3 mm Pb | Main $^{228}$Ra substitute for interstitial LDR<br>Main HDR source<br>Wire, seeds, ribbons |
| $^{125}$I | γ 0.035 MeV | 59.4 days | 0.025 mm Pb | Seeds for prostate implant, lung implant, or eye plaque<br>Low energy requires little shielding<br>Seed models require individual characterization and commissioning<br>Older seed models very anisotropic |
| $^{103}$Pd | X-rays 0.02-0.023 MeV<br>Average 0.021 MeV | 17 days | 0.008 mm Pb | Seeds for prostate implants<br>Faster dose delivery than $^{125}$I |
| $^{131}$Cs | X-rays 0.004-0.034 MeV<br>Average 0.03 MeV | 9.7 days | | Permanent seed implant<br>Higher energy, shorter half-life than $^{125}$I and $^{103}$Pd |
| $^{137}$Cs | γ 0.662 MeV | 30 years | 6.5 mm Pb | $^{228}$Ra substitute: less shielding, no Rn gas<br>Intracavitary and interstitial<br>Tubes or pellets<br>Dose along transverse axis about same as $^{228}$Ra to 10 cm depth<br>Semipermanent stock of sources (exchange ≈ 7 years) |
| $^{90}$Sr/$^{90}$Y | X-ray 2.27 MeV | 28.9 years | | Pterygium applicator<br>IVBT<br>Calibration source |
| $^{90}$Y | | 64 hours | | Liver mets (microspheres) |
| $^{198}$Au | γ 0.412 MeV | 2.7 days | 2.5 mm Pb | Permanent seed implant<br>Replaced $^{222}$Rn seeds<br>High energy required several half-life hospital stay<br>Mostly replaced by $^{125}$I and $^{103}$Pd |
| $^{131}$I | β 0.19 MeV<br>γ 0.38 MeV | 8 days<br>(radiological) | | Unsealed source<br>Hyperthyroidism, thyroid carcinoma |

For more information on unsealed sources such as microspheres, see Chapter 24.

TABLE 8.2 ▦ **Typical Brachytherapy Applicators**

| Type of Implant | Applicators |
| --- | --- |
| Gyn | Tandem and ovoids, cylinder, tandem and cylinder |
| Prostate | Needles |
| Endobronchial | Thin, flexible catheter (5F or 6F diameter) |
| Esophageal | 5-8 mm flexible catheter |
| Breast | Needles or balloon applicators (single or multilumen) |

TABLE 8.3 ▦ **Summary of Typical Brachytherapy Applications**

| | Type of Implant | | |
| --- | --- | --- | --- |
| Time | Interstitial | Intracavitary | Surface |
| Temporary | Prostate (HDR)<br>Sarcoma (HDR or LDR)<br>Head and neck (HDR or LDR) | Gyn (HDR or LDR)<br>Endobronchial (HDR or LDR)<br>Nasopharynx (HDR or LDR)<br>Esophageal (HDR or LDR) | Skin (HDR)<br>Eye (LDR) |
| Permanent | Prostate<br>Lung | NA | NA |

remote afterloaders are also available. They move source trains into position for treatment, and when staff enters the treatment room, the source train retracts. After the staff leaves the room the treatment is re-initiated. Although LDR is included here it is mainly for historical purposes as most facilities have converted to HDR. For example, in a 2009 survey of practice HDR represented 62% of the patients treated for carcinoma of the cervix compared to 13% in 1999.[6] The trend will continue to advance toward 100% as the last $^{137}$Cs manufacturer ceased operation in 2002.[1] Despite this, when describing the process, differences between LDR and HDR will be highlighted.

# 8.5 Brachytherapy Workflow

A generic brachytherapy workflow is shown in Figure 8.2. The steps are common to HDR and LDR with the exception of the source ordering, receipt, and assay for LDR.

## INITIAL PLANNING AND TREATMENT PRESCRIPTION

The initial planning will involve a discussion on applicator selection and treatment goals. The prescription will be based on the stage of the patient and the combination with external beam radiotherapy and/or chemotherapy.

## ORDER, RECEIPT, AND ASSAY OF SOURCES

For LDR treatments, time must be allowed for the procurement of sources. To order seeds in the United States the vendor must have a current copy of the radioactive material license for the facility on file. Some radionuclides are only produced in limited quantities once per month (e.g., $^{125}$I seeds in suture for lung implants), so some lead time may be required. Vendors may also have a limited supply of the rarer types of seeds (e.g., the high-activity $^{125}$I seeds used in eye plaques). Once received, the package must be surveyed and determined not to have contamination as

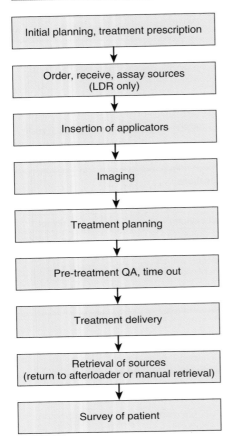

**Figure 8.2** Brachytherapy workflow.

described in Chapter 10. The sources must be assayed as described in Chapter 1. As mentioned in Chapter 1, there are special considerations when assaying sterile sources; either sterility must be maintained during the assay or extra seeds from the same batch can be ordered for assay purposes.

## INSERTION OF APPLICATORS

Applicator insertion is usually a team effort between the surgeon and the radiation oncologist, although the implants are increasingly performed only by the radiation oncologist. For LDR it is crucial to have a quality implant because there is no possibility for optimization. HDR treatments can take advantage of dwell position and time optimization to overcome suboptimal geometry, but it is still advisable to use good technique in the placement of the applicators as there are limits to the amount of optimization that can be done. For instance, if the distance to a critical structure is less than the distance to the prescription point for a dwell position, the dose to the critical structure will always be higher than the prescription dose. Other dwells can be given higher weights to counteract this, but it may cause hot spots in other locations. When performing planar or volume implants, it is important to keep the catheters at a uniform distance apart and parallel to each other to minimize local hot or cold spots. Templates are sometimes used to assist with catheter or needle spacing. Prostate seed implants utilize templates, for instance. For soft tissue masses or breast implants, a rigid hollow needle can be used to make a path through the tissue, and then a flexible catheter with a button end can be threaded through and the needle removed. More details are given in Chapters 20 through 22.

## IMAGING FOR BRACHYTHERAPY

Imaging was traditionally done with 2D radiographs. This made it somewhat difficult to determine the catheter positions if there were many, and soft tissue structures were not visible unless contrast was used. The contrast sometimes obscured the applicators so images were taken pre- and post contrast. In addition, for gyn brachytherapy it is recommended that a Foley catheter be inserted and a small amount of contrast injected into the Foley balloon to aid in identifying the bladder. The accurate reconstruction from 2D radiographs requires precise knowledge of the beam center, magnification factor, and angulation of the imager to the x-ray source. Reconstruction jigs can be used to aid in the accurate reconstruction from orthogonal 2D images. These jigs have reference markings that define the projection geometry and magnification. By digitizing known points into the system, the source geometry can be defined. The use of CT and US has become the standard for imaging in brachytherapy cases. MR imaging is also becoming more common.[7]

Slice thickness is important in delineating the entire length of an applicator. If the tip of an applicator is fully within a slice versus part way, errors on the order of half the slice thickness could be introduced.[8] Slice spacing for CT of 2.5 mm to 3 mm is common. For multiple channel plans, it is important to uniquely identify each channel. This could be done by using dummy radiographic markers with a unique pattern of short and long markers. For applicators such as multilumen balloons used in breast brachytherapy, consistent orientation is important. For example, if the channel closest to the skin is not used to minimize skin dose, it should be confirmed prior to every treatment that the proper orientation is maintained.

## TREATMENT PLANNING FOR BRACHYTHERAPY

Treatment planning for LDR involves the determination of dose rate. With the applicators in place in a fixed geometry, the only variables to optimize are the availability of different $^{137}$Cs-source strengths for gyn applicators and their arrangement within the applicators or the number of seeds and position within the catheters for $^{192}$Ir planar implants, for instance. For volume or planar implants the maximum contiguous-contour dose is used to determine the treatment dose rate.[4] This is the highest isodose line that encompasses the target without breaking up. The treatment time is determined by simply dividing the total dose by the dose rate. Care should be taken to keep the dose rates to acceptable levels, historically 40 to 70 cGy/hour.

Treatment planning for HDR can take advantage of the ability to optimize the source position and dwell time anywhere along the applicator length. The Thomadsen paper has a discussion of optimization techniques.[2] The paper lists some general principles for optimizing interstitial implants. These are not unique to HDR, but HDR does have more flexibility to optimize as mentioned above. The principles for interstitial brachytherapy are:

1. To achieve the most uniform dose distributions, the concentration of sources or dwell positions needs to be higher near the periphery (i.e., peripheral loading). As much as 75% of the activity could be in peripheral locations but will depend on the shape of the clinical target volume (CTV) and the source positions.
2. Needles in the corners of implants should be moved inward to avoid breaks in the isodose lines. Reducing the distance to about two thirds of the distance for a regular geometric pattern usually suffices.
3. When using small seeds, the strength at the ends of the needles needs to be twice that of the other locations in the needle. For prostate seed implants this is achieved by placing sources back to back at the distal and proximal ends of the needle.

The principles for intracavitary brachytherapy are:

1. When the goal is to project the dose to points distant to the applicator, the source locations should be far from the applicator–tissue interface. This is due to the inverse square effect. Just as a greater source-to-surface distance (SSD) in external beam radiotherapy yields a higher fractional depth dose, a greater source-to-tissue distance in brachytherapy does also. For example, choosing a larger diameter cylinder will result in higher doses at distance relative to the surface of the cylinder.
2. If possible, the applicator arrangement should place sources around the target (i.e., use tandem and ovoids vs. tandem and cylinder).
3. The dose distribution will not be uniform but will be continually decreasing with distance from the sources.

For HDR applicator-based planning (e.g., cylinders) the prescription distance should be greater than the source spacing to limit undulation in the isodose lines.

## BRACHYTHERAPY PRETREATMENT QA AND TIME-OUT

AAPM TG-59, High Dose-Rate Brachytherapy Treatment Delivery,[9] describes pretreatment QA for an HDR procedure. Although these steps are specific to HDR, the general principles would apply to LDR as well.

1. Two people should check proper connection of catheters to the HDR unit and that the transfer tubes are free of kinks.
2. The emergency kit and source container are available.
3. Survey meter is present and operational. (Not mentioned in AAPM TG-59 but recommended is to survey the patient prior to the treatment to confirm background. The patient may have had a nuclear medicine scan prior to the treatment, causing an elevated reading. If not known prior to the treatment, there could be confusion when performing the post-treatment survey).
4. Transfer tube lengths are correct.
5. Check applicator positioning. This can be done by check of measurements taken at the time of insertion (i.e., distance from template to proximal end of needle) or tandem positioning against marks on patient skin.
6. Treatment documentation review.
   a. Signed prescription and plan.
   b. Second check has been performed.
   c. Plan agrees with prescription.
   d. Plan is consistent with previous fractions if applicable.
   e. Dwell positions and times in plan agree with what is programmed on the treatment console. (Verification of source loading by second person for LDR.)
7. Patient identity confirmed by two methods.

In addition, it is good practice to conduct a time-out prior to initiating the treatment to ensure that all staff participating in the delivery agree that the intended parameters are correct, the correct patient is being treated to the correct site, that staff have their exposure badges, and that the emergency responders have been identified.

## TREATMENT DELIVERY

LDR treatments can be delivered using a remote afterloading device, as mentioned, but manual loading is more common. The loading should be well thought out to minimize the time and thereby minimize exposure. As mentioned in the previous section, the source loading should be verified by two people. This would include laying out the appropriate tools within easy reach ahead of time, removing applicator caps, and ensuring an unobstructed work space. LDR deliveries can be 1 to 3 days in length. This requires that the patient be confined to a shielded room. Portable shields can be used to augment room shielding. Staff should be instructed as to safe practice when caring for these patients. One key is to limit the amount of time at the bedside. Unless direct patient care is being given there is no need to be at the bedside. Taking several steps back when communicating with the patient will greatly reduce the exposure. As mentioned above, afterloading units eliminate this issue since the sources are removed when staff is in the room. A survey of the surrounding areas should be done to confirm that all levels are acceptable.

An HDR treatment typically takes from 5 to 15 minutes, depending on the source strength and type of treatment, though interoperative treatments can be much longer. According to U.S. NRC regulations an authorized medical physicist and an authorized user (radiation oncologist) must be present during the treatment. If an emergency occurs where the source becomes stuck inside an applicator, the staff must be trained how to respond. The first course of action is to press the emergency stop in an attempt to force the source retraction. If that does not work then the emergency responder should enter the room and attempt to return the source to the shielded position using the manual retraction method (hand crank). If that does not work the physician would then enter the room and remove the applicator with the source still in it and place it in the emergency container. The patient should be removed from the room and immediately surveyed to confirm that the source has been removed from the patient. The room should be secured (marked "do not enter") and the vendor notified. The unintended exposure to staff should be estimated. The actual readings can be obtained when the staff exposure badges are read. AAPM TG-59 gives estimated exposures from a 10 Ci source for various times and distances. For example, in 10 minutes an individual would receive 750 mGy at 10 cm from the source, 30 mGy at 50 cm, and 7.5 mGy at 100 cm. By comparing these to the allowable annual limit of 50 mSv (mSv = mGy for photons) it can be seen that an efficient emergency response will not result in excessive exposure to the staff but could result in significant unintended dose to the patient. To minimize the chance of a stuck source, all HDR units have a dummy wire that is sent out prior to the radioactive source to confirm that the path is open. If any resistance is encountered during the dummy run an alarm is activated. There may be options regarding how the dummy runs are configured. For a multiple channel implant it would be desirable to confirm all channels are open prior to treating any channel. This would prevent a partial treatment being delivered if one channel had a constriction. Some units offer a double-check configuration that checks all channels prior to treating the first channel and then again prior to treating each channel. Care should be taken to keep the transfer tubes as straight as possible to minimize the chance of kinking a tube and causing a constriction.

## RETRIEVAL OF SOURCES, POST-TREATMENT SURVEY, AND RECORDS REVIEW

For manual LDR treatments, the sources are simply removed from the applicators. As with the loading, the process should be well thought out and efficient. The storage container should be placed close with an unobstructed work area. After source removal, the applicators are removed. For HDR treatments the source returns to the shielded position after the treatment is complete. The transfer tubes can then be disconnected and the applicators removed.

A post-treatment survey of the patient and immediate area is required by the NRC (10 CFR 35.604 for remote afterloaders and 10 CFR 35.404 for manual brachytherapy) to confirm that no sources remain inside the patient and that sources were not inadvertently dropped. A review of all records should then be done to ensure that everything is complete. For remote afterloader treatments the post-treatment log should be reviewed to confirm that it matches the planned delivery.

## 8.6 QA of the Brachytherapy Process

AAPM TG-56, Code of Practice for Brachytherapy,[4] recommends the creation of a QA program for the entire brachytherapy process. The stated goals of the QA program are:

1. To ensure that each individual treatment is administered consistently.
2. To ensure that each treatment accurately reflects the radiation oncologist's clinical intent.
3. To ensure that each treatment is executed with regard to the safety of the patient and staff.

The QA program should address three basic processes: applicator insertion, implant design and evaluation, and the treatment delivery process. They describe four categories of QA program end points.

1. Safety of the patient, public, and institution. This includes the control of exposure, provision of adequate shielding, and procedures to maintain control of all radioactive sources. The users must have the ability to recognize a hazard and know how to respond in an emergency. For remote afterloaders the QA will involve verifying the operation of all interlocks. Regulatory compliance, while required, does not necessarily address safety.
2. Positional accuracy. The source position or active dwell position as defined by the physician must be verified. This is often done relative to dummy markers, so staff must understand how each system determines dwell positions. For instance, one system, Varian, may need to have the most distal point in a catheter identified, while another, Elekta, may need the center of the most distal source position. The NRC requires ±1 mm accuracy for source position tests, but this may not be achievable in clinical practice due to catheter localization uncertainties.
3. Temporal accuracy. A goal of ±2% is easily achievable. Transit dose should be evaluated and corrections made if necessary.[10]
4. Dose delivery accuracy. The core requirement is an accurate calibration of the source activity. In addition, the proper source calculation parameters should be used. Applicator attenuation and the effect of shields should be addressed if possible. The accuracy of the 3D reconstruction of the applicators should be confirmed. The accuracy of dose reference points (i.e., Point A) and critical structure points (i.e., rectum and bladder) will also have an impact on plan quality.

AAPM TG-56 stresses that every institution will need to design its own QA process but that these factors should be addressed. For procedure-specific QA, rules and guidelines should be developed to define the chronology of the process and to restrict the range of actions at each step to minimize the chance of error. Redundant checks and a carefully designed workflow should also be developed. It further describes a step-by-step process for developing procedure-specific QA.

1. Define the workflow. At each step identify the team members involved, the critical activities, and the information to be captured.
2. Use carefully designed documentation to ensure accurate communication and to form the basis of the permanent treatment record.
3. Identify vulnerable points in the treatment delivery process and design redundant checks.

4. Develop a written procedure outlining the chronology, team member functions, QA checks, and associated documentation. Checklists are recommended.
5. Integrate with the overall QA program. Institute a random independent audit of sample patient records and a review of any errors. Develop a formal clinical quality improvement (CQI) process.

## 8.7 Brachytherapy Dose Calculations, Dose Specification, and Dose Reporting

Chapter 1 describes the calibration of a brachytherapy source, and Chapter 5 describes the testing of brachytherapy dose calculations. The dose calculation formalism will be described here. The current generally accepted dose calculation method is that described by AAPM TG-43 and the follow-up documents.[11-13] The general 2D dose rate equation is:

$$D(r,\theta) = S_K \, \Lambda \, (G_L(r,\theta)/G_L(r_0,\theta_0)) \, g_L(r) \, F(r,\theta)$$

where $S_K$ = air kerma strength in unit of U (i.e., $\mu Gy \, m^2 \, h^{-1} = cGy \, cm^2 \, h^{-1}$)

$\Lambda$ = dose rate constant in water (in units of $cGy \, h^{-1} \, U^{-1}$)

r = distance in cm

$r_0$ = reference distance = 1 cm

$\theta$ = the polar angle relative to the longitudinal axis of the line source

$G_L(r,\theta)$ = the geometry function (approximate model of effective inverse square)

$G_L(r_0,\theta_0)$ = the geometry function at the reference distance and angle (90 degrees)

$g_L(r)$ = radial dose function (dose fall-off due to scattering and attenuation)

$F(r,\theta)$ = anisotropy function (variation in dose as a function of polar angle to account for source encapsulation and design, = 1 for $\theta_0$)

All of the parameters are specific to a source model and care should be taken to ensure that the correct values are used. As mentioned in Chapter 5, consensus values are available on the IROC-Houston (formerly RPC) website.

For a point source, the equation becomes:

$$D(r) = S_K \, \Lambda \, (G_L(r,\theta_0)/G_L(r_0,\theta_0)) \, g_L(r) \, \phi_{an}(r)$$

where $\phi_{an}(r)$ = 1D anisotropy function (solid angle-weighted average dose rate over entire $4\pi$ solid angle). The original AAPM TG-43 report called for an isotropy constant independent of r, but is no longer recommended.

The geometry function is given by:

$\beta/Lr \sin\theta$     if $\theta \neq 0$

$(r^2 - L^2/4)^{-1}$     if $\theta = 0$

$r^{-2}$                     for a point source

where $\beta$ is the angle in radians subtended by the tips of the line source with respect to the calculation point and $L$ is the active length of the source. The radial dose function is tabulated by distance and interpolation is used to derive the value needed. The anisotropy function is tabulated by distance and angle.

At distances close to a line source the fall-off of dose is less than would be expected by the inverse square law due to the fact that photons from the tips of the source travel a farther distance and pass through more filtration with oblique incidence. As a rule of thumb, at distances >2 times source length the line source will follow the inverse square law.

Again it should be reiterated that all of these values are source model dependent and that the line and point source formulas are approximate models for the distribution of activity in a source. They do not include effects such as differential absorption in the capsule. In addition, dose

TABLE 8.4 ▓ **Implant Dose Specifications**

| Type of Implant | Dose Specification |
| --- | --- |
| Vaginal cylinder | At surface or 5 mm |
| Tandem and ovoids | Average of point A left and right (2 cm superior and 2 cm lateral to cervical os) |
| Endobronchial | 0.5 or 1.0 cm from center of catheter |
| Breast balloon | 1.0 cm from surface of the balloon |

calculations based on the above formalism do not allow for source-to-source attenuation or corrections for inhomogeneity in tissue.

## 8.8 Dose Specification and Dose Reporting

Table 8.4 shows typical dose specification points for various types of implants. The use of 3D planning will ultimately replace simple point dose specifications with volume specifications similar to external beam radiotherapy.

For intracavitary brachytherapy ICRU-38 recommends reporting the following quantities:[5]

1. The dimensions of the 60 Gy isodose contour including external beam dose
2. The dose at a bladder point at the posterior surface of the Foley balloon on the anterior/posterior line through the center of the balloon
3. The dose at a rectal point 0.5 cm posterior to the vaginal cavity at an anterior/posterior line midway between the vaginal sources
4. Doses at points representing the lower para-aortic, common, and external iliac lymph nodes
5. Doses representing the distal parametrium and obturator lymph nodes

As pointed out in AAPM TG-56, the volume of the 60 Gy isodose contour has not been shown to correlate with individual dimensions but rather with total activity implanted. AAPM TG-56 recommends that the integrated reference air kerma (IRAK) be reported. IRAK is the total air kerma strength in the implant multiplied by the treatment time for each source used. The time should be in seconds for HDR and hours for LDR. The dose specification process at a facility should be well described and understood by all staff members involved in the planning process. Conventions for localizing reference points should be well documented. Mixing of dose specification and treatment planning practices is not recommended. These factors are designed to work as a system, and results cannot be predicted if the system in its entirety is not used.

ICRU-58 specifies guidelines for interstitial brachytherapy as shown in Table 8.5.[14] In addition, the ABS recommends reporting of the planning methodology (i.e., Manchester, Paris, Memorial nomogram, custom template, optimization, etc.).[15]

## 8.9 Personnel and Qualifications

The NRC specifies the qualifications for an authorized user (10 CFR 35 parts 35.59, 35.190(a), 35.290(a), 35.390(a), 35.392(a), 35.394(a), 35.490(a), 35.590(a), 35.690(a)) and an authorized medical physicist (AMP) (10 CFR 35.51). The qualifications for an AMP are:

Except as provided in §35.57, the licensee shall require the authorized medical physicist to be an individual who

TABLE 8.5 ■ **ICRU Recommendations for Dose Reporting in Interstitial Brachytherapy**

| Parameter | Description |
|---|---|
| Description of target volumes | Gross tumor volume (GTV), clinical target volume (CTV), etc. |
| Treated volume | Volume of tissue encompassed by prescription isodose |
| Radionuclide | Type of source |
| Source size and shape, source pattern | Implant geometry |
| Reference air kerma rate | |
| Description of time pattern | |
| Total reference air kerma (TRAK) | Sum of air kerma strength × treatment time for each source |
| Prescription dose | Location of point or surface |
| Reference dose in the central plane | Largest plane at the center of the implant |
| Mean central dose | |
| Minimum target dose | |
| High dose volume | V150% |
| Low dose volume | V90% |
| Uniformity parameters | |
| Dose rates at point or surface of Rx | |

(a) Is certified by a specialty board whose certification process has been recognized by the Commission or an Agreement State and who meets the requirements in paragraphs (b) (2) and (c) of this section. (The names of board certifications that have been recognized by the Commission or an Agreement State will be posted on the NRC's Web page.) To have its certification process recognized, a specialty board shall require all candidates for certification to:

  (1) Hold a master's or doctor's degree in physics, medical physics, other physical science, engineering, or applied mathematics from an accredited college or university;

  (2) Have 2 years of full-time practical training and/or supervised experience in medical physics—

   (i)  Under the supervision of a medical physicist who is certified in medical physics by a specialty board recognized by the Commission or an Agreement State; or

   (ii) In clinical radiation facilities providing high-energy, external beam therapy (photons and electrons with energies greater than or equal to 1 million electron volts) and brachytherapy services under the direction of physicians who meet the requirements in §35.57, 35.490, or 35.690; and

  (3) Pass an examination, administered by diplomates of the specialty board, that assesses knowledge and competence in clinical radiation therapy, radiation safety, calibration, quality assurance, and treatment planning for external beam therapy, brachytherapy, and stereotactic radiosurgery; or

(b) (1) Holds a master's or doctor's degree in physics, medical physics, other physical science, engineering, or applied mathematics from an accredited college or university; and has completed 1 year of full-time training in medical physics and an additional year of full-time work experience under the supervision of an individual who meets the requirements for an authorized medical physicist for the type(s) of use for which the individual is seeking authorization. This training and work experience must be conducted in clinical radiation facilities that provide high-energy, external beam therapy (photons and electrons with energies greater than or equal to 1 million electron volts) and brachy-therapy services and must include:

    (i) Performing sealed source leak tests and inventories;

    (ii) Performing decay corrections;

    (iii) Performing full calibration and periodic spot checks of external beam treat-ment units, stereotactic radiosurgery units, and remote afterloading units as appli-cable; and

    (iv) Conducting radiation surveys around external beam treatment units, stereotactic radiosurgery units, and remote afterloading units as applicable; and

  (2) Has obtained written attestation that the individual has satisfactorily completed the requirements in paragraphs (c) and (a)(1) and (a)(2), or (b)(1) and (c) of this section, and has achieved a level of competency sufficient to function independently as an authorized medical physicist for each type of therapeutic medical unit for which the individual is requesting authorized medical physicist status. The written attestation must be signed by a preceptor authorized medical physicist who meets the requirements in §§35.51, 35.57, or equivalent Agreement State requirements for an authorized medical physicist for each type of therapeutic medical unit for which the individual is requesting authorized medical physicist status; and

(c) Has training for the type(s) of use for which authorization is sought that includes hands-on device operation, safety procedures, clinical use, and the operation of a treatment planning system. This training requirement may be satisfied by satisfactorily completing either a training program provided by the vendor or by training supervised by an authorized medical physicist authorized for the type(s) of use for which the individual is seeking authorization.

## 8.10 Source Handling, Transport, Storage, and Inventory

The dose rate at the surface of a radioactive source can be extremely high, and therefore sources should never be handled directly. Long-handled forceps or tweezers should be used. Sources must be shipped in accordance with U.S. Department of Transportation (DOT) regulations as discussed in Chapter 10. To be able to transport radioactive materials outside the facility, a license is required. See 10 CFR 71.5. There is an exemption for physicians in 10 CFR 71.13:

> Any physician licensed by a State to dispense drugs in the practice of medicine is exempt from §71.5 with respect to transport by the physician of licensed material for use in the practice of medicine. However, any physician operating under this exemption must be licensed under 10 CFR part 35 or the equivalent Agreement State regulations.

Radioactive materials must be under control by the facility at all times. This means under direct control or by securing in a locked area. In addition, the facility must have strict inventory control and document the location of all radioactive materials at all times. When shipments are received, the sources are logged into an inventory. If sources are removed from the storage area to take to the treatment area, the log should reflect what sources were taken, the destination, the date, the time, and who took them. If not all the sources were used for the treatment, any returned sources to the storage area must be logged back in. Similarly, after completion of the treatment the sources must be returned to the storage area and logged back in to inventory. Short-lived radionuclides can be returned to the vendor for disposal or decayed in storage for 10 half-lives before disposal as normal waste. If a source is shipped back to the vendor, the facility must receive and keep the confirmation of receipt by the vendor.

## FOR THE PHYSICIAN

Brachytherapy has the advantage of delivering high dose radiation to a localized area with rapid dose fall-off. A variety of sources with differing energies and half-lives are available for use commercially, as seeds, wires, ribbons, plaques, and microspheres. The process of brachytherapy differs for LDR (≤2 Gy/hr) versus HDR (>12 Gy/hr) and by body site. The workflow starts with selection of treatment course and prescription depending on clinical scenario. Then seeds must be ordered and assayed, applicators inserted, and patients imaged to ascertain correct positioning. Treatment plans are generated with pretreatment QA and time-out. Then treatment is delivered, sources must be retrieved with post-treatment survey for safety, and all proceedings recorded. Both LDR and HDR require shielded rooms.

With technological advances, it has become standard to use 3D imaging for treatment planning (CT, US, MRI, etc.) instead of plain films. Scan slice thickness must be small enough to detect the entire applicator, and typically 2.5 mm to 3 mm is used. Planning principles are different for interstitial versus intracavitary brachytherapy; whereas interstitial treatment aims for uniform dose across a volume by peripherally loading the sources, intracavitary treatment aims for dose distant to the applicator, with as much distance between the source and tissue as possible to minimize relative hot spots at the surface of the applicator.

Prior to treatment, QA must check for proper connection of catheters and source transfer tubes, correct tube lengths, applicator positioning, patient identity, survey meter function, and treatment documentation. The main goals of the QA process are to ensure patient and public safety, positional and temporal accuracy of treatment, and dose delivery accuracy. Treatment delivery is through remote afterloaders for HDR and some LDR, although most LDR is still performed with manual loading. LDR treatment typically takes days (1 to 3), while HDR treatment times vary by clinical scenario but can be as short as 5 to 15 minutes to over an hour, especially with intraoperative treatments. For dose recording, the prescription point must be specified for the dose to be meaningful (such as prescribing to surface of implant or 5 mm depth). ICRU has guidelines for dose reporting.

A physicist and radiation oncologist must be present during treatment per NRC regulations. Given the high risk nature of brachytherapy treatments, NRC specifies qualifications for physicists performing brachytherapy, including formal training, experience, and accreditations. There are also regulations for source handling, transport, storage, and inventory. Due to the short half-life of HDR sources ([192]Ir is most common), they typically need to be replaced about every 3 months because treatment time increases as source strength decreases.

## References

1. Williamson JF. Brachytherapy technology and physics practice since 1950: A half-century of progress. Phys Med Biol 2006;51:R303–25.
2. Thomadsen BR, Williansom JF, Rivard MJ, et al. Anniversary paper: Past and current issues, and trends in brachytherapy physics. Med Phys 2008;35(10):4708–23.
3. Ibbott G, Ma CM, Rogers DW, et al. Anniversary paper: Fifty years of AAPM involvement in radiation dosimetry. Med Phys 2008;35(4):1418–27.
4. Nath R, Andeerson LL, Meli JA, et al. Code of practice for brachytherapy physics: Report of AAPM Radiation Therapy Committee Task Group No. 56. Med Phys 1997;24(10):1557–98.
5. Chassagne D, Dutreix A, Almond P, et al. Dose and volume specification for reporting intracavitary therapy in gynecology, ICRU Report No. 38. Bethesda, MD: International Commission on Radiation Units and Measurements; 1985.
6. Viswanathan AN, Beriwal S, De Los Santos JF, et al. American Brachytherapy Society consensus guidelines for locally advanced carcinoma of the cervix. Part II: High dose-rate brachytherapy. Brachytherapy 2012;11:47–52.
7. Haie-Meder C, Pötter R, Van Limbergen E, et al. Recommendations from Gynaecological (GYN) GEC-ESTRO Working Group (I); concepts and terms in 3D image based 3D treatment planning in cervix cancer brachytherapy with emphasis on MRI assessment of GTV and CTV. Radiother Oncol 2005;74(3):235–45.

8. Slessinger ED. Practical considerations for prostate HDR brachytherapy. Brachytherapy 2010;9(3): 282–7.
9. Kubo HD, Glasgow GP, Pethel TD, et al. High dose-rate brachytherapy treatment delivery: Report of AAPM Radiation Therapy Committee Task Group No. 59. Med Phys 1998;25(4):375–403.
10. Fonseca GP, Landry G, Reniers B, et al. The contribution from transit dose for $^{192}$Ir HDR brachytherapy treatments. Phys Med Biol 2014;59(7):1831–44.
11. Nath R, Anderson LL, Luxton G, et al. Dosimetry of interstitial brachytherapy sources: Recommendations of the AAPM Radiation Therapy Committee Task Group No. 43. Med Phys 1995;22:209–34.
12. Rivard MJ, Coursey BM, DeWerd LA, et al. Update of AAPM Task Group No. 43 report: A revised AAPM protocol for brachytherapy dose calculations. Med Phys 2004;31(3):633–74.
13. Rivard MJ, Butler WM, DeWerd LA, et al. Supplement to the 2004 update of the AAPM Task Group No. 43 report. Med Phys 2007;34(6):2187–205.
14. Dose and volume specification for reporting interstitial therapy, ICRU Report No. 58. Bethesda, MD: International Commission on Radiation Units and Measurements; 1997.
15. Anderson LL, Nath R, Olch AJ, et al. American Endocurie Society recommendations on dose specification in brachytherapy. Endocuri/Hyperther Oncol 1991;7:1–12.

# CHAPTER 9

# Proton Radiotherapy

## 9.1 Introduction

First proposed by Robert Wilson in 1946, radiation therapy with proton beams quickly became a reality with the first patient treatments performed in 1954 at Lawrence Berkeley National Labs. Starting in 1961 the Harvard Cyclotron Lab began treating patients (and continued up to 2002), and in 1990 the first hospital-based system became operational at Loma Linda University Medical Center, California, which featured the first gantry unit. As of 2014 there are 42 facilities in operation worldwide (14 in the USA), 25 under construction (9 in the USA), and at least 11 in the planning stages, according to statistics from the Particle Therapy Cooperative Group (PTCOG).[1] Further historical background can be found in International Commission on Radiation Units Report 78 (ICRU-78)[2] and a personalized history in Smith.[3]

Though numerous planning studies suggest dosimetric advantages to proton versus photon radiotherapy, support in the form of clinical trials has been lagging. 2007 saw the publication of three large systematic reviews of clinical experience.[4-6] One of these was updated in 2012 and determined that the conclusions had not changed from the original report. Also published in 2012 was a report from the Emerging Technologies Committee of the American Society for Radiation Oncology (ASTRO).[7]

One of the major issues identified in these reports is lack of prospective clinical trials. Randomized controlled trials (RCTs) are an important tool for evaluating health technology, and they address the inherent biases in retrospective studies. There are, however, few RCTs of proton radiotherapy. The review by Olsen et al. identified only four RCTs involving proton radiotherapy.[6] RCTs in proton radiotherapy have included fewer than 700 patients or approximately 1% to 2% of all patients who have received proton radiotherapy.[6] Further studies are under way, an example being Radiation Therapy Oncology Group (RTOG) 1308, which is a phase III trial of photon versus proton chemoradiotherapy in inoperable Stage II-IIIB non-small cell lung cancer with an endpoint of overall survival.

There is a lively debate as to the feasibility and even ethics of randomized trials with proton radiotherapy, given that a better dose distribution often can be achieved with particle beams compared to photons. The ethics of such trials are driven by the need for "clinical equipoise"— that is, a genuine uncertainty as to which method of treatment is superior. Although perhaps not everything need be tested in phase III trials, it has been suggested that more convincing data are needed for proton radiotherapy and that further clinical trials and/or registry data will be crucial.[8]

Based on the balance of evidence, the review studies noted above conclude that proton radiotherapy has a rationale in some situations. The ASTRO emerging technologies report[7] highlights the following disease sites where proton radiotherapy may provide an advantage:

- **Central nervous system (CNS):** Potential sparing of critical structures and reduced overall integral dose to brain tissue are key advantages. Protons have been shown to be effective for meningiomas and skull base tumors such as chordomas and chondrosarcomas.

- **Ocular melanoma:** Local control rates of approximately 95% have been shown and there is particular benefit for large and/or posterior lesions where brachytherapy is more challenging. Special low energy beam lines (≤70 MeV) have been developed for this application.
- **Lung cancer:** Use of proton radiotherapy may reduce dose to normal lung (essentially no dose to the contralateral lung) and also spare the esophagus. It may offer some advantage for stereotactic body radiation therapy (SBRT). Respiratory motion and associated density changes are a particular challenge for proton radiotherapy of lung.
- **Gastrointestinal:** Though largely untested outside of hepatocellular carcinoma, there is a rationale for proton radiotherapy in esophageal and pancreatic cancer for decreasing dose to duodenum, liver, stomach, and kidneys, since these are dose limiting structures.
- **Prostate cancer:** Though this site has the most patients treated with proton radiotherapy, the possible advantages are still not proven in clinical trials. Two of the 4 phase III proton trials mentioned above involved prostate cancer, but they were not designed to directly compare proton and photon radiotherapy so no firm conclusions can be drawn. Proton radiotherapy represents an option for this site though it is not proven superior to photons.[5]
- **Head and neck cancers:** Proton radiotherapy offers potential sparing of critical structures, especially in targets near the base of the skull. It must be noted that air cavities/heterogeneities in the head and neck region make planning challenging.
- **Pediatric cancers:** The reduction of integral dose makes proton therapy very attractive for pediatric patients because this may lower the rate of secondary malignancy and spare the developing tissues. Homogeneous doses can also prevent growth-related malformation (e.g., uneven vertebral growth). In the pediatric population over 50% of solid tumors arise within the CNS.

Given the lack of level I evidence for the use of proton therapy, much attention has been given to its cost-effectiveness. In a widely cited study in 2003, Goitein and Jermann[9] estimated that proton therapy is 2.4 times as expensive per fraction as intensity-modulated radiation therapy (IMRT) using photons, with costs being dominated by business costs associated with facility construction (estimated to be 42% of operations costs versus 28% for a photon facility), though if the recovery of initial costs was not an issue the total cost ratio could drop to 1.6 to 1.3. In the USA, under the reimbursement rates currently dictated by insurance, a relatively limited number of proton facilities may be independently viable, and these may be restricted to major population centers.[10] It must be noted, however, that the technology continues to evolve rapidly and compact single-room devices have now appeared.[11] Costs may come down, which would change the equation.

Finally, in addition to proton beam radiotherapy, therapeutic beams with heavier ions are also in use (helium, carbon, and others). These may provide biological as well as dosimetric advantages due to the higher relative biological effectiveness (RBE) compared to protons and photons. As of this writing there are at least six facilities in operation, the newest being HIT in Heidelberg, Germany (2009), and CNAO in Pavia, Italy (2011). Compared to proton radiotherapy, however, there is less well-established clinical experience with heavy ion therapy.

## FURTHER RESOURCES

There are several textbooks dedicated to particle and proton radiotherapy.[12-14] Another standard reference is ICRU-78 from 2007.[2] ICRU-78 has definitive recommendations on some aspects of proton radiotherapy and provides excellent background. PTCOG operates a website that has useful resources (www.ptcog.ch), and a North America spin-off group has been formed (PTCOG-NA; www.ptcog-na.org). The official journal of PTCOG is the *International Journal of Particle Therapy* (www.theijpt.org), which began publication in 2014.

## 9.2 Physics of Clinical Particle Beams

Unlike electrons, which are roughly 2000 times less massive, protons travel in relatively straight lines as they penetrate through tissue. As they travel they gradually slow down. As a proton slows down it loses energy, slowing down even further. (Recall that the energy loss per unit length, or stopping power, is proportional to $1/v^2$ to first order.) Through this energy-loss process the proton slows down continuously as it penetrates through tissue. When the proton reaches the end of its range it becomes very slow, and the stopping power correspondingly becomes very large. This results in a sharp rise in deposited dose near the end of the proton range, called the "Bragg peak." The energy of the proton determines where this Bragg peak is and how far the proton penetrates, or its range. Distal to this point essentially no dose is delivered. Data tables showing proton ranges and stopping powers for the continuous slowing down approximation can be found on the PSTAR section of the National Institute of Standards and Technology (NIST) website.[15]

A typical "pristine" Bragg peak is shown in Figure 9.1 (colored curves). Because a single pristine Bragg peak is typically not large enough in extent to irradiate an entire target volume, clinical systems create a spread-out Bragg peak (SOBP) by essentially adding many pristine Bragg peaks together. This principle is illustrated in Figure 9.1. The highest energy proton beam used determines the distal-most extent of the SOBP (red) while lower energy beams penetrate less deeply (e.g., violet). The end result of adding these beams together, each with the appropriate weight, is the SOBP (black). The SOBP irradiates a large "plateau" region to a uniform dose. From this figure the main advantage of proton beams is clear: that is, essentially no dose is deposited distal to the end of the SOBP. This results in greater normal tissue sparing in the intermediate to low dose range.

In actual practice the creation of an SOBP is achieved with a rotating stepped wheel or a filter with ridges (see the following description). The wheel acts to produce many pristine Bragg peaks with varying ranges. By selecting the appropriate maximum beam energy and modulation wheels one can control the shape of the SOBP as illustrated in Figure 9.2. One disadvantage to note, however, is that skin sparing may be almost completely absent in a proton beam. The magnitude of skin dose depends on the modulation and other factors but the effect can be appreciated in Figure 9.2. In some shallow target sites such as sacral chordoma, the skin dose is so high (close to 100%) that a combined proton plus photon plan is sometimes used.[2]

The nomenclature of proton beam parameters is an important consideration, and a valuable reference is ICRU-78 Section 3.4.[2] One key parameter is the range of the beam. The d90% depth is commonly used, though ICRU-78 advocates the use of d100%. Another parameter is the amount of ripple in the flat plateau portion of the SOBP and also potential bumps or dips on the leading or distal edge of the SOBP.

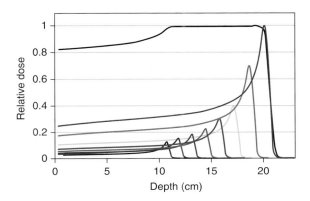

**Figure 9.1** Depth dose curves for proton radiotherapy beams. The pristine Bragg peaks (colored curves) are added together to form a spread-out Bragg peak (SOBP, black). The pristine Bragg peak beams with protons of gradually decreasing energy (red-to-violet) and therefore decreasing range in tissue.

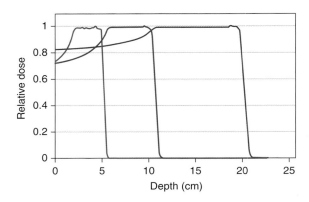

**Figure 9.2** Three representative SOBP curves with different ranges (R in cm) and modulation factors (M in cm). Red: R20M10, green: R10M5, blue: R5M3.

Beams of heavier ions such as carbon display many of the same characteristics as proton beams outlined above. They exhibit a Bragg peak that is even more enhanced than a proton beam, but they also deliver a small dose beyond the Bragg peak due to nuclear spallation products along the beam path. One important difference is the higher linear energy transfer (LET) throughout the entire depth that results in potentially more biological damage. Heavier ion beams also display a sharper penumbra due to less scatter (for a study of this see Kempe et al.[16]).

## 9.3 Proton Beam Clinical Delivery Technologies

### ACCELERATOR SYSTEMS

Most clinical systems produce a maximum beam energy of approximately 250 MeV which, after passing through the various beam devices, is degraded down to approximately 215 MeV. This corresponds to a range of approximately 30 cm in tissue, which provides for treatment of the most deep-seated tumors. An average extracted beam current of approximately 5 nA to 10 nA is required for a dose rate of 2 Gy/min to a 1 L (1000 cm$^3$) target volume, though approximately 50 times as much is possible with some accelerator designs.

To achieve these requirements proton therapy accelerators currently come in two designs: 1) a cyclotron, in which protons are accelerated in a plane between two poles of a magnet, and 2) a synchrotron, in which proton bunches are guided around a ring via magnetic bending and focusing, gaining energy on each pass through an acceleration cavity. Some differences between these two technologies are outlined in Table 9.1. Facilities generally have one accelerator but multiple treatment rooms, so only one treatment room can have beam at any time. The classic

TABLE 9.1 ▓ **Summary of Some Key Differences Between Cyclotron- and Synchrotron-Based Proton Therapy Systems**

| Cyclotron | Synchrotron |
|---|---|
| Continuous wave | Pulsed bunches. Lower current (due to space-charge effects) |
| Smaller size (e.g., ≈4 m diameter ring) | Larger size (e.g., ≈7 m diameter ring) |
| Single energy produced. Energy selection via physical modulator and energy slit selection | Discrete energies produced by accelerator (via timing of extraction from the acceleration ring) |
| Slow energy change (physical modulator change) | Fast energy change. Minimizes range modulation required |

cyclotron design that one might remember from freshman physics (i.e., the proton tracing out a spiral path of ever increasing radius as its energy increases) does not work above about 15 MeV because of the relativistic mass increase of the proton at high energies. Medical cyclotrons operating at up to 250 MeV therefore commonly use an "isosynchronous" cyclotron design in which the magnetic field increases with radius to compensate for relativistic mass increase. Alternatively, the magnetic field can be kept constant and the RF frequency changed to achieve the same effect. This so-called synchrocyclotron was the design used at the Harvard Cyclotron Lab. This design fell out of favor in the intervening decades because of the large size required with conventional magnets but is now being revived in new compact systems that employ superconducting magnets. A technology review can be found in Alonso and Antaya.[17]

## PASSIVE SCATTERING SYSTEMS

Clinical proton therapy beam delivery systems come in two general types: passive scattering systems and dynamic beam delivery systems (or "spot scanning"). The main components of a passive system are shown in Figure 9.3. Scatterers are used upstream to create a dose that is uniform over a large (e.g., 40 × 40 cm field). The two-scatterer design uses the beam particles more efficiently than a single scatterer would (a single scatterer would have to be made very thick and spread the beam into a very wide quasi-gaussian in order to achieve a uniform dose distribution over the beam). The range shifter is selected to provide protons with a range that corresponds to the most distal depth of the planning target volume (PTV). The range modulator (a stepped propeller wheel that rotates or a ridge filter) creates the SOBP. The amount of modulation needed can be selected by using the appropriate modulator. The patient-specific aperture (often brass) collimates the beam to the shape of the PTV in the beam's-eye view (Figure 9.4, left). Finally, a patient-specific compensator (wax or acrylic) makes the dose distribution conform to the PTV at its distal edge (Figure 9.4, right). The compensator can also be designed to accommodate inhomogeneities in the patient. If a bone is in the beam path, for example, the range compensator would be made thinner to ensure the high dose region extends to the distal edge of the PTV that lies in the shadow of the bone.

Passive scatter systems are by far the more prevalent technology to date. Several issues are worth noting:

- Although the dose distribution conforms to the distal edge of the PTV, it cannot be made to conform to the proximal edge. In the optic nerve sheath meningioma case shown in Figure 9.2, the high dose region is observed to extend back into the temporal lobe.

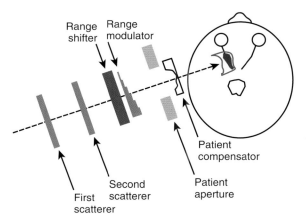

**Figure 9.3** Beamline components for proton beam delivery in a passive scattering system. A compensator shapes the beam so the dose distribution (blue) conforms at the distal edge of the PTV (red).

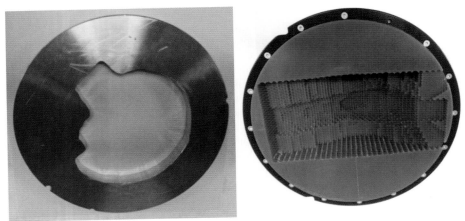

**Figure 9.4** Beamline components, brass aperture (left) and wax patient compensator (right).

- The penumbra of these systems is relatively larger due to the large effective source size with a double scatterer. Penumbra depends sensitively on the depth and the particular beam parameters (e.g., air gaps used) but is typically not smaller for a proton beam than for a photon beam. For studies of this see Oozeer et al. and Rana et al.[18,19]
- If the compensator is constructed to account for heterogeneities in the field (e.g., air pocket or bone), then the alignment of these heterogeneities with respect to the compensator is crucial, and scattering effects also come into play. Algorithms have been developed to design compensator shapes that are less sensitive to the exact alignment and scattering.[20]
- There is an additional dose to the patient from neutrons (with quality factors of 5 to 20 depending on energy). These neutrons are created largely in the devices in the pathway of the beam and contribute an exposure to the whole body. It has been argued that this represents an increased risk for secondary malignancies, particularly for pediatric patients,[21] though these initial estimates were based on a theoretical consideration of the neutron contamination in the beam. Neutron contamination has been measured and simulated in a proton beam and found to depend sensitively on the irradiation technique, with orders of magnitude variation among various studies.[22] Most of the contribution comes from the treatment head and increases with decreasing aperture size.

## DYNAMIC BEAM DELIVERY SYSTEMS

In this method a small spot is magnetically scanned across the target to form a layer. The spot is approximately 10 mm full width half maximum (FWHM), though this is energy- and depth-dependent. Scanning is performed either continuously (a method introduced in the 1960s) or in spot scanning voxel-by-voxel.[23] Scanning is usually performed with no compensator. Once the deepest layer in the PTV is painted, the beam energy is reduced (which requires approximately 1 sec depending on the accelerator system) and then the next layer is scanned. This proceeds until the entire PTV is irradiated. With this technique the dose can be made to conform to both the distal and the proximal aspects of the PTV. The technique also provides for the possibility of intensity-modulated proton therapy (IMPT) in which the intensity of each voxel is controlled independently. The contribution of neutron dose is also reduced because there are fewer components in the beam path.[22] One potential pitfall of dynamic delivery is that it is more sensitive to organ motion than passive systems. In the context of lung tumors, for example, there is an "interplay" effect in which the dose to a given part of the tumor will depend on its location when the particular spot was irradiated. One way to manage this problem is to "repaint" the dose, delivering the beam in multiple scans of the target.

## COMMISSIONING AND QA

Reports for commissioning of proton radiotherapy are under development: AAPM TG-185, Clinical Commissioning of Proton Therapy Systems, and AAPM TG-224, Proton Machine Quality Assurance. In the meantime a relevant benchmark is AAPM TG-53 on therapy planning systems.[24] Chapter 9 of ICRU-78[2] briefly describes QA of a proton beam radiotherapy and lists tables of QA tests and frequencies that are roughly consistent with other reports such as AAPM TG-142, Quality Assurance of Medical Accelerators.

## IMAGE GUIDANCE

X-ray imaging systems have been used in proton treatment rooms from the very earliest systems. This is by necessity since, unlike photon therapy, the proton beam itself typically does not penetrate the patient and an image cannot be formed. Early systems used orthogonal kV sources with films, and modern installations have continued this with use of flat-panel detectors (e.g., MD Anderson Cancer Center and University of Florida Proton Therapy Institute, among others). Because of the accuracy requirements, the patient is often imaged prior to each field. Though the use of in-room imaging systems was pioneered in proton facilities, most centers do not have in-room volumetric computed tomography (CT) imaging, which is now common for photon therapy (cf. Chapter 7), though there are exceptions such as the compact system from Mevion Inc.[11] and the Heidelberg Heavy Ion Facility.[25] A brief overview of in-room imaging systems in proton therapy can be found in AAPM TG-104, The Role of In-Room kV X-Ray Imaging for Patient Setup and Target Localization.[26]

Developments are under way for alternative imaging technologies specific to proton and particle beams. These include the following: positron emission tomography (PET) to image the positron-emitting isotopes activated by the proton beam (typically $^{11}C$ and $^{15}O$),[27] "prompt gamma cameras" in the room to image photons emitted by the beam,[28] and finally proton CT, which uses a high energy beam that penetrates all the way through the patient to form CT images.

# 9.4 Proton Dose Calibration and Dose Reporting

As with photon beams, dose calibration protocols in proton beams are based on dose to water using a calibrated ion chamber under standard conditions (e.g., Farmer chamber in the center of a range 16 cm/modulation 10 cm SOBP). The International Atomic Energy Agency (IAEA) TRS-398 protocol is typically used for proton beams. A full description is found in Chapter 1 on reference dosimetry.

Doses in proton radiotherapy are most often reported as equivalent dose: the dose required to achieve the same biological effect as a standard reference beam (typically $^{60}Co$). The RBE of a proton beam is somewhat enhanced over a photon beam due to the differing dynamic of dose deposition related to slightly higher LET. A full review of RBE in proton beams can be found in Paganetti[29] and Skarsgard[30] and ICRU-78 Chapter 22 and will be the subject of the upcoming AAPM TG-256, Proton Relative Biological Effectiveness (RBE). RBE is also known to vary somewhat along the Bragg peak, particularly at the distal end where LET is high. For simplicity, however, ICRU-78 advocates that an overall RBE factor of 1.1 be applied (ICRU-78 Section 2.5.1). This factor is grossly consistent with in-vitro and in-vivo laboratory data and applies to both early- and late-responding tissue. ICRU-78 advocates that this equivalent dose be reported as $D_{RBE}$, RBE-weighted proton absorbed dose, using the notation "Gy (RBE)." This is meant to replace older definitions and symbols such as cobalt-gray equivalent (CGE), GyE, or Gy(E).

As advocated by ICRU-78, a prescription might read "70 Gy (RBE)"; it would be derived by multiplying the absorbed dose (in Gy) by a factor of 1.1. For heavier ion beams such as carbon, the RBE is greatly enhanced over that of a proton or photon beam due to the higher LET. Because the magnitude of the effect depends on the depth along the beam, treatment planning systems for particle therapy must explicitly include the biological effects in calculations.

## 9.5 Proton Treatment Planning

Though treatment planning for proton radiotherapy shares many similarities with photon radiotherapy, there are some important differences. There are also differences in planning between spot scanning beams versus passive scatter or uniform scanning beams. This section focuses on the latter, though many principles apply equally.

Generally, fewer beams are used for proton plans. Normal tissue sparing is possible even with a single beam. There is also less need to have wide angular spacing between beams. The design of the compensator is important. It is typically kept close to the patient to keep the penumbra small (but too close may increase the low energy scattered proton contaminants and the chance of collision).

Figure 9.5 shows example plans for treating a brain ependymoma in a pediatric patient (from MacDonald et al.[31]). In this case two beams were used for the proton plans. The dose to normal tissue was greatly reduced (e.g., mean dose to cochlea: 2 Gy (RBE) versus 37 Gy and temporal lobes: 4 Gy (RBE) versus 16 Gy). The plan using IMPT is more conformal than that with passive scattering. This illustrates an important point: the conformality of dose to the target can be worse for a proton plan versus a photon plan, particularly if passive scattering is used.

Heterogeneities are also very important to proton planning, and CT-based planning is essentially required. Proton 2D planning is very uncommon. Due to scattering and other effects, heterogeneities are also much more complex in proton beams. Many commercial dose calculation methods do not account for these effects and Monte Carlo is required. In practice, heterogeneous regions of the patient are avoided to the extent possible when planning.

The concept of a PTV is more complex than it is in photon planning. A simple CTV-to-PTV expansion in all directions does not adequately account for the properties of proton beams. This is because the CTV-to-PTV margin required along the beam direction (for effects like range uncertainty) is different from the margins required in the lateral direction (for setup and beam penumbra). In principle, then, a different PTV is required for each beam direction. Even though

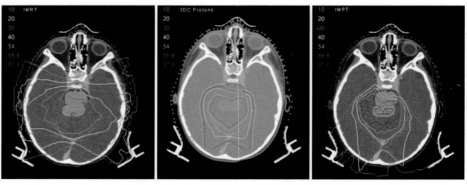

**Figure 9.5** Comparative plans for a pediatric patient with ependymoma with IMRT (left), a passive scatter proton (center), and IMPT (right). *(From MacDonald SM, Safai S, Trofimov A, et al. Proton radiotherapy for childhood ependymoma: initial clinical outcomes and dose comparisons. Int J Radiat Oncol Biol Phys 2008;71:979-986.)*

the concept of a single CTV-to-PTV expansion no longer applies, ICRU-78 advocates that a PTV still be defined for proton plans for the purposes of dose reporting.[2]

Deriving the appropriate PTV margins is a complex process in proton radiotherapy. A commonly used formula follows that of Moyers et al.:[32]

$$\text{Distal margin} = 0.035 \times d_{CTV-distal} + 3 \text{ mm}$$

where $d_{CTV-distal}$ is the depth of the distal edge of the CTV. The 3.5% accounts for uncertainties in relative linear stopping power and heterogeneities and the extra 3 mm is added to account for uncertainty in accelerator energy and thicknesses of beam modifying devices and other uncertainties. For a discussion of PTV especially in the context of IMPT see Lomax.[33,34]

Given these uncertainties, it is best practice to avoid beams that are oriented directly toward an organ at risk that lies close to a PTV (e.g., an AP beam directed toward the prostate). This is especially true since the RBE is known to rise by 5% to 10% at the distal-most end of the SOBP.[2] Some centers stipulate that no more than one third of the dose should be directed through such beams.[2]

Another potential pitfall is beam directions that are tangential to the patient's skin. These are hazardous because the resulting compensator will have relatively steep edges and small shifts in alignment or anatomy can result in large changes in dose distribution.

## FOR THE PHYSICIAN

Proton therapy has distinct dosimetric advantages over photon radiation, although randomized clinical trial data are lacking. There is a rationale for proton radiotherapy in a variety of disease sites as outlined in several recent reviews.[4,7,35] This is driven by the better normal tissue sparing and lower integral dose compared to therapy with photons. The advantages of proton therapy are a result of the fundamental physics of heavy charged particle interactions (i.e., the phenomenon of a Bragg peak beyond which essentially no dose is delivered). The depth of the Bragg peak is determined by the energy of the proton beam (215 MeV penetrates approximately 30 cm). Though this effect offers a dosimetric advantage over photon beams, other aspects of proton beams are not necessarily superior to photon beams: the penumbra is roughly the same, the skin sparing can be worse, and, depending on how the beams are delivered, the target conformality can also be inferior. Biologically, proton beams are not thought to be substantially more effective than photon beams. An overall RBE of 1.1 is used, though this is higher near the distal end of the Bragg peak. The overall RBE factor of 1.1 is typically used to report prescription as dose equivalent (i.e., Gy (RBE), as advocated by ICRU-78). Image guidance with proton therapy is also potentially inferior to photon therapy, since most proton therapy facilities use planar kV x-ray radiographs, whereas CT guidance is increasingly common in photon therapy.

The technology for delivering clinical proton beams is complex. One of two accelerator designs is used: a cyclotron or a synchrotron. Bending magnets are used to steer the beam from the accelerator into the treatment room. One of the largest and highest cost items in a proton facility is the gantry; some treatment rooms use fixed beams with no gantry. Because of magnet weight and design requirements, gantries can be 10 m in diameter and weigh over 200 tons. Newer designs are emerging, however, and one unit has become available (Mevion S250) that uses a 10 T superconducting magnet to put a compact gantry-mounted proton accelerator in a single (10 × 10 × 10 m) room.

The high energy proton beam must be modified for each patient treatment. One method for doing this is "passive scattering" in which range modulators and compensators are used to control the energy and depth of the beam and thereby make it conform to the distal edge of the target. An SOBP is generated by superimposing multiple Bragg peaks at different depths. The other delivery method is spot scanning, a "paint-by-numbers" technique in which the target is irradiated voxel-by-voxel. This method is becoming more common and allows for IMPT, which provides improved dose conformality.

Clinical proton beams are subject to an inherent uncertainty in the range of penetration. This is due to uncertainty in the conversion of CT number to linear stopping power, uncertainty in beam energy, and other effects. This complicates the process of treatment planning because the margin required along the beam direction is different from the margins required in the lateral direction (for beam penumbra). This muddles the concept of a PTV, since, in principle, a different PTV is required for each beam direction. Nevertheless, ICRU-78 advocates that a PTV still be defined for the purposes of dose reporting. Proton therapy is also more sensitive to tissue heterogeneity than photon therapy, and small shifts in areas of changing tissue density can have large impacts on dose. These uncertainties must all be accounted for as part of treatment planning and QA.

## References

1. Particle Therapy Co-Operative Group (PTCOG); 2014.
2. ICRU. ICRU Report 78. Prescribing, recording and reporting proton-beam therapy. In: Agency ICoRUaMIAE, editor. vol. 7. Oxford, UK; 2007. p. 210.
3. Smith AR. Proton therapy. Phys Med Biol 2006;51:R491–504.
4. Brada M, Pijls-Johannesma M, De Ruysscher D. Proton therapy in clinical practice: Current clinical evidence. J Clin Oncol 2007;25:965–70.
5. Lodge M, Pijls-Johannesma M, Stirk L, et al. A systematic literature review of the clinical and cost-effectiveness of hadron therapy in cancer. Radiother Oncol 2007;83:110–22.
6. Olsen DR, Bruland OS, Frykholm G, et al. Proton therapy: A systematic review of clinical effectiveness. Radiother Oncol 2007;83:123–32.
7. Allen AM, Pawlicki T, Dong L, et al. An evidence based review of proton beam therapy: The report of ASTRO's Emerging Technology Committee. Radiother Oncol 2012;103:8–11.
8. Tepper JE. Protons and parachutes. J Clin Oncol 2008;26:2436–7.
9. Goitein M, Jermann M. The relative costs of proton and x-ray radiation therapy. Clin Oncol 2003;15:S37–50.
10. Kerstiens J, Johnstone PAS. Proton therapy expansion under current United States reimbursement models. Int J Radiation Oncol Biol Phys 2014;89:235–40.
11. Bloch C, Hill PM, Chen KL, et al. Startup of the Kling Center for proton therapy, vol. 1525. AIP Conference Proceedings; 2013. p. 314–218.
12. DeLaney TF, Kooy H. Proton and charged particle radiotherapy. Philadelphia, PA: Lippincott Williams & Wilkins; 2007.
13. Paganetti H. Proton therapy physics. Boca Raton, FL: CRC Press/Taylor & Francis; 2012.
14. Linz U. Ion beam therapy: Fundamentals, technology, clinical applications. Berlin: Springer-Verlag; 2012.
15. NIST. Stopping Power and Range Tables for Protons (PSTAR). National Institute of Standards and Technology (NIST); 2014.
16. Kempe J, Gudowska I, Brahme A. Depth absorbed dose and LET distributions of therapeutic H-1, He-4, Li-7, and C-12 beams. Med Phys 2007;34:183–92.
17. Alonso JR, Antaya TA. Superconductivity in medicine. Rev Accel Sci Tech 2012;5:227–63.
18. Oozeer R, Mazal A, Rosenwald JC, et al. A model for the lateral penumbra in water of a 200-MeV proton beam devoted to clinical applications. Med Phys 1997;24:1599–604.
19. Rana S, Zeidan O, Ramirez E, et al. Measurements of lateral penumbra for uniform scanning proton beams under various beam delivery conditions and comparison to the XiO treatment planning system. Med Phys 2013;40(9):091708.
20. Urie M, Goitein M, Wagner M. Compensating for heterogeneities in proton radiation-therapy. Phys Med Biol 1984;29:553–66.
21. Hall EJ. Intensity-modulated radiation therapy, protons, and the risk of second cancers. Int J Radiation Oncol Biol Phys 2006;65:1–7.
22. Xu XG, Bednarz B, Paganetti H. A review of dosimetry studies on external-beam radiation treatment with respect to second cancer induction. Phys Med Biol 2008;53:R193–241.
23. Lomax AJ, Bohringer T, Bolsi A, et al. Treatment planning and verification of proton therapy using spot scanning: Initial experiences. Med Phys 2004;31:3150–7.

24. Fraass B, Doppke K, Hunt M, et al. American Association of Physicists in Medicine Radiation Therapy Committee Task Group 53: Quality assurance for clinical radiotherapy treatment planning. Med Phys 1998;25:1773–829.

25. Haberer T, Debus J, Eickhoff H, et al. The Heidelberg Ion Therapy Center. Radiother Oncol 2004;73(Suppl. 2):S186–90.

26. Yin F, Wong J. The role of in-room kv x-ray imaging for patient setup and target localization: Report of Task Group 104. College Park, MD: AAPM; 2009.

27. Grogg K, Alpert NM, Zhu X, et al. Mapping $^{15}$O Production Rate for Proton Therapy Verification. Int J Radiat Oncol Biol Phys 2015. pii: S0360-3016(15)00070-X. doi:10.1016/j.ijrobp.2015.01.023; [Epub ahead of print].

28. Perali I, Celani A, Bombelli L, et al. Prompt gamma imaging of proton pencil beams at clinical dose rate. Phys Med Biol 2014;59(19):5849–71. doi:10.1088/0031-9155/59/19/5849; [Epub 2014 Sep 10].

29. Paganetti H. Significance and implementation of RBE variations in proton beam therapy. Technol Cancer Res Treatment 2003;2:413–26.

30. Skarsgard LD. Radiobiology with heavy charged particles: A historical review (vol. 14, p. 1, 1998). Phys Med 1998;14:179–80.

31. MacDonald SM, Safai S, Trofimov A, et al. Proton radiotherapy for childhood ependymoma: Initial clinical outcomes and dose comparisons. Int J Radiat Oncol Biol Phys 2008;71:979–86.

32. Moyers MF, Miller DW, Bush DA, et al. Methodologies and tools for proton beam design for lung tumors. Int J Radiat Oncol Biol Phys 2001;49:1429–38.

33. Lomax AJ. Intensity modulated proton therapy and its sensitivity to treatment uncertainties 1: The potential effects of calculational uncertainties. Phys Med Biol 2008;53:1027–42.

34. Lomax AJ. Intensity modulated proton therapy and its sensitivity to treatment uncertainties 2: The potential effects of inter-fraction and inter-field motions. Phys Med Biol 2008;53:1043–56.

35. De Ruysscher D, Lodge MM, Jones B, et al. Charged particles in radiotherapy: A 5-year update of a systematic review. Radiother Oncol 2012;103:5–7.

# CHAPTER 10

# Radiation Safety and Shielding in Radiotherapy

## 10.1 Introduction

The National Council on Radiation Protection (NCRP) Report No. 116, Limitation of Exposure to Ionizing Radiation, outlines the goals and philosophies of radiation protection in Chapter 2 of that document.[1] The specific objectives are:

1. "To prevent the occurrence of clinically significant radiation-induced deterministic effects by adhering to dose limits that are below the apparent threshold levels and
2. "To limit the risk of stochastic effects, cancer, and genetic effects, to a reasonable level in relation to societal needs, values, benefits gained, and economic factors."

The goal is not to reduce exposures to zero or near zero levels but rather to reduce levels to ALARA (as low as (is) reasonably achievable) (as defined in Title 10, Section 20.1003, of the U.S. Nuclear Regulatory Commission (NRC) Code of Federal Regulations (10 CFR 20.1003)). The concept of ALARA clearly includes using a risk/benefit approach incorporating societal needs and economic factors to reduce exposures to a reasonable level. The money spent on excessive shielding could be better used to provide direct care to patients with known conditions that can be treated. The risks of radiation exposure largely involve the possibility of an injury that can be immediate or delayed for months or years. It is more beneficial to improve the care for patients with a known condition than to further reduce the possibility of radiation injury to the patient or to others as long as the risk is acceptably low. For example, spending an extra $200,000 on shielding will take away capital that could have been spent on upgrading the treatment planning system (TPS) to a more accurate dose calculation algorithm that would immediately benefit patients.

To develop the exposure limits that are used to keep the risks at a reasonable level, several international agencies regularly review the available data on radiation risk. Among them are the United Nations Scientific Committee on the Effects of Atomic Radiation (UNSCEAR), the International Commission on Radiation Protection (ICRP), and the National Academy of Sciences/National Research Council Committee on the Biological Effects of Ionizing Radiation (BEIR), the most recent report being BEIR VII.[2] UNSCEAR and BEIR develop risk estimates which the ICRP uses to establish recommended dose limits. The NCRP determines how those recommendations will be implemented in the United States.

The dose limits for radiation workers is higher than those for a member of the general public. This is based on the fact that they have received special training in radiation protection, are aware of the associated radiation risks, and have decided to accept them. To determine compliance with the dose limits a facility must either assign a dose monitor to the staff member or perform calculations that show that the worker will not exceed 10% of the annual limit. There are some exceptions to this; staff who work in high risk areas such as interventional radiology, nuclear medicine, and Radiation Oncology should be monitored regardless of their expected annual dose level. This is because of the potential for unexpected incidents, particularly with regard to brachytherapy in Radiation Oncology. To ensure the continued safe use of radiation in medicine, staff should receive periodic radiation safety training.[3] This training should include basic radiation safety principles, details specific to their job function, and communication of risk estimates.

To determine compliance with dose limits for the general public, shielding calculations and surveys are done to show that individuals in the areas surrounding the radiation source will not exceed the regulatory limits. The calculations must be confirmed by performing a survey of dose levels surrounding the radiation source after installation using an appropriate instrument. These calculations should be reviewed on a regular basis to confirm that the assumptions made during the design process are still valid.

## 10.2 Risk Levels and Radiation

The BEIR VII report is a standard reference for understanding the risks of radiation exposure. At very high doses the risks are deterministic in nature with the following endpoints and D50 levels (the dose at which 50% of exposed individuals would be expected to reach a particular endpoint, such as death): central nervous system (CNS) death (>20 Sv), gastrointestinal (GI) death (>10 Sv), and bone-marrow death (>5 Sv). At lower doses stochastic effects occur, the main concern being excess cancer risk with the main types being lung, liver, breast, prostate, stomach, colon, thyroid, and leukemia. BEIR VII quotes the excess number of cases per 100 mSv as being 800 per 100,000 people for men and 1300 per 100,000 people for women. There is a threefold higher risk for small children, with females having a twice higher risk as males. A feature of the BEIR VII report is that it distinguishes between incidence rates (the above numbers) versus mortality, which are, of course, not the same thing. BEIR VII notes that the former is approximately twice the latter. In looking at models of stochastic risk there is active debate as to whether there is a threshold of dose below which there is no risk. The BEIR VII report suggests that there is no evidence for a lower threshold and, as such, used the linear no-threshold (LNT) model for radiation risk.

## 10.3 Units

The estimation of risk for a given organ is determined by the biological sensitivity to radiation of that organ and the type of radiation. To account for the different density of ionization caused by each type of radiation, a weighting factor is used to modify the physical dose. This **equivalent dose (H)** is defined as:

$$H = W_R \times D$$

where $W_R$ is the radiation weighting factor and D is the physical dose in Gy. The radiation weighting factor, $W_R$, is defined and used by the ICRP, but an older terminology and calculation method was the quality (or "Q") factor, a term that is still used by the U.S. NRC. Weighting factors are shown in Table 10.1.

The SI unit for H is the Sievert (Sv), and an older non-SI unit is the roentgen equivalent man (rem), which is 0.01 Sv. Internationally there is some slight disagreement in the accepted values for the weighting factors as shown in Table 10.1. The values for neutrons and protons have changed over time to reflect new risk estimates.

Another weighting factor is used to account for the radiation sensitivity of each organ. These factors have also changed over time. Current values are shown in Table 10.2. **Effective dose (E)** is defined as:

$$E = \Sigma_T \left( W_T \times H_T \right)$$

where $W_T$ is the weighting factor and $H_T$ the equivalent dose for organ T. Units of E are also Sv. Also by definition, $\Sigma_T W_T = 1$.

TABLE 10.1 ■ Radiation Weighting Factors

| Radiation Type | W$_R$ from NCRP-116 | W$_R$ from ICRP-103 (4) | U.S. NRC (10 CFR 21.0004, Uses Terminology of Quality Factor) |
|---|---|---|---|
| Photons, electrons | 1 | 1 | 1 |
| Neutrons | 5-20, energy dependent (peak value of 20 at approximately 1 MeV) | Energy dependent, 2.5-5 | Energy dependent, 2-11 (peak value at approximately 1 MeV) |
| Protons | 2 | 2 | Not listed |
| Alpha | 20 | 20 | 20 |

TABLE 10.2 ■ Organ Weighting Factors

| Organ | W$_T$ from NCRP-116 | W$_T$ from ICRP-103 |
|---|---|---|
| Gonads | 0.2 | 0.08 |
| Red bone marrow | 0.12 | 0.12 |
| Colon | 0.12 | 0.12 |
| Lung | 0.12 | 0.12 |
| Stomach | 0.12 | 0.12 |
| Bladder | 0.05 | 0.04 |
| Breast | 0.05 | 0.12 |
| Liver | 0.05 | 0.04 |
| Esophagus | 0.05 | 0.04 |
| Thyroid | 0.05 | 0.04 |
| Skin | 0.01 | 0.01 |
| Brain | Included in remaining organs | 0.01 |
| Salivary glands | Not specifically included | 0.01 |
| Bone surfaces | 0.01 | 0.01 |
| Remaining organs | 0.05* | 0.12** |

*Adrenals, brain, upper large intestine, small intestine, kidney, muscle pancreas, spleen, thymus, uterus
**Adrenals, airways, gallbladder, heart wall, kidneys, lymphatic nodes, muscle, oral mucosa, pancreas, prostate, small intestine, spleen, thymus, uterus/cervix

Some authors have suggested that the concept of effective dose is flawed in that it is based on highly subjective judgments, does not reflect age and gender dependencies, and can be confusing and hard to interpret.[5,6]

# 10.4 Regulatory Limits

NCRP Report No. 116 from 1993 lists the effective dose limits for radiation workers and the general public. NCRP-116 supersedes the earlier NCRP Report No. 91 from 1987. NCRP-116 dose limits are summarized in Table 10.3.

The NCRP initially recommended that the annual effective dose limit for the general public should be 0.25 mSv, but a clarification in 2004 stated that the 1.0 mSv per year was justified because of the conservative estimates built into the shielding design methodology (NCRP Statement 10).[7] The NCRP-116 report calls for remedial action for public exposure to natural sources above 5 mSv and states that there is negligible risk below 0.01 mSv.

TABLE 10.3  ▦  **Allowable Dose Limits per NCRP Report No. 116**

|  | **Basis** | **Annual Limit** |
| --- | --- | --- |
| **Occupational Limits** | Stochastic effects | 50 mSv (5 rem) and cumulative limit of 10 mSv × age |
|  | Deterministic effects | Lens: 150 mSv (15 rem) |
|  |  | Skin, hands, and feet: 500 mSv (50 rem) |
| **Public Dose Limits** | Stochastic effects | Continuous exposure: 1 mSv (0.1 rem) |
|  |  | Infrequent exposure: 5 mSv (0.5 rem) |
|  | Deterministic effects | Lens and extremities: 50 mSv (5 rem) |
|  | Embryo-fetus | 0.5 mSv (0.05 rem) equivalent dose limit in a month once pregnancy is known |

To put these limits in context, the natural background radiation is approximately 3.1 mSv/year, which is 3 times higher than the public dose limit. The amount of natural background can vary significantly depending on factors such as altitude and radon gas concentrations. In addition, the average person in the United States is exposed to approximately 3 mSv/year in medical uses of radiation. The majority of that exposure comes from computed tomography (CT), although there is also a contribution from procedures performed in nuclear medicine and interventional radiology.[8]

## 10.5 Release of Patients with Radioactive Materials

In addition to shielding design limits, there are limits to the exposure levels at which a patient who has been injected or implanted with radioactive material may be released. The U.S. NRC NUREG-1556 documents three methods by which patient release criteria may be calculated.[9] If the activity administered is less than the activity listed in column 1 of Table U1 or the measured dose rate at 1 m is less than the value listed in column 2 of Table U1 in NUREG-1556, then the patient may be released. Table 10.4 lists the values from NUREG Table U1 for some common radionuclides used in Radiation Oncology. The levels listed in Table U1 are not intended to apply to infants or children who are being breast fed by the patient. In this case it is necessary to give special instructions to the patient. These instructions must specify the discontinuation or interruption of breastfeeding and the consequences for failing to do so if the levels exceed those listed in Table U3. Selected data from Table U3 are shown in Table 10.5. These apply to injected radionuclides used in nuclear medicine and are not relevant in Radiation Oncology. The third method is to perform patient-specific calculations to ensure that no individual will receive more than 5 mSv (0.5 rem). Factors such as the effective half-life, retained activity, occupancy factors <0.25, or shielding by tissue may be used in the calculation. A record of the calculation must be retained. In addition, it is good practice to give patients documentation of the administered activity so that they can address any questions that may arise, such as in the event that a portal radiation alarm in a public place is set off. A wallet card is a convenient way to do this.

Instructions on how to maintain acceptable dose limits for other individuals must be given to the patient if the activities or dose rate at 1 m exceeds the levels in Table U2 of NUREG-1556. They are on the order of 20% of the values listed in Table U1 and are shown in Table 10.6. Sample instructions are shown in sections U.2.3.1 and U.2.3.2 of NUREG-1556.

## 10.6 Personnel Monitoring

NCRP Report No. 102, Medical X-Ray, Electron Beam and Gamma-Ray Protection, states that "personnel monitoring is a valuable means of checking the adequacy of a radiation protection program. Its use can disclose inadequate or improper radiation protection practices and

TABLE 10.4 ▦ Release Criteria for Common Radionuclides from NUREG Table U1

| Radionuclide | Column 1 Activity Limit (Gbq) | Column 1 Activity Limit (mCi) | Column 2 Dose Rate Limit (mSv/hr) | Column 2 Dose Rate Limit (mrem/hr) |
|---|---|---|---|---|
| $^{125}$I implant | 0.33 | 9 | 0.01 | 1 |
| $^{192}$Ir implant | 0.074 | 2 | 0.008 | 0.8 |
| $^{103}$Pd implant | 1.5 | 40 | 0.03 | 3 |

TABLE 10.5 ▦ Activities of Radiopharmaceuticals That Require Instructions and Records When Administered to Patients Who Are Breastfeeding from NUREG Table U3

| Radionuclide | Activity Above Which Instructions Are Required (mBq) | Activity Above Which Instructions Are Required (mCi) | Activity Above Which a Record Is Required (mBq) | Activity Above Which a Record Is Required (mCi) | Examples of Recommended Duration of Interruption of Breastfeeding |
|---|---|---|---|---|---|
| $^{131}$I Sodium iodide | 0.01 | 0.0004 | 0.07 | 0.002 | Complete cessation (for this infant or child) |
| $^{99m}$Tc sulfur colloid | 300 | 7 | 1000 | 35 | 6 hours for 440 mBq (12 mCi) |

TABLE 10.6 ▦ Activity and Dose Rate Levels for Determination of Patient Instruction Requirement from NUREG Table U2

| Radionuclide | Column 1 Activity Limit (Bq) | Column 1 Activity Limit (mCi) | Column 2 Dose Rate Limit (mSv/hr) | Column 2 Dose Rate Limit (mrem/hr) |
|---|---|---|---|---|
| $^{125}$I implant | 0.074 | 2 | 0.002 | 0.2 |
| $^{192}$Ir implant | 0.011 | 0.3 | 0.002 | 0.2 |
| $^{103}$Pd implant | 0.3 | 8 | 0.007 | 0.7 |

potentially serious radiation exposure situations."[10] A summary of the program recommendations in that document is as follows:

1. A qualified expert should be consulted when establishing or evaluating the program.
2. Personnel monitoring should be performed for occupationally exposed individuals who have a reasonable possibility of exceeding 10% of the applicable dose limits.
3. All reported cases where the doses exceed the occupational limits shall be investigated by the radiation safety officer.
4. Devices worn for monitoring occupational exposure shall not be worn when the individual is exposed to radiation as a patient.
5. Dosimeters should be worn so that they are visible at all times except when they are deliberately covered by a shield.
6. In Radiation Oncology, the dosimeter should be worn on the trunk of the body above the waist. Extremity dosimeters should be worn when handling radioactive material.
7. Consideration should be given to the monitoring of pregnant personnel.

Some regulatory bodies require that any staff exceeding 10% of the applicable dose limit be notified in writing. Further, if the dose exceeds 30% an investigation should be performed. Local regulations (e.g., in an agreement state in the U.S.) may be different and should be followed.

In addition to monitoring individual staff, it is a good idea to place area monitors around new equipment for a period of time to confirm adequate shielding. This may also be done if the assumptions in the shielding design change such as the workload or the implementation of a new technology such as IMRT.

## 10.7 Shielding

The areas around radiation sources must be shielded to ensure that radiation workers and the general public are not exposed to dose levels that exceed those discussed in Section 10.3. A key reference for shielding of an MV linac is NCRP-151.[11] According to the NCRP, shielding calculations should only be performed by a qualified expert (QE), which they define as a person who is certified by the American Board of Radiology, American Board of Medical Physics, American Board of Health Physics, or Canadian College of Physicists in Medicine.

The nature of the shielding will be determined by the following:

1. How often the radiation source is used (workload, W)
2. How often it is aimed in a particular direction (use factor, U)
3. Whether the primary beam directly strikes the barrier or not (primary vs. secondary barrier)
4. How often the adjoining area is occupied (occupancy factor, T)
5. Who occupies the area (radiation worker, controlled area, or general public, uncontrolled area which will determine the design goal (P) usually expressed in effective dose per week)
6. The distance (d) to the area of interest
7. The type of radiation source (kV x-ray, MV x-ray, radioisotope, particle beam)

The workload (W) will be determined by the number of patients being treated or imaged per week and the treatment or imaging times.

The use factor (U) will be determined by the equipment capabilities and the types of treatments or imaging exams being performed.

The basic equation to calculate the transmission factor for the barrier (B) required to reduce the effective dose in an area to the design goal is:

$$B = P\, d^2 / WUT$$

P is the design goal, usually expressed as effective dose per week. From the transmission factor (B), the number of tenth value layers (the thickness required to reduce the transmission by a factor of 10, TVL) is:

$$n = -\log(B)$$

The thickness (X) is then calculated by:

$$X = TVL_1 + (n-1)TVL_e$$

$TVL_1$ is the first TVL. Subsequent TVLs are different due to spectral changes in the beam as it penetrates the barrier and are designated $TVL_e$.

Secondary barriers are exposed to scatter radiation from the patient, patient support devices, and room structures or leakage radiation from the radiation source. In general, only scatter from the patient is considered. The energy and intensity depend on the angle from the primary beam. The primary beam will have a much higher intensity and energy than the scatter radiation. The leakage radiation will have a higher energy than the primary beam due to a hardening effect as the radiation passes through the source housing but will have a much lower intensity. IEC

TABLE 10.7 ■ Occupancy Factors As Recommended in NCRP-151

| Type of Area | Occupancy Factor (T) |
| --- | --- |
| Office, lab, pharmacy, reception area, attended waiting room, kid's play areas, x-ray rooms, nursing stations, x-ray control rooms, treatment planning areas | 1 |
| Patient exam and treatment rooms | 1/2 |
| Corridors, employee lounges, staff rest rooms, patient rooms | 1/5 |
| Corridor doors (to treatment or imaging room) | 1/8 |
| Public toilets, vending areas, storage rooms, outdoor areas with seating, unattended waiting rooms, patient holding areas | 1/20 |
| Outdoor areas with transient traffic, unattended parking lots, stairways, unattended elevators | 1/40 |

standard 60601-2-1 limits the leakage radiation around the head of a linac to less than 0.1% of the primary beam at 1 m from the head.[12] The use factor for scatter and leakage radiation is taken to be 1 (i.e., the scatter and leakage radiation are not directed primarily to any particular direction).

Occupancy factors (T) are designed to reduce shielding in areas with a low probability of a person occupying that area. When performing shielding calculations for a low occupancy area such as a public toilet, the dose should also be evaluated for high occupancy areas beyond it. For example, there may be a fully occupied office just beyond the bathroom that will ultimately determine the shielding needed in that direction. Recommended occupancy factors from NCRP-151 are shown in Table 10.7.

It should be noted that no barrier will completely eliminate the radiation dose surrounding a radiation source but it should be reduced to safe levels. The ALARA principle is relevant here. The NCRP recommends using a design goal (P) of 0.1 mSv/week (10 mrem) for controlled areas and for 0.02 mSv/week (2 mrem) in uncontrolled areas. This corresponds to a dose level of approximately 10 times lower than the maximum permissible dose for an occupational worker.

In addition to the calculations above, the dose rate in a public area needs to be kept below a certain level as well, regardless of the occupation factor. This is to prevent the exposure of individuals who happen to be occupying the space when the beam is directed at them. In such a situation the effective dose could exceed the weekly limit in a short period of time. The relevant limits are 0.02 mSV (2 mR) in any one hour.[7] This sometimes ends up being the main determinant of a shielding calculation.

The following sections discuss shielding specifics related to the types of equipment used in Radiation Oncology.

## MV SHIELDING

NCRP-151, Structural Shielding Design and Evaluation for Megavoltage X- and Gamma-Ray Radiotherapy Facilities, is the primary resource for MV shielding. The International Atomic Energy Agency (IAEA) has also issued a report, Radiation Protection in the Design of Radiotherapy Facilities.[13] There are four sources that must be considered when designing shielding barriers for MV linear accelerators.

1. Primary beam ($B_{pri}$)
2. Patient scatter ($B_{ps}$)
3. Head leakage ($B_L$)
4 Neutrons (if > 10 MV)

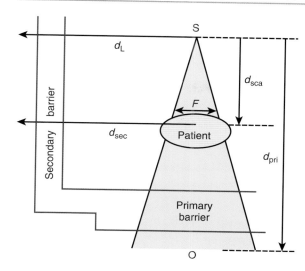

**Figure 10.1** Room layout showing distances associated with patient-scattered and leakage radiations. *(Adapted from NCRP Report No. 151, Structural shielding design and evaluation for megavoltage x- and gamma-ray radiotherapy facilities, National Council on Radiation Protection and Measurements, Bethesda, MD, 2005.)*

TABLE 10.8 ■ Scatter Fractions from NCRP-151

| Angle (degrees) | Scatter Fraction $\alpha$ | | |
|---|---|---|---|
| | **6 MV** | **10 MV** | **18 MV** |
| 10 | $1.04 \times 10^{-2}$ | $1.66 \times 10^{-2}$ | $1.42 \times 10^{-2}$ |
| 20 | $6.73 \times 10^{-3}$ | $5.79 \times 10^{-3}$ | $5.39 \times 10^{-3}$ |
| 30 | $2.77 \times 10^{-3}$ | $3.18 \times 10^{-3}$ | $2.53 \times 10^{-3}$ |
| 45 | $1.39 \times 10^{-3}$ | $1.35 \times 10^{-3}$ | $8.64 \times 10^{-4}$ |
| 60 | $8.24 \times 10^{-4}$ | $7.46 \times 10^{-4}$ | $4.24 \times 10^{-4}$ |
| 90 | $4.26 \times 10^{-4}$ | $3.81 \times 10^{-4}$ | $1.89 \times 10^{-4}$ |
| 135 | $3.00 \times 10^{-4}$ | $3.02 \times 10^{-4}$ | $1.24 \times 10^{-4}$ |
| 150 | $2.87 \times 10^{-4}$ | $2.74 \times 10^{-4}$ | $1.20 \times 10^{-4}$ |

The relevant equations for the photon components are:

$$B_{pri} = P\, d_{pri}{}^2 / WUT$$

$$B_{ps} = P\, d_{sca}{}^2\, d_{sec}{}^2\, 400/\alpha WTF$$

$$B_L = Pd_L{}^2 / 10^{-3}\,WT$$

where

$d_{pri}$, $d_{sca}$, $d_{sec}$, and $d_L$ are as described in Figure 10.1. The distances are 30 cm from the outside surface of the wall or door to represent an occupyable space.

$\alpha$ = scatter fraction for a given angle

F = field area at mid-depth of the patient at 1 m.

The $10^{-3}$ factor in BL is to account for the leakage radiation being <0.1% of primary beam at 1 m.

For $d_{sca} = 1$ m, which is typical, and a $20 \times 20$ field = 400 cm$^2$, which cancels the factor of 400, the equation for $B_{ps}$ becomes $P\, d_{sec}{}^2/\alpha WT$. Therefore if $\alpha$ is much less than the $10^{-3}$ factor in the leakage formula, the leakage radiation will dominate the secondary barrier calculation. The scatter fractions shown in Table 10.8 show this to be true in many cases.

**TABLE 10.9 ▪ Use Factors by Gantry Angle**

| Angle Interval Used to Calculate | Gantry Angle | Use Factor, U |
|---|---|---|
| 90 degrees | 0 | 0.31 |
| | 90 and 270 | 0.213 each |
| | 180 | 0.263 |
| 45 degrees | 0 | 0.256 |
| | 45 and 315 | 0.058 each |
| | 90 and 270 | 0.159 each |
| | 135 and 225 | 0.04 each |
| | 180 | 0.23 |

Rearranging any of these equations, the dose equivalent (H) can be calculated. For example:

$$H_{pri} = WUTB_{pri}/d^2,$$

where $H_{pri}$ is uSv/week.

It should be noted that workload, W, for $B_{pri}$ and $B_{ps}$ are based on the weekly dose at isocenter while W for $B_L$ is based on the total beam on-time. In the case of IMRT or volumetric-modulated arc therapy (VMAT), more monitor units (MU) are delivered per unit dose (and total beam on-times are longer) so $B_L$ in the leakage equation has to be divided by a factor to account for this. This "IMRT factor," designated $C_I$, is equal to $MU_{IMRT}/MU_{conventional}$. Typical values are 3 to 5. It will be higher (10 to 15) for special cases such as TomoTherapy and CyberKnife.

The primary barrier use factor (U) for a modern linac is detailed in NCRP-151 and is shown in Table 10.9. Values are given depending on whether one uses the 4 cardinal angles for calculation versus a more detailed interval of 45°. This differs from the historical methodology of using 0.25 for each of the cardinal angles (0, 90, 180, 270). The width of the primary barrier should be the width of the maximum field size projected at the barrier distance plus 30 cm on either side. The width of the maximum field size is usually the diagonal of the maximum field size. The distance used to calculate the maximum field size projection varies based on whether or not the barrier protrudes into the room (see Figure 10.2). Using this formula, the barrier will also usually encompass the 20° scatter area that contains the maximum scatter contribution. If the amount of space occupied by the primary barrier needs to be reduced, a combination of concrete and lead or steel can be used. If the energy is greater than 10 MV, the amount of concrete must be sufficient to absorb the neutrons or equal to the secondary barrier as is discussed below. Primary barrier tenth value layers (TVLs) for various energies and materials are shown in Table 10.10.

Secondary barriers need to account for both leakage and scatter. In practice the secondary barrier is calculated independently for leakage and scatter. If the two values are within 1 half value layer (HVL) of each other, then 1 HVL should be added to the larger and used as the barrier thickness. An HVL equals 0.3 TVL. Leakage and scatter TVLs are shown in Tables 10.11 and 10.12.

As discussed previously, there is a limit of 0.02 mSv in any one hour.[4] Because linacs have pulsed beams and patients are usually treated in 10 to 20 minute time slots with the actual beam on-time being a small fraction of that time, the instantaneous dose rate (IDR) can be well above 0.02 mSv/hour and still meet the 0.02 mSv in any one hour rule as long as W is not exceedingly low. The concept of time-averaged dose-equivalent rate (TADR) helps explain this. TADR, denoted $R_W$, is calculated by:

$$R_W = IDR\ W_{pri}\ U_{pri}/D_0,$$

where $D_0$ is the output at 1 m.

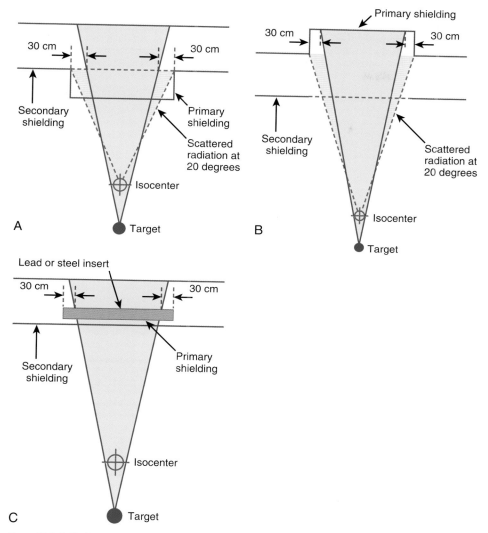

**Figure 10.2 A-C,** Determination of primary barrier width for various barrier configurations. *(Adapted from NCRP Report No. 151, Structural shielding design and evaluation for megavoltage x- and gamma-ray radiotherapy facilities, National Council on Radiation Protection and Measurements, Bethesda, MD, 2005.)*

Conceptually, $R_W$ is always less than or equal to P/hours of operation (i.e., 40 hour work week). If $R_W \times T$ is less than P, then the barrier is adequate. Rearranging the formula gives the following result:

$$\text{IDR} < P\, D_0 / WUT$$

For example, if P = 0.02 mSv/week, $D_0$ = 4 Gy/min, W = 750 Gy/week, and U = 0.213, then IDR must be less than 0.0005 mSv/min or 0.03 mSv/hour. In practice, regulatory agencies may limit the maximum IDR even if the 0.02 mSv in any one hour is met. In the UK, for example, there is a limit of 7.5 μSv/hour in uncontrolled areas.[14]

TABLE 10.10 ▤ **Primary Barrier TVLs from NCRP-151**

| Energy (MV) | Material | TVL$_1$ (cm) | TVL$_e$ (cm) |
|---|---|---|---|
| 4 | Concrete | 35 | 30 |
|  | Lead | 9.9 | 9.9 |
|  | Steel | 5.7 | 5.7 |
| 6 | Concrete | 37 | 33 |
|  | Lead | 10 | 10 |
|  | Steel | 5.7 | 5.7 |
| 10 | Concrete | 41 | 37 |
|  | Lead | 11 | 11 |
|  | Steel | 5.7 | 5.7 |
| 15 | Concrete | 44 | 41 |
|  | Lead | 11 | 11 |
|  | Steel | 5.7 | 5.7 |
| 18 | Concrete | 45 | 43 |
|  | Lead | 11 | 11 |
|  | Steel | 5.7 | 5.7 |
| 20 | Concrete | 46 | 44 |
|  | Lead | 11 | 11 |
|  | Steel | 5.7 | 5.7 |
| $^{60}$Co | Concrete | 21 | 21 |
|  | Lead | 7 | 7 |
|  | Steel | 4 | 4 |

TABLE 10.11 ▤ **Leakage Barrier TVLs in Concrete from NCRP-151**

| Energy (MV) | TVL$_1$ (cm) | TVL$_e$ (cm) |
|---|---|---|
| 4 | 33 | 28 |
| 6 | 34 | 29 |
| 10 | 35 | 31 |
| 15 | 36 | 33 |
| 18 | 36 | 34 |
| 20 | 36 | 34 |
| $^{60}$Co | 21 | 21 |

TABLE 10.12 ▤ **Scatter Barrier TVLs from NCRP-151**

| Scatter Angle (degrees) | TVL (cm) | | | | | | |
|---|---|---|---|---|---|---|---|
|  | $^{60}$Co | 4 MV | 6 MV | 10 MV | 15 MV | 18 MV | 20 MV |
| 15 | 22 | 30 | 34 | 39 | 42 | 44 | 46 |
| 30 | 21 | 25 | 26 | 28 | 31 | 32 | 33 |
| 45 | 20 | 22 | 23 | 25 | 26 | 27 | 27 |
| 60 | 19 | 21 | 21 | 22 | 23 | 23 | 24 |
| 90 | 15 | 17 | 17 | 18 | 18 | 19 | 19 |
| 135 | 13 | 14 | 15 | 15 | 15 | 15 | 15 |

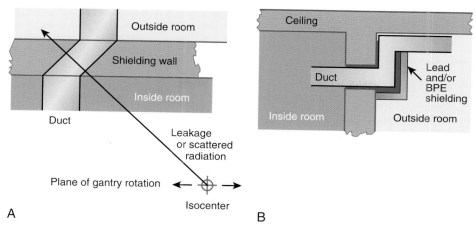

**Figure 10.3 A** and **B**, Duct penetration methods. *(Adapted from NCRP Report No. 151, Structural shielding design and evaluation for megavoltage x- and gamma-ray radiotherapy facilities, National Council on Radiation Protection and Measurements, Bethesda, MD, 2005.)*

Special consideration should be given to wall penetrations for conduits and air ducts. When possible the wall penetrations should be angled so that there is not a direct path through them. It is advisable to have a bend in the penetration. This may not be possible for large air ducts, and so they will require shielding baffles (see Figure 10.3). In addition, special procedures such as TBI will need to be specifically addressed. Because of the long beam on-times, the IDR may need to be lower.

If there is no occupancy above the vault, the roof shielding may be relatively thin. In this case the shielding thickness requirements may be determined by scatter through the roof and back down on the other side of a wall or to an adjacent area or building. This is called *skyshine*. NCRP-151 gives the following equation to calculate skyshine dose equivalent rate (H):

$$H = 2.5 \times 10^7 \ (B_{xs} \ D_0 \ \Omega^{1.3})/(d_i \ d_s)^2$$

where

$2.5 \times 10^7$ converts Gy to nSv

$B_{XS}$ = roof shielding transmission factor for photons

$D_0$ = output at 1 m (Gy/hour)

$\Omega$ = solid angle of the maximum beam (steradians)

$d_I$ = distance from the target to a point 2 m above the roof

$d_S$ = distance from isocenter to the point of calculation on the other side of the wall

Skyshine is particularly important to consider for vaults in which there is no occupied space above. If this space is a roof with maintenance access, it may need to be considered a public area and/or controlled in some fashion. A similar phenomenon can occur through the floor, called *groundshine*.

Shielding for neutrons is in some ways simpler and in other ways much more complicated. Materials with a high hydrogen concentration are particularly effective at shielding thermal neutrons due to the high neutron cross section. For the main walls of the vault, if there is enough concrete to shield for high energy (>10 MV) scatter and leakage, there will be enough shielding for the neutrons. Concrete has high water content and hydrogen. Lead is mostly transparent to neutrons. If lead is used as the primary shielding material in a high energy vault, it will need concrete or steel support because it lacks structural integrity. If steel is used as the support or if there is not enough concrete to shield for the photon scatter and leakage, a neutron shielding material such as polyethylene can be used. The polyethylene can be doped with boron to increase the neutron shielding efficiency.

The most complicated aspect to shielding a megavoltage room is the maze and door. Three components are considered:

1. Photon scatter and leakage ($H_{Tot}$)
2. Neutron capture gamma production ($H_{cg}$)
3. Neutrons ($H_n$)

The equations are quite involved and the reader is advised to consult NCRP-151 directly for the details. In general, factors such as the number of scatter paths required to reach the door, the cross-sectional area of the maze entrance to the maze corridor, and the use of absorbing materials at the end of the maze (borated polyethylene) all contribute to the calculation. If neutron shielding is required for a door, then boronated polyethylene is typically recommended on the vault side of the door with lead or steel on the outside to shield for photons produced by the thermal neutron interactions in the plastic.

Special considerations need to be made for units such as TomoTherapy and CyberKnife. In addition to the increase in MU as mentioned above, the primary beam characteristics are different. TomoTherapy has a beam stopper that attenuates a significant portion of the primary beam. NCRP-151 quotes an attenuation value of $4.1 \times 10^{-3}$ as measured by the vendor. The robotic arm of the CyberKnife system allows for a nearly isotropic arrangement of beam directions, making every wall, the floor, and the ceiling a primary barrier. The isocenter distances for both units are nonstandard, 85 cm for TomoTherapy and 90 to 100 cm for CyberKnife. NCRP discusses both of these units, as do other references.[15-16] In addition, the site planning guides, available from the vendor (Accuray), for these units contain useful information regarding shielding.

---

### Sample MV Calculations

To get an idea of typical shielding thicknesses let's look at some examples. For workload, let us assume 40 patients/day on a dual energy linac, 6 and 18 MV, with half the patients on each energy. That yields W = 20 patients/day × 5 days/week × 3 Gy/patient = 300 Gy/week at isocenter for each energy. For a primary barrier, let us assume a fully occupied (T = 1) uncontrolled area (P = 0.02 mGy/week) and a 90° use factor (U = 0.213). For a distance of 5 m the required thickness would be 221.6 cm (87″) of concrete. For a distance of 7 m the required thickness would be 209 cm (82″) of concrete. Thus we see that distance (inverse square law) can be an effective shield. Larger rooms, in addition to being more functional, are less expensive to shield. The same calculation for 6 MV yields 172.5 cm (68″) of concrete at 5 m, or a difference of 49 cm. This is approximately 1.4 TVLs for 6 MV. Therefore the dose from 6 MV will be a factor of $1/10^{1.4}$ less than the 18 MV dose, or 4% of the 18 MV dose. This is a negligible contribution given all of the overly cautious assumptions such as 3 Gy/patient, so shielding for the higher energy beam using a 50/50 split will be sufficient for the lower energy beam as well. Some factors to consider are not placing fully occupied uncontrolled areas adjacent to a primary barrier. Having a controlled area or a corridor at 5 m would drop the thickness to 191.5 cm (75″), a 30 cm (12″) difference.

Performing the leakage barrier using the same assumptions as above yields a thickness of 95 cm (37″) for a fully occupied uncontrolled area at 5 m. Again, by switching to a controlled area or a corridor the thickness can be reduced, to 72 cm (28″) in this case.

---

## KV SHIELDING

In Radiation Oncology, a dedicated computed tomography (CT) simulator may require shielding. If needed, it is typically 1.5 mm (1/16″) or 0.75 mm (1/32″) of lead embedded in drywall. The lead should extend to at least 7 ft from the floor if there is no occupancy above the unit. All door frames, door knobs, electrical boxes, and so on must have the same lead equivalency or be backed with lead. CT scanners are self-shielded with regard to the primary beam since it is completely intercepted by the detectors. The scatter from the patient is the main source of exposure. NCRP-147 details the shielding methodology.[17]

The general equation to calculate the required attenuation (B) for a barrier is:

$$B = \kappa \times (\text{factors to account for peripheral dose, pitch, contrast use}) \times DLP/d^2$$

The scatter fraction ($\kappa$) at 1 m is typically taken as $9 \times 10^{-5}$ for head scans and $3 \times 10^{-4}$ for body scans. To obtain the scatter dose at 1 m ($K^1$), the dose length product (DLP) is multiplied by $\kappa$. Typical DLPs are 1200 mGy for head scans and 550 mGy for body scans, but exact values should be obtained from the manufacturer. A factor of 1.2 is applied to the scatter fraction for body scans to account for the increased peripheral dose for body scans and the pitch for helical scans (assumed to be 1.35). The pitch for head scans is assumed to be 1. Therefore:

$$K^1_{head} \text{ (mGy)} = 9 \times 10^{-5} \times 1200 \text{ mGy} = 0.108 \text{ mGy}$$

$$K^1_{body} \text{ (mGy)} = 3 \times 10^{-4} \times 1.2 \times 550 \text{ mGy} = 0.198 \text{ mGy}$$

If 20 head scans and 40 body scans are done per week, the total unshielded weekly kerma is 10.08 mGy at 1 m. If IV contrast is used and pre- and postcontrast scans are done, the value should be multiplied by a factor 1+fraction of pre-/postcontrast scan studies. For example, if 40% of the scans are pre-/post contrast, the factor would be 1.4. The total weekly unshielded kerma at the distance of the area to be shielded ($K_0$) is then calculated from the inverse square law. So if the distance (d) is 3 m, $K_0$ for the above example is 10.08 mGy $\times (1/3)^2$, or 1.12 mGy/week. The barrier transmission required (B) is calculated by dividing the design goal (P) by $K_0$. So if the area is an uncontrolled area, P = 0.02 mGy, B = 0.018 for this example. NCRP-147 figures A.2 and A.3 give the material thickness needed based on the attenuation (B) for lead and concrete, respectively. Using this value for B, a barrier thickness of 0.6 mm ($\approx 1/32''$) of lead or 65 mm ($\approx 2.6''$) of concrete is obtained. The thickness can also be found by fitting the data in Figures A.2 and A.3 to Equation A.2 in the report:

$$B = [(1+\beta/\alpha)e^{a\gamma x} - \beta/\alpha]^{-1/\gamma}$$

where x is the material thickness.

Solving the equation for x yields:

$$X = (1/\alpha\gamma) \ln[(B^{-\gamma} + \beta/\alpha)/(1+\beta/\alpha)]$$

The equation parameters are shown in Table 10.13 for lead and concrete.

TABLE 10.13 ■ **Transmission Equation Parameters from NCRP-147**

| Material | kVp | α | β | γ |
|---|---|---|---|---|
| Lead | 120 | 2.246 | 5.73 | 0.547 |
| Lead | 140 | 2.009 | 3.99 | 0.342 |
| Concrete | 120 | 0.0383 | 0.0142 | 0.658 |
| Concrete | 140 | 0.0336 | 0.0122 | 0.519 |

## POSITRON EMISSION TOMOGRAPHY/CT SHIELDING

AAPM Report 108 discusses the shielding requirements for a positron emission tomography (PET)/CT unit.[18] The annihilation photons of PET radionuclides have an energy of 511 keV, which is much higher than other diagnostic imaging modalities. In addition, because the radionuclide is injected into the patient, the patient becomes the source of radiation, which presents challenges as the patient moves through the clinic. In a PET study the patient is injected with the radionuclide followed by a wait time of approximately 60 minutes to allow for uptake. During this time the patient is placed in a quiet resting area to reduce the non-specific uptake. A designated uptake room, which must be shielded (unless the room is unusually large), is used for this. The patient is then taken into the imaging room. Because PET radionuclides have very short half-lives, the shielding requirement is less due to decay. The decay factor for 60 minutes for the most common PET radionuclide, fluorodeoxyglucose (FDG), is 0.68. Further, if the patient is asked to void prior to imaging, approximately another 15% will be removed from the body.

Because of the high energy of the annihilation photons, ceiling and floor shielding must be carefully evaluated. Other considerations for PET/CT shielding are the location of other imaging devices and sensitive instruments such as scintillation counters and thyroid uptake probes. Scintillation cameras should be positioned such that the detectors are never pointed directly at an uptake or imaging room. Sensitive counters should not have an ambient background above 1000 cpm and should be located in isolated areas away from the uptake and imaging rooms. The doors to the imaging and uptake rooms should be carefully positioned to minimize the amount of lead needed (i.e., as far away as possible and toward areas with low occupancy).

The equations for the required attenuation (B) are as follows:

$$\text{Uptake room: } B = 218 \times d^2 / [T \times N_W \times A_0 \times t_U \times R_{tU}] \text{ for uncontrolled areas}$$

$$\text{Imaging room: } B = 256 \times d^2 / [T \times N_W \times A_0 \times F_U \times t_I \times R_{tI}] \text{ for uncontrolled areas}$$

where:

$T$ = occupancy factor

$N_W$ = number of patients per week

$A_0$ = administered activity (MBq)

$t_U$ = uptake time (hours)

$R_{tU}$ = dose reduction factor over uptake time = $1.443 \times (T_{1/2}/t_U) \times [1 - \exp(-0.693 t_U/T_{1/2})]$

$T_{1/2}$ = PET radionuclide half-life (hours)

$F_U$ = uptake decay factor = $\exp[-0.693 t_U/T_{1/2}]$

$t_I$ = imaging time (hours)

$R_{tI}$ = dose reduction factor over imaging time = $1.443 \times (T_{1/2}/t_I) \times [1 - \exp(-0.693 t_I/T_{1/2})]$

The factors of 218 and 256 are derived from the assumption that the dose rate from the patient is 0.092 $\mu$Sv m$^2$/MBq hr immediately after injection. For uncontrolled areas P = 20 mSv; therefore, for the uptake room, 20/0.092 = 218. For the imaging room the dose rate is modified by the 0.85 voiding factor, yielding 218/0.85 = 256.

The values of B for controlled areas are a factor of 5 or higher. The resulting barriers for controlled and uncontrolled areas around the rooms typically range from 2 to 12 mm of lead. The value of the required material thickness for a given value of B can be determined using the equation in the section on kV shielding in this chapter. The parameters for 511 keV photons are listed in Table 10.14.

The shielding for the CT component is generally less than for the PET component but should be evaluated to confirm that no additional shielding is required. The DLP will be much higher than for a conventional CT since the scan length is much greater (1.25 to 1.5 m).

TABLE 10.14 ▓ **Transmission Equation Parameters for PET (511 keV)**

| Material | $\alpha$ | $\beta$ | $\gamma$ |
|---|---|---|---|
| Lead | 1.543 | −0.4408 | 2.136 |
| Concrete | 0.1539 | −0.1161 | 2.0752 |
| Iron | 0.5704 | −0.3063 | 0.6326 |

TABLE 10.15 ▓ **TVLs for Common LDR Sources from IAEA Report 47**

| Source | Lead (mm) | Steel (mm) | Concrete (mm) |
|---|---|---|---|
| $^{137}$Cs | 22 | 53 | 175 |
| $^{192}$Ir | 16 | 43 | 152 |

## LDR SHIELDING

Although now rare, there are facilities that do use $^{137}$Cs or $^{192}$Ir for low dose rate (LDR) implants over 1 to 2 days. IAEA Report 47 describes the shielding methodology.[13]
The equation for B is:

$$B = P \times 1000 \times d^2 / S_K \times t \times n \times T$$

where
P = design goal (mSv/week)
1000 uSv/mSv
d = distance (m)
$S_K$ = air kerma strength (uGy m$^2$ h$^{-1}$ or U)
t = average time of an implant (h)
n = number of implants per week
T = occupancy factor
For photons, Gy = Sv.

---

**Example Calculation (LDR) for an Uncontrolled Area at a Distance of 3 m with T = 1**

An activity of 500 U per implant is used with 50 hours per implant and 2 implants per week. The equation above yields B = 0.0036. To calculate the shielding required, the number of tenth value layers is calculated by −log$_{10}$(B), which equals 2.44 in this case.
Table 10.15 shows the TVL in various materials for $^{192}$Ir and $^{137}$Cs. Using the values for lead, a thickness of 54 mm (≈2″) would be required for $^{137}$Cs and 39 mm (≈1.5″) for $^{192}$Ir.

---

In practice, to shield a patient room with this amount of lead would be very expensive. Typically portable shields are used and placed close to the patient to eliminate the need to shield the entire room. It is advisable to situate LDR rooms adjacent to corridors or rest rooms to take advantage of the lower occupancy. In addition to the weekly design goal, since these implants are several days long and the use factor = 1, the IDR needs to be limited. IAEA Report 47 suggests a value of 2.5 μSv/hour (0.25 mR/hour) for uncontrolled areas and 7.5 μSv/hour (0.75 mR/hour) for controlled areas.

## HDR SHIELDING

The high dose-rate (HDR) shielding calculation is the same as for LDR.[13] HDR sources are typically 41,000 U when installed, and the treatment times are on the order of 15 minutes. If 20 treatments are delivered per week, the shielding required for an uncontrolled area at 3 m with occupancy of 1 would be 49 mm ($\approx$2″) of lead. Similarly, the calculation for a controlled area at 3 m with occupancy of 1 would be 38 mm ($\approx$1.5″) of lead.

## PROTON AND HEAVY ION SHIELDING

The Particle Therapy Cooperative Group (PTCOG) has produced a report on shielding for particle accelerators.[19] The report is available on their website, http://www.ptcog.ch/index.php/ptcog-publications. Since the installation of these units is handled by a dedicated team with experience in this area, it is unlikely that a general medical physicist would become involved in the shielding design. Therefore only a brief overview is given here.

Particle accelerators produce secondary radiation whenever there are beam losses. These occur "in the synchrotron and cyclotron along the beam line during injection, acceleration, extraction, energy degradation, and transport of the particles in the beam line to the treatment room, and in the beam shaping devices in the treatment nozzle."[19] In addition, interactions within the patient or beam stop also produce secondary radiation. Because of this, the entire facility must be shielded. Heavy particles produce a complex cascade of secondary radiation as they traverse the shielding material. It is a combination of neutrons, charged particles, and photons. These charged particles will be well shielded by any barrier used to attenuate the neutrons and do not need to be considered. The neutron component dominates the shielding calculation. Cyclotrons require more shielding than synchrotrons because they use a beam degrader to achieve beam energies lower than the output of the cyclotron. Passive scattering beams require more shielding than pencil beam scanning beams because of the secondary radiation produced during the scattering.

One of the differences between particle shielding and photon shielding is that the neutron production is forward directed versus the nearly isotropic pattern from linacs. The very high energy neutrons are more efficiently shielded with steel rather than concrete but must be backed with a hydrogenous material to absorb the lower energy neutrons. The report shows the shielding for various facilities, and the concrete thicknesses range from 1.2 to 4 m. One issue that must be considered with particle facilities is the activation of materials in the beam path, particularly beam apertures and range compensators that are handled by the staff.

## SHIELDING EVALUATION

NCRP-151 states that a shielding evaluation must be performed for each new installation or upon any changes to the assumptions of an existing shielding calculation such as the addition of IMRT or TBI treatments. The report must have the following components:

1. Title page describing the radiation source, facility name, and person(s) performing the calculations and measurements and who prepared the report
2. A review of the calculations used to determine the shielding
3. Inspection during construction
4. Description of the survey methods, including technique and instrumentation, machine operating parameters for each measurement, and method used to calculate H from the measurements
5. Floor plans showing locations of measurements
6. Instruments used, with serial numbers and calibration certificates

7. Results for each location around the vault including H, TADR, IDR, and maximum dose in any one hour
8. Conclusions and recommendations
9. A copy of the report must remain at the facility.
10. If shielding modifications are required, a follow-up survey must be performed.

## RADIATION PROTECTION SURVEY

Immediately after the linac is able to produce radiation, a survey must be performed in all occupied areas to ensure that they are within limits. The survey is done by using a GM detector or other instrument that has a fast response to scan for defects in the shielding and to find the area of maximum dose rate. Once that area is identified, a calibrated ion chamber or other instrument with a small energy dependence should be used to document the dose rate at 1 foot from the wall (30 cm). For facilities with beams above 10 MV, a neutron meter will also be needed. Remember that because of differences in occupancy factors and skyshine, the area immediately adjacent to the vault may not be the limiting factor for that barrier.

For the primary barriers, the measurements should be made with the maximum field size and no phantom. Gantry angles that impinge on floor and ceiling corners are of particular concern because of skyshine and groundshine. The measurements should be made at 30 cm from the wall or floor. Secondary barriers are measured with the maximum field size with a phantom in the beam. In the case of a linac with no occupied building structure above it, surveys will need to be performed on the roof.

# 10.8 Source Receipt, Inventory, and Return

Whenever radioactive sources are received in the department, procedures must be followed to ensure the safety and accountability of the source. Regulations will vary by locale but some features will be constant. The package must be surveyed within 3 hours of receipt to ensure that the exposure levels are acceptable.[20] The U.S. Department of Transportation (DOT) categorizes exposure levels based on the readings at the package surface and at 1 m. There are three categories of radioactive source shipments based on these readings; the details are shown in Table 10.16. Yellow II and Yellow III packages require what is called a transport index (TI). The TI is equal to the exposure reading at 1 m in mR/hr rounded up to the nearest tenth with no units. A package reading 0.26 mR/hr at 1 m would have a TI of 0.3. In addition, the surface of the package should be checked for removable contamination by performing a wipe test. For example, the NRC requires a wipe over 300 $cm^2$ with a limit of 6600 dpm/300 $cm^2$ (NRC 10 CFR 20). Radioactive materials should be secured at all times to ensure inventory control. A log of the receipt, use, and disposal of all radioactive material must be maintained.

TABLE 10.16 ▪ **U.S. DOT Shipping Label Categories**

| Category | Surface Reading | One Meter Reading |
|---|---|---|
| WHITE I | <0.005 mSv/hr (0.5 mR/hr) | Background |
| YELLOW II | 0.005-0.5 mSv/hr (0.5-50 mR/hr) | <0.01 mSv/hr (1 mR/hr) |
| YELLOW III | 0.5-2.0 mSv/hr (50-200 mR/hr) | 0.01-0.1 mSv/hr (1-10 mR/hr) |
| YELLOW III (exclusive use only) | 2-10 mSv/hr (200-1000 mR/hr) | >0.1 mSv/hr (10 mR/hr) |

# 10.9 Radiation Safety Training

NCRP-134 lists four reasons to provide radiation safety training:[21]

1. The development of skills through training allows staff to perform tasks more efficiently and with confidence.
2. When individuals are aware that there is some risk associated with radiation exposure, they become active participants in accepting that risk and where possible to reduce that risk.
3. The number and seriousness of accidents can be reduced through training.
4. Workers who are properly trained will become aware of the regulatory requirements.

Management has a responsibility to provide qualified trainers, to evaluate the performance of the trainers, and to maintain records of the training.

There are many factors to consider when identifying training requirements. They include:

1. The potential for exposure
2. The complexity of the task
3. Regulatory requirements
4. The level of physics knowledge
5. The level of supervision of the staff: less supervised staff need more training
6. More training for individuals who provide supervision.
7. Any previous training
8. Specific concerns of the staff

There are six steps in developing a training program:

1. Perform a job task analysis. Analyze the competencies needed to perform the task safely.
2. Training design and development. What is the nature of the radiation hazard? What is the size of the group to be trained? What skills, knowledge, and attitudes are needed? What are the previous experience and training? What budget and staff are available for training? What are the training objectives? What will be the testing criteria? What will be the course structure?
3. Develop the course outline and training materials.
4. Develop the evaluation plan. There are four types: 1) reaction evaluation given immediately following the training to get immediate feedback on what went well and what did not; 2) learning evaluation in the form of a written or oral test; 3) performance evaluation of the task; 4) results evaluation to determine relative success of the training (i.e., monitor accident rates or collective doses).
5. Provide the training instruction.
6. Follow the evaluation plan and get feedback.

The training can be provided in different formats ranging from individual study of materials, to group instruction, to mentoring, to on the job training (OJT). OJT may be most effective for complex tasks.

Once the training program is developed, it should be audited periodically to confirm that proper records are being kept and that the evaluations demonstrate the effectiveness of the program and the trainers. Table 10.17 lists the suggested topics for radiation safety training from NCRP.

TABLE 10.17 ■ **Suggested Topics for Radiation Safety Training**

| Essential Elements | Optional Elements | Additional Elements for Radiation Safety Technicians |
|---|---|---|
| Risks related to radiation exposure | Waste management | Inspections/audits |
| Dose limits and site-specific administrative controls | Radiation safety manual | Packing/shipping/labeling for transport |
| Modes of exposure<br>External<br>Internal | Contamination control | Leak testing |
| Basic protective measures including engineering and administrative controls | Work area decontamination | Use and calibration of survey equipment |
| Security | License/regulations | Record keeping |
| Emergency notification and response | Characteristics of ionizing and nonionizing radiation | Principles and practices for reducing radiation exposure |
| Warning signs, postings, labels, and alarms | Radioactive materials and decay | Radiation and radioactive contamination survey techniques |
| Responsibility of employees and organizations | Radiation producing equipment<br>Natural and manufactured sources | Emergency response and personal decontamination |
| Interaction with radiation safety staff | Acute and chronic effects | Radioactive waste disposal |
| Overall safety | Determination of dose | Bioassay requirements |
| Description of and requirements related to specific facility hazards | Basic radiation survey instrumentation | Radiation accident control |
| Basic monitoring for radiation exposure | Radiation monitoring program and procedures | Proper selection of personnal protective equipment |
| Procedures for maintaining ALARA | Identification and control of radiation sources | |
| | Selection and proper use of personal radiation dosimeters | |

# 10.10 Regulatory Oversight

Various governmental agencies control the regulations surrounding the use of radiation in medicine. For instance, in the United States, the NRC governs the use of by-product materials, which would include $^{60}$Co, $^{137}$Cs, and $^{125}$I. Certain sections of the Code of Federal Regulations (CFR) apply to the use of by-product materials, such as 10 CFR 20 and 10 CFR 35. These can be found on the NRC website (http://www.nrc.gov/). The use of electrically produced radiation (x-ray units, CT scanners, linacs, etc.) is regulated by the individual states. The Conference of Radiation Control Program Directors (CRCPD) produces suggested state regulations that many states adopt. Their website is a good source of information (http://www.crcpd.org/).

A component of the regulatory process is routine inspections of the facilities. In all cases with the NRC and many cases with individual states, the facility is required to obtain a license to use radiation in medicine. The license will specify the exact conditions under which the facility can use radiation, including who is authorized to prescribe its use, what types of uses are approved, who can handle the radiation sources, and who can calibrate the radiation sources. The facility is required to appoint a radiation safety officer and have a radiation safety committee to ensure the safe use of radiation and to monitor the exposures to staff, patients, and the general public. This is described in 10 CFR 35. The routine inspections will confirm that these activities are being performed according to regulations, license conditions, and recommended best practices.

There are resources that can help prepare an institution for inspections and audits. The CRCPD has an inspection protocol for medical linacs that is available on their website. In addition, Ritter et al. have published an audit tool for external beam radiotherapy departments.[22] In fact, an onsite inspection may be required on a new installation prior to the treatment of patients, depending on local regulations. Sometimes the approval to treat patients may just be in the form of a letter from the appropriate regulatory body. It is advisable to check with local regulations as part of the installation planning process.

### FOR THE PHYSICIAN

The goal of radiation protection is to prevent the occurrence of serious radiation-induced conditions and to reduce stochastic effects (such as carcinogenesis) to a degree that is acceptable relative to the benefits of the activities that generate radiation exposure. Specifically, the objectives are to prevent radiation-induced deterministic effects (such as infertility and bone marrow suppression) by adhering to dose limits that are below apparent thresholds and to limit the risk of stochastic effects to a reasonable level.

Regulatory limits are based on equivalent dose (H), which accounts for the biological effectiveness of the type of radiation by applying a weighting factor ranging from 1 for photons and electrons to as high as 20 for neutrons and alpha particles. Further, to account for irradiation to parts of the body, an effective dose (E) is calculated by multiplying H by an organ-specific weighting factor. The total, E, is obtained by summing E for each organ.

The basic annual limits for occupational workers is 50 mSv (5 rem) to the whole body, 150 mSv (15 rem) to the lens, and 500 mSv (50 rem) to the hands, skin, and feet. For the general public the values are 1 mSv (0.1 rem) for the whole body and 50 mSv (5 rem) to the lens and extremities. The dose limits for radiation workers are higher than those for members of the general public. This is based on the fact that radiation workers have received special training in radiation protection, are aware of the associated radiation risks, and have decided to accept them. Areas occupied by the general public or nonradiation workers (uncontrolled areas) are subject to stricter dose limits compared to areas occupied by radiation workers (controlled area).

To determine compliance with dose limits for the general public, shielding calculations are done to show that individuals in the areas surrounding the radiation source will not exceed the regulatory limits. When designing a radiotherapy treatment room, several considerations should be made to minimize the amount of material required:

1. If an area is not occupied full-time, the dose levels can be higher since the calculations take into account how long someone might be exposed.
2. Avoid placing fully occupied uncontrolled areas adjacent to the treatment room.
3. Special procedures such as IMRT and TBI can significantly affect the shielding calculations due to higher beam on-times.
4. Distance can be used to help reduce shielding thickness (inverse square law), and larger rooms require less shielding.

The calculations must be confirmed by performing a survey of dose levels surrounding the radiation source after installation, using an appropriate instrument. The calculations should be reviewed on a regular basis to confirm that the assumptions made during the design process are still valid. According to the NCRP, shielding calculations should only be performed by a qualified expert whom they define as a person who is certified by the American Board of Radiology, American Board of Medical Physics, American Board of Health Physics, or Canadian College of Physicists in Medicine. If the use of a treatment unit changes, the shielding should be reevaluated.

For example, if an IMRT program is started on a linac, secondary shielding may need to be increased because 3 to 5 times more monitor units will be used in a typical treatment, resulting in more leakage radiation from the head of the machine.

To ensure the continued safe use of radiation in medicine, staff should receive annual radiation safety training. This training should include basic radiation safety principles, details specific to their job functions, and communication of risk estimates.

## *References*

1. NCRP Report No. 116, Limitation of exposure to ionizing radiation. Bethesda, MD: National Council on Radiation Protection and Measurements; 1993.
2. BEIR VII. Health Risks from Exposure to Low Levels of Ionizing Radiation: BEIR VII. Washington D.C.: The National Academies Press; 2006.
3. IAEA safety standards series, Occupational radiation protection. Vienna: IAEA; 1999.
4. ICRP. The 2007 Recommendations of the International Commission on Radiological Protection. ICRP Publication 103. Ann ICRP 2007;37(2–4).
5. Brenner DJ. Effective dose: a flawed concept that could and should be replaced. Br J Radiol 2008;81(967):521–3.
6. Li X, Samei E, Segars WP, et al. Patient-specific radiation dose and cancer risk for pediatric chest CT. Radiology 2011;259(3):862–74.
7. NCRP Statement No. 10, Recent applications of the NCRP public dose limit recommendation for ionizing radiation. Bethesda, MD: National Council on Radiation Protection and Measurements; 2004.
8. NCRP Report No. 160, Ionizing radiation exposure of the population of the United States. Bethesda, MD: National Council on Radiation Protection and Measurements; 2009.
9. NUREG-1556, Consolidated guidance about materials licenses. Rockville, MD: US NRC; 2008.
10. NCRP Report No. 102, Medical x-ray, electron beam and gamma-ray protection for energies up to 50 MeV. Bethesda, MD: National Council on Radiation Protection and Measurements; 1989.
11. NCRP Report No.151, Structural shielding design and evaluation for megavoltage x- and gamma-ray radiotherapy facilities. Bethesda, MD: National Council on Radiation Protection and Measurements; 2005.
12. IEC 60601-2-1. Medical electrical equipment – Part 2-1: Particular requirements for the basic safety and essential performance of electron accelerators in the range 1 MeV to 50 MeV, IEC 60601-2-1, International Electromechanical Commission, 2009.
13. IAEA Safety Reports Series No. 47, Radiation protection in the design of radiotherapy facilities. Vienna: International Atomic Energy Agency; 2006.
14. Institute of Physics and Engineering in Medicine (IPEM), Medical and dental guidance notes, a good practice guide to implement ionising radiation protection legislation in the clinical environment. York, England: IPEM; 2002.
15. Balog J, Lucas D, DeSouza C, et al. Helical TomoTherapy radiation leakage and shielding considerations. Med Phys 2005;32(3):710–19.
16. Baechler S, Bochud FO, Verellen D, et al. Shielding requirements in helical TomoTherapy. Phys Med Biol 2007;52(16):5057–67.
17. NCRP Report No. 147, Structural shielding design for medical x-ray imaging facilities. Bethesda, MD: National Council on Radiation Protection and Measurements; 2004, rev 2005.
18. Madsen MT, Anderson JA, Halama JR, et al. AAPM Task Group 108: PET and PET/CT shielding requirements. Med Phys 2006;33(1):4–15.
19. PTCOG Report 1, PTCOG publications sub-committee task group on shielding design and radiation safety of charged particle therapy facilities. Particle Therapy Co-Operative Group; 2010.
20. US NRC Code of Federal Regulations, 10 CFR 1906.
21. NCRP Report No. 134, Operational radiation safety training. Bethesda, MD: National Council on Radiation Protection and Measurements; 2000.
22. Ritter T, Balter JM, Lee C, et al. Audit tool for external beam radiation therapy departments. Practical Radiat Oncol 2012;2:e39–44.

# CHAPTER 11

# Information Technology in Radiation Oncology

## 11.1 Introduction

Information technology (IT) in Radiation Oncology has developed into highly complex networks driving much of treatment delivery and other safety-critical tasks in the department. Based on the size of a Radiation Oncology clinic, the role of the physicist in IT can range from being the system administrator with all the responsibilities to being the liaison of the Radiation Oncology department to a large IT group supporting all hospital IT systems.

The American College of Radiology (ACR)-American Association of Physicists in Medicine (AAPM)-Society for Imaging Informatics in Medicine (SIIM) Practice Parameter for Electronic Medical Record Information Privacy and Security[1] summarized current best practices in radiology and Radiation Oncology. The document emphasizes that security awareness and security training should be integral parts of initial and periodic staff training. The document also contains recommendations on the definition of responsibilities, risk analysis, backup, storage, and system down time/recovery planning. A preliminary report from AAPM TG-201, "Information on Technology Resource Management in Radiation Oncology",[2] provides a broad overview on the central topics in this area. The core challenge in the interaction of the different specialties is that the IT needs of Radiation Oncology are dissimilar to those in other departments within a hospital (e.g., software such as a record and verify system does not exist). It is therefore essential that there is mutual flow of information and education between the Radiation Oncology physicist and the IT specialists about the use of IT resources as well as the impact of resource failure on patient treatments. It must be well understood by all parties that the continued operation of treatment planning systems, Radiation Oncology information systems, and record and verify systems is mission critical (i.e., patient treatments cannot proceed without these systems).

## 11.2 Networks and Network Safety

IT systems are networked both within a Radiation Oncology department as well as to the outside. Beyond Internet and email functionality, other network connections may include HL7 interfaces to outside providers or insurance companies, connection to device vendors for diagnostic purposes, remote backup and archive servers, picture archiving and communication system (PACS) access, and others.

The main safety risks are theft of mobile devices, theft of protected health information (PHI) data through network safety breaches, viruses, and loss of data or functionality due to hardware failure or catastrophic events. Protecting against loss of data is discussed in the context of database backup in Section 11.7. The theft of mobile devices (laptops, tablets, cell phones, and Universal Serial Bus (USB) sticks can be safeguarded against using several safety precautions including controlling access to the department, password-protecting devices, and encrypting data on the devices. Some cell phone carriers provide a remote kill-switch for stolen devices; these should be enabled where available. The amount of PHI stored on mobile devices should be minimized as much as possible.

All hardware (PCs, servers, and mobile devices) should have up-to-date antivirus software installed when permissible. Clinical workstations for which installation of antivirus software is prohibited (e.g., due to restrictions associated with the Food and Drug Administration (FDA) 510k clearance process) must be protected as securely as possible. This includes limiting connections to the network through firewalls, removing internet access except for secure remote login tools used by the vendor for diagnostic purposes, and limiting USB access to USB devices that have been scanned for malware immediately before use. Workstations that are classified as medical devices should be made exempt from automatic updates as they may inadvertently affect functionality.

## 11.3 Electronic Health Records Systems

### ELECTRONIC HEALTH RECORDS

Electronic health records (EHR), sometimes also referred to as electronic medical records (EMR), are rapidly replacing paper charts in the hospital setting. One of the advantages of EHR is easy availability of healthcare information to all providers, including sharing of health records with patients through web-based secure access. Integrated database analysis allows graphing health trends, reconciling medications, and even flagging of potentially negative pharmacological interactions. In addition, there is increased safety because an EHR can be backed up remotely, which provides redundancy in case of catastrophic loss of the primary record.

However, in addition to being a retainer of information, a paper chart has additional functions which may not be immediately obvious but need to be integrated into the EHR for a successful transition. The following list includes a sample of paper chart functions that need to be transferred to EHR:

- **Information repository:** Charts contain information in an organized manner. The EHR must be able to categorize information in a systematic manner such that the care team can easily find and retrieve important information, especially from scanned documents such as pdf files. Search functions should include the ability to search document titles and file contents. The ability to view multiple documents simultaneously is highly desirable.
- **Checklist:** The paper chart contains written treatment records, which include checkboxes or signature lines for completed second check, weekly chart check, MD signature, imaging protocol and imaging review, and use of accessories such as bolus. These items provide an easy visual check on performance of quality control processes according to the policies and procedures implemented in the department. Transferring these checks to the EHR system can be challenging, because those paper chart functions were not obvious for the initial software designs in EHR (e.g., missing initials from a physicist indicating the completion of a weekly chart check might not be as obvious in an EHR). Another example is the ordering and recording of the different bolus regimens: bolus qod can be easily verified by the radiation therapist's initials in a paper chart, but equivalent functionality is still missing in most EHR systems. One way to address this is to schedule bolus and no bolus treatments into the treatment calendar of the EHR.
- **Workflow task:** A handover of a paper chart from one member of a patient care team to another initiates a workflow task (e.g., a paper chart would move from the dosimetrist to a physicist to indicate plan completion and initiate the second check process). Most EHR systems have several tools to communicate workflow tasks; in addition, tools outside the EHR such as pages, emails, or texts can be used. It is recommended that the department standardize the workflow task method used at each step in the patient treatment workflow to avoid delays in communicating tasks. Task cascading, which automatically notifies the next step in the workflow upon completion of a task, is available in some EHRs.

- **Communication:** A paper chart is also used as a tool to communicate essential information among caregivers (e.g., a handwritten note on the treatment record can indicate "please discontinue bolus starting today"). As for workflow tasks, EHR systems may contain multiple possible channels of communication among caregivers. The communication channels among caregivers need to be clearly defined in the paperless policies and procedures to avoid failure of communication resulting in possible negative treatment outcomes. There should be only one location in the EHR for each type of information. Allowing multiple locations will ultimately lead to errors due to missed information.

AAPM TG-262, Electronic Charting of Radiation Therapy Planning and Treatment (in progress), is charged with providing guidance on electronic charting, safe clinical practices for transitioning to electronic charting, implementation in the context of other IT systems (e.g., hospital EHR), and common pitfalls.

## RECORD AND VERIFY SYSTEM

One particular form of EHR in Radiation Oncology is the record and verify (R&V) system. Originally R&V systems were designed to do just that: record and verify the correct delivery of a treatment. This was especially important and useful in an era when manual actions and entry of data were more common. R&V systems could verify, for example, that the correct monitor unit (MU) were input or that the intended wedge or block was applied during treatment. In some parts of the developing world R&V systems are still not in use.

The role of R&V systems has evolved toward controlling all technical aspects of the delivery system. Some systems now serve as an entire EHR with additional operational functions such as scheduling, communication, and billing. As such, these systems are now often referred to as oncology information systems (OIS) or treatment management systems (TMS), though the term R&V is still in common use.

## INTEGRATION AND COMMUNICATION ACROSS EHR AND R&V SYSTEMS

In smaller Radiation Oncology clinics and freestanding centers, the R&V system provides double functionality as the EHR system as well. If the Radiation Oncology department is part of a larger hospital system, the hospital has its own EHR software in place (e.g., EPIC or Cerner). These systems often do not have good functionality for the extended treatment courses and types of records needed in Radiation Oncology. As a result, software tools have been developed using the HL7 standard (http://www.hl7.org) to integrate Radiation Oncology R&V systems with hospital EHR, although some of these efforts are still works in progress and many challenges still exist.

The scope of the integration and procedural details should be discussed in detail to outline the information flow clearly and avoid miscommunication. Specific sectors of integration are:

- **Billing:** This is typically the most straightforward integration project. Charges are collected within the Radiation Oncology EHR and transferred to the hospital EHR. The main decision required is whether charges get reviewed by a Radiation Oncology billing expert before being released to the hospital EHR. One issue in the United States is that the charges must be billed under the physician who is on site each day, not the attending physician.
- **Scheduling:** Scheduling integration is more complex than might be obvious at first sight. For example, in Radiation Oncology it is not uncommon to schedule a patient as a "placeholder" to reserve a requested time on the machine, while the actual treatment start might fluctuate depending on treatment plan completion or timing of chemotherapy. This may not be immediately obvious to schedulers in other departments, who might convey incorrect scheduling

information to the patient. Similarly, a patient's appointment may be rescheduled in the hospital EHR, but the change may not be communicated to the Radiation Oncology EHR. Therefore, scheduling integration requires in-depth discussion on to what extent schedules are shared, in which direction scheduling information flows (both ways, one way from EHR to R&V or vice versa, etc.), and who has permission to change Radiation Oncology appointments. In addition, the patient may have multiple appointments in the department on a given day (i.e., nurse visit, treatment, nutrition counseling, etc.), and changing one time will affect the others.

- **Documentation:** A patient chart includes various types of documents, such as pathology reports, the history and physical, treatment plan, and special physics consult requests. These documents are not always easily exchanged between systems and can have the potential to clutter a patient's EHR with information which might make it more difficult for care providers outside Radiation Oncology to find relevant information. An integration of document exchange requires answering questions of which types of documents should be shared and when, how accurate document labeling will be accomplished, or, in the case where documents will not be exchanged, which document will be filed in which of the two EHR systems.

- **Imaging:** An increasing amount of imaging data is generated in Radiation Oncology for treatment planning, treatment verification, and adaptive planning purposes. Some of the imaging might contain valuable information for outside departments (e.g., an Emergency Room (ER) physician might gain important information from a simulation computed tomography (CT) showing the treatment target if a patient is admitted through the ER during a course of radiation). Other imaging information (e.g., port films or setup images) is not useful to caregivers outside of Radiation Oncology. Therefore, it should be well defined which imaging information is shared across EHR systems. In some countries or states, there might also be legal considerations if images that have not been assessed by a radiologist or are not intended for diagnostic purposes are shared across departments.

## 11.4 Integrating the Healthcare Enterprise—Radiation Oncology

To efficiently share healthcare information across EHR systems, the Integrating the Healthcare Enterprise (IHE) International (http://www.ihe.net) initiative was founded. IHE promotes the use of established health information standards such as DICOM (see Section 11.5) and HL7. American Society for Radiation Oncology (ASTRO) sponsors the IHE Radiation Oncology (IHE-RO) subgroup focusing on safe and efficient sharing of healthcare information across Radiation Oncology platforms. An example would be the transfer of data between a treatment planning system from one vendor to an R&V system from another vendor. IHE-RO manages the Radiation Oncology Profiles and the Radiation Oncology Technical Framework.

One major tool for connectivity testing organized by IHE-RO is the annual Connectathon. During this event, vendors meet to test the connectivity of their products using different challenge scenarios encountered in a typical Radiation Oncology practice. When a vendor passes the tests posed at the Connectathon, the product can be labeled as "IHE-RO Compliant." Integration statements are available from vendors to describe the IHE-RO compatibility on a technical level. All requests for quotes or proposals from prospective vendors should inquire as to the IHE-RO compliance level.

## 11.5 Digital Imaging and Communications in Medicine

Digital Imaging and Communications in Medicine (DICOM) was developed as a standard for handling, storing, printing, and transmitting information in medical imaging (http://dicom.nema.org). DICOM includes a file format definition and a network communication protocol. The communication protocol is an application protocol that uses transmission control protocol/internet protocol (TCP/IP) to communicate among systems. DICOM files can be exchanged between any two entities that are capable of receiving image and patient data in DICOM format.

As the DICOM standards developed over time, supplements were added to include Radiation Oncology information such as contouring, dose, and beam files. Supplement 11 contains DICOM radiotherapy (RT) extensions for RT Image, RT Dose, RT Structure Set, and RT Plan. Supplement 29 added RT Treatment Record. They contain the following information object definitions:

- **RT Image:** Digitally reconstructed radiograph (DRR), portal imaging, simulator
- **RT Dose:** Dose matrix, dose points, isodoses, dose-volume histogram (DVH)
- **RT Structure Set:** Volume of interest, dose reference points, observations/characterizations
- **RT Plan:** External beam and brachytherapy plan, tolerance table, fractionation scheme, patient setup
- **RT Treatment Record:** External beam and brachytherapy session/summary recording information

A DICOM object or data set contains a number of data elements. Each data element in turn consists of (1) a unique tag defined in the DICOM data dictionary, (2) a value representation dependent on the transfer syntax (optional), (3) the value length, and (4) the value field. Figure 11.1 shows part of a DICOM file including tag, value length, and value field information. A dictionary of tags and values is available from the National Electric Manufacturer's Association (NEMA) website. Various commercial packages are available that read DICOM files (e.g., products from MIM or Velocity Inc.). In addition, there are numerous free DICOM file readers available, including ImageJ (from NIH), Slicer3 (from Brigham and Women's Hospital), ezDICOM, microDICOM, and OsiriX. MATLAB is also capable of reading and outputing DICOM files. DICOM-RT files are somewhat more challenging.

## 11.6 Database and Database Management

Issues of database management and security are discussed in detail in the ACR-AAPM-SIIM Practice Parameter for Electronic Medical Record Information. The following sections provide a brief overview.

### FALLBACK SYSTEMS AND TESTING OF FALLBACK SYSTEMS

R&V systems drive day-to-day clinical operations for modern linacs. While planned outages of R&V systems can be anticipated by loading the RT plan files onto a local disk driving the treatment machine delivery and later recording the delivered dose manually, unanticipated R&V system down time can cause major interruptions in the treatment schedule. Because extended treatment interruptions have been shown to negatively affect treatment outcomes in some disease sites, it is essential to have a fallback system in place. A fallback system is designed to automatically take over after the main R&V system exceeds a user-defined down time interval such as 1 hour.

Fallback systems are designed to be an exact hardware and software mirror of the main R&V system and are typically located in the same server room or in close proximity to the R&V server. Each night a copy or update of the main R&V database is made to the fallback R&V system. With this setup, any engagement of the fallback system will ensure that the data are at most 24 hours old. Though the most recent changes to patient plans and new patient plans might not be available, the majority of patients will be able to be treated from the fallback R&V database.

The fallback database should be tested at installation, with each software upgrade, and at regular intervals. The testing has to be performed outside of regular treatment hours, ideally

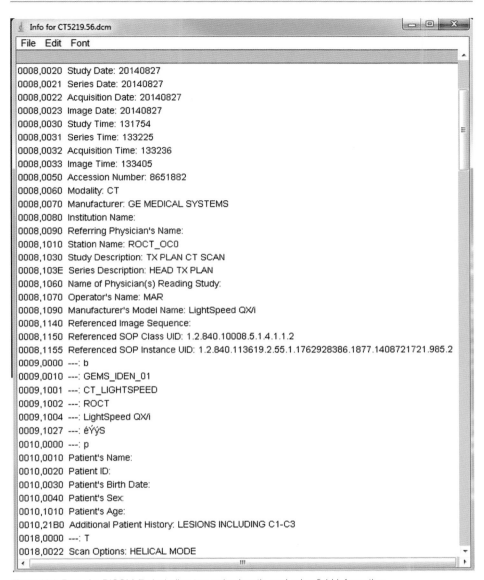

**Figure 11.1** Part of a DICOM file including tag, value length, and value field information.

starting at the end of a work week to allow sufficient time for recovery efforts if needed. Correctly accounting for the number of phantoms (as stand-in for patients) treated during the fallback and recovery phase should be included in the testing, because these are safety-critical processes to deliver the accurate total dose across software fallback and recovery.

## 11.7 Database Backup

Each database within the department should be backed up locally and also remotely to safeguard against a catastrophic event (e.g., earthquake). A good backup system has two levels: one that is immediately available locally to initiate the restore of a failed database, and a second level of backup located on servers at a large physical distance and in a different geophysical/climatic environment from the main database. This requirement serves to protect the backup database from being affected by the same catastrophic environmental event as the primary database. Examples of large-scale catastrophic events are hurricanes Katrina and Sandy or a major earth-quake hitting large population centers on the West Coast. Database restoration from the backup database should be tested at install, with each software upgrade, and at regular intervals.

## 11.8 Storage and Archive

As part of the installation of new software including a new database, storage needs for the expected lifetime of the software must be evaluated. In the example of a new R&V or treatment planning system (TPS), the typical file size per patient treatment course should be assessed. In some software systems, data can be archived (i.e., removed) from the working database to an archive database and restored as needed. Archive functionality should be tested at install, with each software upgrade, and at regular intervals.

## 11.9 Safety and Data Integrity

### DATA TRANSFER SAFETY

During the course of a radiation treatment, a patient's data set is transferred across the network and among different software packets and databases multiple times. For example:

- Patient PHI is imported from the hospital EHR to the Radiation Oncology R&V.
- Simulation images are acquired and transferred to the TPS or a third-party image fusion software.
- Additional diagnostic studies are downloaded from the hospital PACS to the TPS or a third-party image fusion software.
- The patient plan is transferred from the TPS through the R&V system onto the treatment machine.
- Treatment records are transferred from the treatment machine to the R&V system.

At each step, the file transfer integrity must be maintained. The most common tool used for this purpose is a checksum. In addition to checking the integrity of files after transfer, the routine checking of static files such as beam data files on a TPS is also recommended. If checksum functionality is not available, then confirming the file date and time stamp and file size is an alternative.

### ACCESS

Because much of the software used in Radiation Oncology contains PHI or directly drives patient treatments, access needs to be well thought out and managed. As a general rule, it is recommended that only staff who are required to use specific software for their work function are granted access. Additionally, user rights within the software should be configured such that only staff trained to use those rights within the software are permitted to use them. Typically, user rights are designed by groups of people; for example, in the TPS user groups would be designed for dosimetry, physics, attending physicians, and residents. Each software application should have two to three administrators: one main administrator and one or two other people familiar with the software and administrative functions to back up or cover in case the main administrator is not available.

Under certain circumstances (e.g., for the diagnostics of errors or system recovery), outside vendors need to be granted access to IT resources containing protected patient information. Before such access is granted, a contract such as a business associate agreement (BAA) or trust agreement must be in place.

## INSTALL CONFIGURATIONS

Many software solutions offer the choice between standalone installation on individual workstations or access through a centralized database through the Internet or Citrix servers. The advantage of a server-based installation, especially in larger departments, is that changes in software settings and software updates are standardized across all users. For example, in case of a second MU calculation check software, an update to beam data or tolerance levels made on a server-based version immediately transfers to all users, which minimizes the risk of users using old or outdated data.

## RESEARCH SOFTWARE

A special case of software safety is the instance in which research software used for similar purposes as standard software installs is present in the department. The safety risk in those situations is that software that is not intended for patient use is accidentally used for that purpose. Examples are CT image acquisition protocols, custom-designed brachytherapy planning software, or research scripts used in TPS. Before research software is installed, the medical physicist and IT support must verify that any install will not void warranties or violate FDA or other applicable regulations. Furthermore, research software must be tested for noninterference with clinical software; there should be no possibility of treatment-relevant data being changed by the research software. Ideally, research software should not be installed on the same workstations as clinical software if at all possible; this allows access to research software to be restricted by workstation and software password protection. All research involving access to patient data must be approved by an institutional review board (IRB) in the United States or by similar regulatory bodies in other countries.

## NEW VERSION UPGRADE AND TESTING

Each software upgrade must be thoroughly validated and tested before clinical release. Chapters 4 and 5 discuss the commissioning of new equipment and testing of TPS software. Similar principles apply to all other software used in Radiation Oncology. Software upgrade and testing projects can have vastly different scales, ranging from relatively short projects such as upgrading secondary MU calculation check software to multiday endeavors such as upgrading the R&V system. There are different strategies for minimizing interruption to the clinical workflow:

- For small software upgrades only requiring a few hours of QA, the upgrade can be scheduled to allow sufficient time for thorough testing with the option to revert to the original software version.
- In some situations it is possible to set up a testing environment simulating the install environment. New software can be tested in this environment first before the install goes clinical. One example is using a mirrored database server for the R&V system to test an R&V software upgrade.
- Running software in parallel: In this situation, the clinic continues to work on the current software while the new software is installed in parallel. Access to the new software should be password protected and limited to the commissioning team. Once commissioning and testing are completed, the new software can be released while at the same time access to the old software is removed.

**FOR THE PHYSICIAN**

IT is an integral part of radiation treatment delivery, and Radiation Oncology departments typically have IT needs that are distinct from general hospital systems (such as treatment planning and R&V systems). ACR and AAPM have guidelines for privacy and security, as well as reports that provide an overview of IT needs. As more clinics move away from paper charts to EHR, it is important to be mindful of key components of a successful EHR, including a good organizational structure for locating information quickly, ability to generate checklists, and workflow tracking. In addition, all staff members should be able to access the software and data required for their job performance, but access should be limited to protect system integrity.

One essential IT component for Radiation Oncology is a R&V system to ensure documentation of radiation treatment delivered. Depending on the exact systems used, there are often challenges associated with integrating the R&V system with the Radiation Oncology EHR and overall hospital EHR. Specific areas of challenge include billing, scheduling, documentation, and imaging. Since major treatment interruptions have negative clinical impact, there should be a fallback system for the R&V database. There should also be regular backups for all departmental data. System upgrades must be thoroughly tested prior to release.

IHE-RO is a group focusing on effective data sharing between systems. In support of these goals, DICOM was developed as a standard for exchanging imaging data among systems and sites. There is also functionality for storing radiation dose, contours/structures, plans, and treatment records. When data are being sent between different systems (such as hospital EHR to TPS, or TPS to R&V), the data reliability and security must remain intact.

## References

1. ACR-AAPM-SIIM Practice Parameter for Electronic Medical Information Privacy and Security Res. 37-2014.   http://www.acr.org/Quality-Safety/Standards-Guidelines/Practice-Guidelines-by-Modality/Documentation-Reporting.
2. Siochi RA, Blater P, Bloch CD, et al. Information technology resource management in Radiation Oncology. J Appl Clin Med Phys 2009;10(4):16–35.

# CHAPTER 12

# Quality and Safety Improvement in Radiation Oncology

## 12.1 Introduction

### WATERSHED ACCIDENTS IN RADIATION ONCOLOGY

One way to view the issue of quality and safety in radiotherapy is to consider the serious accidents that have garnered the attention of the community and occasionally the media. The purpose of such an exercise is to understand the error pathways involved and prevent such events in the future. To this end, Table 12.1 summarizes selected watershed accidents in Radiation Oncology. Of particular note is the tragic death of Scott Jerome Parks, a patient with oropharyngeal cancer who received treatment in New York and was given a large radiation overdose. His story was reported in the U.S. national news media in 2010 and galvanized support for improved safety in radiation therapy.

Further material and information on accidents in radiation therapy can be found in International Atomic Energy Agency (IAEA) Safety Report No. 17 from 2000,[9] which gives a brief account of 92 incidents. In the United States various public records are available, including through the U.S. Nuclear Regulatory Commission (NRC) Agencywide Documents Access and Management System (ADAMS), a searchable repository of public documents of medical events involving by-product materials (https://forms.nrc.gov/reading-rm/adams.html# web-based-adams), and the Manufacturer and User Device Experience (MAUDE) database (http://www.accessdata.fda.gov/scripts/cdrh/cfdocs/cfmaude/search.cfm) from the Food and Drug Administration (FDA), where information on reported device errors is held.

The overview in Table 12.1 focuses on serious radiation therapy accidents (i.e., catastrophic failures), but it must be recognized that less serious failures are much more common in clinical practice. Such errors are often discussed in the context of "quality of care" as opposed to patient safety. "Quality" and "safety," however, are intermixed concepts in medicine. That is, "low quality care" (care that is deficient in some way) is usually also unsafe care, and vice versa. This is different from many other industries where one can deliver a low quality product (e.g., a car) that may not be, in itself, unsafe. Dunscombe et al.[10] have argued that quality and safety are part of a Gaussian-like spectrum (the most unsafe care lying on the tails of the distribution) and have estimated that in the United States "approximately 20,000 patients per year have their outcome compromised to some unknown extent by poor-quality radiotherapy." Objective estimates of error rates in Radiation Oncology are difficult to formulate. Approximate estimates indicate a rate of misadministrations of 0.2%, though this is likely an underestimate.[11]

### THE QUALITY GAP AND OUTCOMES DATA

Regardless of the terms one uses to describe the situation, there are compelling data in radiotherapy that link quality and safety to patient outcomes. For example, in the Trans Tasman

TABLE 12.1 ▪ Select Watershed Accidents in Radiation Oncology

| Dates | Location | Incident Description | Reference |
|-------|----------|----------------------|-----------|
| 1972-1976 | Columbus, OH | Miscalibration of $^{60}$Co machine output due to linear extrapolation of decay. 40% overdose after 4 years. 10 deaths, 78 serious injuries. | [1] |
| 1985-1987 | Four U.S. sites | Therac-25 treatment unit from AECL. Latent software error causes high current of photon mode to be used in electron treatment. 160-180 Gy to six patients. | [2] |
| 1990 | Zargoza, Spain | Miscalibration of electron beam on Sagittaire linac during a technician service repair. 35 MeV for all beams with up to nine times the intended output. Energy dial indicator interpreted as "stuck." 15 deaths. | [3] |
| 2004-2009 | Springfield, MO | Error commissioning stereotactic radiosurgery (SRS) system results in 50% output deviation. Farmer chamber used to measure field sizes <1.1 cm. 127 patients treated, 76 receive >50% overdose. | [4,5] |
| 2004-2005 | Tampa, FL | Error commissioning SRS system. Percent depth dose (PDD) factor not used in AAPM TG-51 output due to corrupted Excel file. 77 patients receive >50% overdose. | [6] |
| 2005 | New York, NY | Patient Scott Jerome Parks receiving Intensity modulated radiation therapy (IMRT) for head and neck (H&N), receives 13 Gy x 3 to open field (no modulation) due to computer crash during replanning in which multi-leaf collimator (MLC) files were lost. Patient died in 2007. | [3,7] |
| 2006 | Glasgow, Scotland | Patient Lisa Norris receiving whole central nervous system (CNS) irradiation for pineoblastoma receives 58% overdose to brain fields due to plan calculation error (2.92 Gy x 19 vs. an intended 1.75 Gy x 20). Patient died 6 months later. | [3,8] |

A brief description of the incident is provided for learning purposes. Further information on causal factors and other details can be found in the references.

Radiation Oncology Group (TROG) 02.02 trial for head and neck cancer Peters et al.[12] have shown that protocol deviations are significantly correlated with overall survival. Their technique involved a reanalysis of the dosimetric data from the multicenter international trial. Similarly, a recent meta-analysis by Ohri et al.[13] of eight trials showed that protocol deviations resulted in significantly more treatment failures and higher mortality in most cases.

## PRESCRIPTIVE QUALITY ASSURANCE VERSUS SYSTEMS THINKING

In medical physics the traditional approach to addressing quality relies on prescriptive quality assurance (QA) often codified in the form of task group reports and other documents. There are numerous such recommendations (see, e.g., American Association of Physicists in Medicine (AAPM) Task Group (TG) reports listed in Appendix I); indeed, such prescriptive QA measures form a large portion of the present book. It has been realized more recently, however, that prescriptive QA has important limitations. More than 200 steps may be required in a typical modern workflow,[14] and prescriptive QA is ineffective at probing most of them. A more productive approach is that of "systems thinking," which addresses the clinical care delivery process and environment as a whole. This is the subject of the rest of this chapter. Though some aspects of this may fall outside of the traditional purview of the medical physicist, it is still within the scope of practice of the medical physicist as a manager and leader of the departmental quality management program.

## SAFETY CULTURE, JUST CULTURE, AND HUMAN ERROR

The term "safety culture" was first used in the wake of the accident at the Chernobyl nuclear power facility.[15] It is used to signify a "commitment to safety at all levels, from frontline providers to managers and executives" (Agency for Healthcare Research and Quality (AHRQ)). Safety culture has been clearly linked to patient outcomes.[16]

AHRQ is one of the most authoritative sources on the topic of safety culture. The agency administers a patient safety culture survey each year in which thousands of hospitals participate and provides a primer on the topic (http://psnet.ahrq.gov/primer.aspx?primerID=5). Four key features of a safety culture are identified:[17]

1. Acknowledgment of the high-risk nature of an organization's activities and the determination to achieve consistently safe operations
2. A blame-free environment where individuals are able to report errors or near misses without fear of reprimand or punishment
3. Encouragement of collaboration across ranks and disciplines to seek solutions to patient safety problems
4. Organizational commitment of resources to address safety concerns

The last point especially highlights the need for leadership support of safety culture. This is a concept frequently noted in the Radiation Oncology literature as well (e.g., American Society for Radiation Oncology (ASTRO) report Safety Is No Accident).[18] A useful discussion of the role that physicians play can be found in the editorial by Marks et al.,[17] which advocates that physicians must serve as "champions for a safety culture." A specific example of this can be found in Potters and Kapur.[19]

The basis of a positive safety culture is the concept of "just culture," that is, a culture in which staff are empowered to take on safety-critical actions in an environment that supports and encourages this. To fully understand just culture and safety culture one has to appreciate what drives human error. In this regard the work of Sydney Dekker has been widely cited and influential in healthcare (e.g., *The Field Guide to Understanding Human Error*).[20] In Dr. Dekker's view the old model of error held that the major source of medical errors was the (under)performance of individual people, the "bad apples." He calls for a more nuanced and productive approach, however, which is to understand what drives human error. The realization that "most people don't come to work to do a bad job" leads one to focus more productively on the environment and system around the person that lead him or her toward error.

---

**Patient Safety: Further Resources for Learning**

A wealth of information is available regarding patient safety and quality improvement both within Radiation Oncology and beyond. The following is a select list of references for further reading and education:

- AAPM 2013 Summer School and "Quality and Safety on Radiotherapy"[21]
- IAEA Report No. 17, Lessons Learned from Accidental Exposures in Radiotherapy[9]
- Online (fee-based) modules on patient safety education from the National Patient Safety Foundation (NPSF). See npsf.org.

---

## 12.2 Features of an Effective Quality Management System

Though quality management (QM) is an evolving topic, there are several well-established features that should be present in all Radiation Oncology practices as recommended by numerous

TABLE 12.2　■　**Quality Management Approaches as Recommended in Various References**

| Section | QM Approach | Comments | References |
|---------|-------------|----------|------------|
| 12.2.1 | Peer review | Case-oriented review of radiotherapy plans by one or more peers. | 22,23 |
| 12.2.2 | Checklists | Used for safety-critical processes. Value in standardizing practice and ensuring compliance. | 24 |
| 12.2.3 | Physics plan and chart review | Review of initial plan by a qualified medical physicist; also weekly review of chart. | 18,22,25-27 |
| 12.2.4 | Audits | Independent evaluation. Includes audits of commissioning data, beam output, and phantom tests. | 18,25,28,29 |
| 12.2.5 | Staff training and competency | Continuing medical education on procedures and the safe operation of equipment. | 18,25,26,30,31 |
| 12.2.6 | Policies and procedures | Policies and procedures should be carefully described and documented. | 18,30,32,33 |
| 12.3.2 | Incident learning system | A formalized system for logging and evaluating incidents and near-misses. | 18,30,34-37 |

documents endorsed by various professional societies. Table 12.2 provides an overview list of the most common of these. Some are administrative in nature (e.g., the maintenance of policies and procedures) while some refer to specific QM tasks (e.g., plan checks).

## PEER REVIEW

Peer review is a key feature of high quality care. An important reference for physicists is AAPM TG-103 report on peer review in clinical radiaion oncology physics,[22] which describes the peer review of the clinical process from the physics perspective. In clinical operations, "peer review" is often taken to be synonymous with the peer review of patients' plans by physicians at the start of treatment (i.e., "chart rounds" or "QA rounds"), though peer review can be much more general than that. A key reference is the ASTRO safety white paper on peer review.[23] Table 2 in that reference lists different areas for peer review, the highest priority areas being review of target definition and treatment delivery.

## CHECKLISTS

Checklists are an important tool for error reduction and have been featured in popular accounts in healthcare showing their remarkable effectiveness.[38,39] Checklists are a tool for standardizing and enforcing the most safety-critical aspects of operations. While a well-designed checklist can be very impactful, a poorly designed checklist can do little more than create extra work and may even have a negative safety impact. Recognizing this, the AAPM Medical Physics Practice Guideline 3[24] considers the topic of checklists and presents the principles for the design and validation of an effective checklist.

## PHYSICS INITIAL PLAN REVIEW AND WEEKLY CHART REVIEW

Of particular importance to medical physicists are the initial plan review and weekly chart review. Numerous reports recommend that these tasks be performed (see Table 12.3). The work of Ford et al.[40] suggests that initial physics plan review may be the most effective safety practice in the clinical process. Very little information is available, however, as to how to best perform these checks. This represents an area for future development and perhaps the availability of automatic software to check for common errors will become wide spread.[41-43]

TABLE 12.3 ▪ **Society-Level Recommendations for Physics Review of New Plans and Weekly Checks of Charts**

| Source | Recommendation |
|---|---|
| AAPM TG-40[27] | Calls for weekly chart review and specifies what this should consist of (see Section VI.C, Chart Check Protocol) |
| ACR Technical Standards for EBRT[25] | "The medical physicist must review each patient's chart to ensure accuracy of calculation, appropriateness of charting data, and fulfillment of the physicians' written prescription." And "physics chart review must be conducted at least weekly." (Section C.4.a) |
| ACR Practice Guidelines on RO[26] | "Documentation that the treatment record was checked weekly during treatment" |
| ASTRO Report "Safety Is No Accident"[18] | Table 2.1 notes "weekly evaluation" as one of the roles of the medical physicist |
| AAPM TG-103 Peer Review in Clinical Radiation Oncology Physics[22] | "Verify that the chart was reviewed by the physics staff on a weekly basis." (Section B.2) |

## AUDITS

Audits can take many forms, but the broad goal is to provide an independent assessment of a clinical procedure conducted by an objective third party. As an example, AAPM TG-106, Accelerator Beam Data Commissioning Equipment and Procedures,[28] calls for an audit of the collected data by an independent physicist. On the other end of the spectrum, the entire Radiation Oncology practice can be audited through the process of practice accreditation, which has been run through the American College of Radiology (ACR), American College of Radiation Oncology (ACRO), and, as of 2015, ASTRO's APeX program (Accreditation Program for Excellence).

One widely used form of audit is an independent validation of the output of a device under reference conditions. This is accomplished by a mail-in dosimetry service.[44] Both the ASTRO report Safety Is No Accident[18] and the ACR technical standards for external beam radiation therapy (EBRT)[25] call for this audit to be done at commissioning and annually thereafter. The ACR guidelines also allow for a check by an independent physicist. The Imaging and Radiation Oncology Core-Houston (IROC-H) defines a 5% dose agreement between the institution-reported dose and the measured dose. One 2006 study from the IROC-H group showed that 11% of institutions fell outside this range,[45] further underscoring the need for such audits.

Audits can also take the form of credentialing required to participate in cooperative group trials. This is accomplished by means of an anthropomorphic phantom sent from the credentialing agency containing target structures, films, and thermoluminescent dosimeters/optically stimulated luminescent dosimeters (TLDs/OSLDs). The phantom is scanned, planned, and irradiated by the participating institution, and then the results are read at the credentialing agency (see Molineu et al.[29] for details and images of various phantoms). There have been challenges with institutions meeting the phantom irradiation pass criteria set forth by IROC-H; for example, 30% of institutions have not met the 7%/4 mm agreement for the head and neck phantom.[46]

## STAFF COMPETENCY AND TRAINING

Technical competency is a cornerstone of safe operations. Virtually all of the major society-level safety recommendations advocate strongly for staff training. In the World Health Organization (WHO) report Radiotherapy Risk Profile,[31] for example, staff training is recommended nine separate places. The ACR practice guidelines for Radiation Oncology[26] describe continuing medical education programs that "must cover the safe operation of facility equipment as appropriate to the individual's responsibility, and the treatment techniques and new developments in Radiation Oncology. " Similar recommendations are found in the UK report Towards Safer Radiotherapy[30] and the ASTRO report Safety Is No Accident.[18] Training should not be restricted to vendor-provided training of therapists. It should be multidisciplinary in nature, a point that is highlighted in the ACR practice guidelines for Radiation Oncology that note that training should "include the radiation oncologists and the physics, dosimetry, nursing, and radiation therapy staffs."[26]

As techniques and technology evolve, training also needs to be updated regularly. The need for continued (re)training is underscored in the ASTRO report Safety Is No Accident[18] and the ACR practice guidelines for Radiation Oncology.[26] Records of attendance at training events should also be kept.[30]

## POLICIES AND PROCEDURES

Having well-defined and well-documented policies and procedures is a cornerstone of an effective quality management program. A number of reports make the point that policies and procedures should be carefully described and documented.[18,30,32,33] Policies and procedures should be kept in a place that is easily accessible to staff (e.g., online), and any changes must be communicated. Good practice is to document with signatures that changes have been read and understood. Strict version control should be maintained to ensure that everyone has access to the most current policies and procedures. Changes to policy and procedure should have a defined process for approval and implementation. The UK Towards Safer Radiotherapy report specifically calls for these procedures to be reviewed every 2 years or when there are significant changes. While ACR and ASTRO have no specific guidelines in this regard, ACRO calls for policy and procedure manuals to be reviewed once a year and every time a new policy is implemented. The Joint Commission (TJC) recommends they be reviewed during orientation of new employees. The 1998 report from European Society for Radiotherapy and Oncology (ESTRO), Practical Guidelines for the Implementation of a Quality System in Radiotherapy,[33] describes the development of a "quality manual" with reference to ISO9000 certification.

## AAPM SAFETY PROFILE ASSESSMENT TOOL

The vast array of information outlined in the sections above gives an indication of the scope of society-level recommendations. In an attempt to streamline this and provide a practical tool for the community at large, the AAPM has developed an online tool, the Safety Profile Assessment (SPA, spa.aapm.org), which collates all of the safety-critical recommendations. Released in 2013, the SPA consists of 92 questions designed to probe safety-critical aspects of the Radiation Oncology environment. The tool allows participants to save their answers, compare from year to year, and benchmark against other participants in the system. The SPA is free and does not require AAPM membership. SPA has been qualified by the ABR as meeting the criteria for Practice Quality Improvement requirements of the ABR Maintenance of Certification Program (http://www.theabr.org/moc-rp-pqi-projects).

# 12.3 Techniques for Quality Improvement

## FAILURE MODE AND EFFECTS ANALYSIS

Originally developed by the U.S. military and National Aeronautics and Space Administration (NASA), failure mode and effects analysis (FMEA) provides a rational means for identifying and prioritizing risk. FMEA has been widely used in healthcare and is specifically recommended in the United States by TJC. The first report of its use in the Radiation Oncology clinical environment appeared in 2009,[14] and other single institution reports have followed.[47-54] FMEA is the subject of AAPM TG-100[55] which was formed in 2003. AAPM TG-100 will provide a definitive guide of FMEA in Radiation Oncology. As of this writing, the AAPM TG-100 report has been approved by the AAPM and is under review for publication. Further information can be found in the proceedings of the 2013 AAPM Summer School on Quality and Safety in Radiotherapy.[21]

An FMEA exercise consists of identifying a clinical process(es) for evaluation and then identifying all of the "failure modes" that can occur in all the steps in that process. A visual map of the process is often helpful in this regard. A failure mode is essentially anything that can go wrong; each failure mode is associated with one or more antecedent causes. For example, the wrong leg might be identified in treatment planning. Along with each failure mode, a cause is also listed. In this case the wrong site might be due to a left-right reversal because the patient was scanned feet first. Some CT systems have protocols to automatically flip scans to head-first with the goal of standardizing the way that scans are visualized by surgeons. In FMEA, three scores are assigned to each failure mode and cause: severity ($S$), probability of occurrence ($O$), and probability that the failure would go undetected ($D$). Traditionally a ten-point scale is used, and though the absolute values of scores are difficult to quantify, it is the relative values that are of most interest. Finally the $S$, $O$, and $D$ scores are multiplied together to yield a risk priority number (i.e., RPN = $S \times O \times D$). The failure modes are then ranked by RPN, the top-ranked RPN being the failure mode that should be mitigated first. Guidelines on how to score $S$, $O$, and $D$ have been presented previously[14] and can be found in AAPM TG-100. One concern with FMEA is that it is a labor-intensive process, an attitude that may be fueled in part by the 10-year timeline for the completion of AAPM TG-100. This need not be so, however. One of the authors has recently demonstrated a streamlined FMEA process that required 55 hours of staff time and 20 hours of facilitator time for a relatively large-scale FMEA of an entire external beam radiotherapy service.[56]

## INCIDENT LEARNING AND ROOT-CAUSE ANALYSIS

*Incident learning* refers to the identification of problems in the care delivery process and the subsequent investigation of those problems with the aim of uncovering and addressing causal factors and latent conditions for error. There are numerous institutional studies of incident learning in Radiation Oncology dating back to the work of Fraass et al. in the 1990s[57] and continuing on more recently (see the AAPM white paper on incident learning[34] and references therein). The need for incident learning is now well established and specifically recommended in reports approved by various professional societies (see Table 12.4). Though it is possible to use generic hospital reporting systems for incident learning, there are advantages to systems that are tailored for Radiation Oncology. The design and operations of incident learning systems are discussed in detail in the AAPM white paper on incident learning,[34] which focuses particularly on information technology aspects specific to Radiation Oncology.

One key question is what type of information should be entered into the incident learning system. Serious reportable incidents are one type of incident, but these are relatively rare, and incident learning is much broader than just reportable events. AHRQ identifies three categories of safety events (italics denote AHRQ definitions):

1. **Incident:** *A patient safety event that reached the patient, whether or not the patient was harmed.* For example, a wrong isocenter location that is treated for one fraction but then found by a physician reviewing images and corrected for subsequent fractions. This is an error that reached the patient, but depending on the clinical situation this may not cause any harm to the patient.
2. **Near-miss:** *A patient safety event that did not reach the patient.* This is sometimes referred to as a "close call." For example, an error in treatment planning that results in a wrong isocenter location. The error is caught on the initial physics plan review, making this a near-miss.

TABLE 12.4 ■ Society-Level Recommendations for Incident Learning

| Source | Recommendation |
| --- | --- |
| UK Report Towards Safer Radiotherapy[30] | "Each radiotherapy center must operate a quality system, which should ensure best practice is maintained by applying lessons learnt from radiotherapy incidents and near misses from other departments as well as in-house." |
| ASTRO Safety Is No Accident[18] | "Employees should be encouraged to report both errors and near-misses (errors that almost happen)." And: "a quality assurance committee.... should ensure that a mechanism for reporting and monitoring errors and near-misses is in place." |
| ASTRO Safety White Paper on IMRT[36] | Recommends "[an incident reporting structure] to improve error prevention and remediation of events (any unplanned/undocumented deviation from the department's standard process or the patient's expected treatment), the team should discuss potential and actual sources of errors and document all events that occur." |
| ASTRO Safety White Paper on IGRT[35] | "Establish a reporting mechanism for IGRT-related variances in the radiation treatment process." |
| AAPM Consensus White Paper on Incident Learning[34] | "Discipline-specific incident learning systems would significantly improve the practice of Radiation Oncology." |
| ASRT White Paper Radiation Therapy Safety: The Critical Role of the Radiation Therapist[37] | "Reporting of errors is expected and encouraged (of a radiation therapist)." "Radiation therapists should be encouraged to document all errors and exceptions." "It is imperative that radiation therapists feel they can report errors and near-misses—according to the standards and ethics that guide their profession—without fear of negative repercussions." "ASRT rules of ethics for radiological technologists include possible sanctions for any radiation therapist who fails 'to immediately report to his or her supervisor information concerning an error made in connection with imaging, treating, or caring for a patient.'" |

3. **Unsafe condition:** *Any circumstance that increases the probability of a patient safety event.* For example, an unclear set of policies as to when port films are to be checked by physicians.

Near-miss events are particularly useful for incident learning because they are much more numerous than incidents that reach the patient. They offer additional opportunities for learning in a situation with no impact to the patient. Mutic et al.[58] and other groups have advocated for the collection of near-miss events; as many as one incident per patient may be registered. Near-miss incident learning is discussed and advocated in the AAPM white paper on incident learning.[34] Near-miss events are well recognized outside of Radiation Oncology (cf. Albert Wu's textbook on "close calls"[59]).

Root-cause analysis goes hand-in-hand with incident learning. The goal of root-cause analysis is to uncover the underlying causal factors that drive errors. The goal in doing this is to get beyond the simplistic label of "human error," understand what drives errors, and arrive at actionable safety improvement interventions. The concepts of just culture and drivers of human error outlined in a preceding section are particularly relevant in this regard. RCA is typically a very time-intensive process, requiring many hours to complete. It is beyond the scope of this text to fully describe the RCA technique, but useful materials can be found in the 2013 AAPM Summer School, Chapter 6.[21] Protocols for conducting an RCA can be found in the London protocol,[60] the VA system protocol,[61] and TJC framework.[62]

## Reportable Events and Regulatory Agencies

The most serious incidents may rise to the level of an event that must be reported to the patient and to the relevant regulatory agencies. Prompt reporting and investigation are important following any such serious incident (cf. IAEA General Safety Requirements Report Part 3, Requirement #41[63]). Another aspect is the discussion and disclosure of the incident to the patient and his or her family. One recent study explores the attitudes of Radiation Oncology physicians in this regard.[64] The majority of clinicians would disclose errors, though not all were familiar with established best practices for disclosure.

A valuable resource for safety and regulatory issues on the international level is the IAEA's Radiation Protection of Patients (RPOP) program (rpop.iaea.org). In the United States external beam radiotherapy is regulated by the states. Each state agency determines its own rules for what constitutes a reportable event. There are recommended standards, however—in particular, Part X: Therapeutic Radiation Machines from the Congress of Radiation Control Program Directors (CRCPD), which defines a misadministration as (1) the wrong patient, wrong treatment modality, or wrong treatment site, or (2) a 30% deviation from weekly prescribed dose, or (3) a 20% deviation of total dose. The definitions that NRC uses are slightly different, but this is not usually relevant because the NRC does not regulate nonisotope treatment equipment except in VA facilities.

For brachytherapy the situation differs somewhat. CRCPG "Part G" and the NRC currently define a medical event as (1) the wrong radioactive drug, (2) the wrong route of administration, (3) the wrong patient, (4) the wrong mode of treatment, or (5) a leaking sealed source. An excess of 0.5 Sv to an organ or tissue or skin other than the treatment site and exceeding 50% of the dose expected from the written directive is also considered a medical event. The use of radioisotopes in the United States is regulated by the NRC except in "agreement states" (of which there are 37), which take on this responsibility from the NRC. The relevant regulatory statute is 10 CFR 35. The current 10 CFR 35 statutes date back to 2002, but as of 2013 the NRC is proposing an amendment that would change the regulations (http://www.regulations.gov/#!documentDetail;D=NRC-2008-0175-0017). Among other things it would create a separate definition of a medical event for permanent brachytherapy implants as follows: (1) 20% of sources implanted outside the intended site, or (2) 150% dose deviation to 5 cm$^3$ of contiguous normal tissue or target structure, compared to the preimplant written directive.

## Voluntary Incident Learning Systems and the Radiation Oncology Incident Learning System

The above considerations apply to reportable events, but many events do not rise to the level of being reportable but may be of interest to record and analyze. The potential benefit of sharing information about such events among institutions has been appreciated for many years. An early model for this was the ROSIS (Radiation Oncology Safety Information System), led by a group at Trinity College, Dublin.[65] More recently, the SAFRON system developed by the IAEA has come online. Both systems have an organization and database architecture that is consistent with the AAPM white paper on incident learning.

Within the U.S. medical-legal environment, however, voluntary shared incident learning can be a challenge if information is not protected from discovery. Recognizing the need for a protected voluntary incident learning system, ASTRO and AAPM have joined together to sponsor the Radiation Oncology Incident Learning System (RO-ILS, astro.org/roils). This system, launched in June of 2014, is formulated as a patient safety organization (PSO), which is a mechanism within the United States to provide legal protection, made possible by the Patient Safety Quality Improvement Act of 2005. Information in PSO systems is both confidential and privileged. The structure and design of the RO-ILS is consistent with the AAPM white paper on incident learning. The RO-ILS has been qualified by the ABR as meeting the criteria for practice quality improvement requirements of the ABR Maintenance of Certification Program

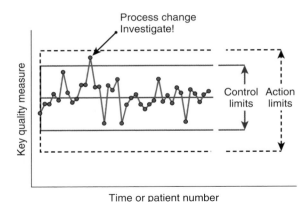

Time or patient number

**Figure 12.1** Control chart used in statistical process control. *(Adapted from Pawlicki T, Chera B, Ning T, et al., The systematic application of quality measures and process control in clinical Radiation Oncology. Semin Radiat Oncol, 2012;22(1):70-6, Fig 2.)*

(http://www.theabr.org/moc-rp-pqi-projects). Currently participation in the RO-ILS is offered as a no-fee contract sponsored by ASTRO and AAPM. Another PSO specifically designed for Radiation Oncology is operated by the nonprofit group the Center for Assessment of Radiological Sciences (CARS). The CARS PSO includes a publicly searchable database with roughly 50 reports as of mid-2013.

## STATISTICAL PROCESS CONTROL

Statistical process control (SPC) is a method to measure and control variability in processes. It relies on control charts to track a data measure of interest, such as the pass rate of IMRT QA plans. Upper and lower control limits are set that are determined by the variability in the process (e.g., 3σ); these are distinct from action limits that are set by an a priori standard of what is clinically acceptable (see Figure 12.1). Measurable endpoints for SPC might include physics-related quality measures (e.g., linac output) and also clinical practice measures (e.g., time from simulation to planning) or patient-related measures (e.g., patient pain levels or treatment breaks). Pawlicki et al.[66] review these and other indicator measures that might be useful in Radiation Oncology.

Though no society-level recommendations exist yet concerning SPC, a number of institutional reports have appeared. SPC has been used in the context of linear accelerator QA.[67] It has also been used to study and control IMRT QA,[68-72] with the suggestion that site-specific tolerances might be required.[71] SPC has been used to study and control clinical workflow. Kapur and Potters[73] studied the number of "slip days" in the planning and delivery process as a measure of process control. The method relies on time stamps of quality checklists in the oncology information system to measure slips. Through various interventions, the average number of slip days was reduced and, more importantly, so was the standard deviation. Further background reading on SPC can be found in Pawlicki et al.[66] and the AAPM 2013 Summer School, Chapter 7.[21]

**FOR THE PHYSICIAN**

From the medical physics perspective, quality and safety improvement have long been tied to performing prescriptive QA measures (e.g., dose calibration checks performed according to well-defined prescriptive protocols). Though such prescriptive QA is no doubt invaluable, it is now recognized that maintaining and improving safety and quality extend far beyond such prescriptive measures. This was driven in part by the watershed accidents in radiation therapy reported in 2010.

Best practices for an effective quality management program are well described in numerous reports approved by national and international societies. Best practices include the following:

- Establish formal policies and procedures
- Employ audits where appropriate (e.g., independent checks of linac output)
- Institute regular peer review of cases
- Perform physics checks of new patient plans and weekly checks of patients on treatment
- Use checklists where appropriate
- Provide ongoing training of staff
- Utilize incident learning with formal review of events including near-misses

A tool developed by the AAPM, the Safety Profile Assessment (spa.aapm.org), provides a means to probe a clinic's performance in these various aspects and benchmark it against data from other participants. Another tool for auditing performance is practice accreditation whereby the entire Radiation Oncology practice is examined by an independent group of experts. The APeX program from ASTRO is one such system in the United States. Internationally, some clinics are employing ISO9000 certification as a certification of good QM practices.

In addition to these QM tools, there are emerging techniques for quality improvement. Voluntary incident learning is one that is strongly encouraged by numerous reports. In the United States a medical-specialty sponsored system is available, the Radiation Oncology Incident Learning System (RO-ILS), sponsored by ASTRO and AAPM. This provides a protected and secure environment for sharing safety-critical information. Other systems are available as well. Another method for risk assessment is failure mode and effects analysis (FMEA), which provides a rational method for assessing risk in a prospective manner. Society-level documents are forthcoming, and a sizable literature of institutional experience with this technique is available. Finally, a valuable emerging tool is statistical process control, which seeks to measure and control process deviations through measurement of various technical or clinical endpoints.

### References

1. Rubin LS. The Riverside radiation tragedy. Columbus Monthly, 52–65, 1978.
2. Leveson NG, Turner CS. An investigation of the Therac-25 accidents. Computer 1993;26(7):18–41.
3. IAEA, IAEA training materials: Module 2, prevention of accidental exposure in radiotherapy. Vienna: International Atomic Energy Agency; 2009.
4. Bogdanich W, Ruiz RR. Radiation errors reported in Missouri. New York Times 2010. Available from: <http://www.nytimes.com/2010/02/25/us/25radiation.html>.
5. CoxHealth. CoxHealth announces some BrainLAB stereotactic radiation therapy patients received increased radiation dose 2010. Available from: <http://www.coxhealth.com/body.cfm?id=3701>.
6. Bogdanich W. As technology surges, radiation safeguards lag. New York Times 2010. Available from: <http://www.nytimes.com/2010/01/27/us/27radiation.html>.
7. Bogdanich W. Radiation offers new cures, and ways to do harm. New York Times 2010. Available from: <http://www.nytimes.com/2010/01/24/health/24radiation.html>.
8. Executive TS. Report into unintended overexposure of Lisa Norris at Beatson. Glasgow: Scottish Govt; 2006.
9. IAEA. Lessons learned from accidental exposures in radiotherapy, in Safety Report Series, International Atomic Energy Agency. Vienna, Austria: IAEA; 2000.
10. Dunscombe P, Evans S, Williamson J, et al. Introduction to quality. In: Thomadsen B, editor. Quality and safety in radiotherapy. Madison, WI: Medical Physics Publishing; 2013. p. 1–30.
11. Ford EC, Terezakis S. How safe is safe?: Risk in radiotherapy. Int J Radiat Oncol Biol Phys 2010;8(2):321.
12. Peters LJ, O'Sullivan B, Giralt J, et al. Critical impact of radiotherapy protocol compliance and quality in the treatment of advanced head and neck cancer: Results from TROG 02.02. J Clin Oncol 2010;28(18):2996–3001.
13. Ohri N, Shen X, Dicker AP, et al. Radiotherapy protocol deviations and clinical outcomes: A meta-analysis of cooperative group clinical trials. J Nat Cancer Instit 2013;105(6):387–93.

14. Ford EC, Gaudette R, Myers L, et al. Evaluation of safety in a Radiation Oncology setting using failure mode and effects analysis. Int J Radiat Oncol Biol Phys 2009;74(3):852–8.

15. IAEA. Ten years after Chernobyl: What do we really know? 1996 Available from: <http://www.iaea.org/Publications/Booklets/Chernoten/index.html>.

16. Mardon RE, Khanna K, Sorra J, et al. Exploring relationships between hospital patient safety culture and adverse events. J Patient Saf 2010;6(4):226–32.

17. Marks LB, Rose CM, Hayman JA, et al. The need for physician leadership in creating a culture of safety. Int J Radiat Oncol Biol Phys 2011;79(5):1287–9.

18. Zeitman A, Palta J, Steinberg M. Safety is no accident: A framework for quality Radiation Oncology and care. ASTRO; 2012.

19. Potters L, Kapur A. Implementation of a "No Fly" safety culture in a multicenter radiation medicine department. Pract Radiat Oncol 2012;2(1):18–26.

20. Dekker S, Dekker S. The field guide to understanding human error. Aldershot, England; Burlington, VT: Ashgate; 2006. p. xv, 236.

21. Thomadsen B, Dunscombe P, Ford E, et al., editors. Quality and safety in radiotherapy: Learning the new approaches in Task Group 100 and beyond. Madison, WI: Medical Physics Publishing; 2013.

22. Halvorsen PH, Das IJ, Fraser M, et al. AAPM Task Group 103 report on peer review in clinical Radiation Oncology physics. J Applied Clin Med Phys/American College of Medical Physics 2005; 6(4):50–64.

23. Marks LB, Adams RD, Pawlicki T, et al. Enhancing the role of case-oriented peer review to improve quality and safety in Radiation Oncology: Executive summary. Pract Radiat Oncol 2013;3(3):149–56.

24. Fong de Los Santos L, et al. Medical Physics Practice Guideline Task Group 3.a: Development, implementation, use and maintenance of safety checklists. J Clin Appl Med Phys 2015; in review.

25. ACR technical standard for the performance of Radiation Oncology physics for external beam therapy. American College of Radiology; 2010.

26. ACR practice guidelines and technical standards: Radiation Oncology. American College of Radiology; 2011.

27. Kutcher GJ, Coia L, Gillin M, et al. Comprehensive QA for Radiation Oncology: Report of AAPM Radiation Therapy Committee Task Group 40. Med Phys 1994;21(4):581–618.

28. Das IJ, Cheng CW, Watts RJ, et al. Accelerator beam data commissioning equipment and procedures: Report of the TG-106 of the Therapy Physics Committee of the AAPM. Med Phys 2008;35(9): 4186–215.

29. Molineu A, Followill DS, Balter PA, et al. Design and implementation of an anthropomorphic quality assurance phantom for intensity-modulated radiation therapy for the radiation therapy oncology group. Int J Radiat Oncol Biol Phys 2005;63(2):577–83.

30. Donaldson L. Towards safer radiotherapy, British Institute of Radiology, Institute of Physics and Engineering in Medicine, National Patient Safety Agency, Society and College of Radiographers. London, UK: The Royal College of Radiologists; 2007.

31. Donaldson L. Radiotherapy risk profile: Technical manual. Geneva, Switzerland: World Health Organization; 2008.

32. Hendee WR, Herman MG. Improving patient safety in Radiation Oncology. Med Phys 2011;38(1): 78–82.

33. Leer JW, McKenzie AL, Scalliet P, et al. Practical guidelines for the implementation of a quality system in radiotherapy. Brussels: ESTRO; 1998.

34. Ford EC, Fong de Los Santos L, Pawlicki T, et al. Consensus recommendations for incident learning database structures in Radiation Oncology. Med Phys 2012;39(12):7272–90.

35. Jaffray D, Langen KM, Mageras G, et al. Safety considerations for IGRT: Executive summary. Pract Radiat Oncol 2013;3(3):167–70.

36. Moran JM, Dempsey M, Eisbruch A, et al. Safety considerations for IMRT: Executive summary. Pract Radiat Oncol 2011;1(3):190–5.

37. Odle TG, Rosier N. Radiation therapy safety: The critical role of the radiation therapist. Albequerque, NM: American Society of Radiologic Technologists Education and Research Foundation; 2012.

38. Gawande A. The checklist manifesto: How to get things right. New York, NY: Metropolitan Books; 2009.

39. Pronovost PJ, Vohr E. Safe patients, smart hospitals: How one doctor's checklist can help us change health care from the inside out. New York: Hudson Street Press; 2010. p. 304.

40. Ford EC, Terezakis S, Souranis A, et al. Quality control quantification (QCQ): A tool to measure the value of quality control checks in Radiation Oncology. Int J Radiat Oncol Biol Phys 2012;84(3): e263–9.

41. Furhang EE, Dolan J, Sillanpaa JK, et al. Automating the initial physics chart-checking process. J Appl Clin Med Phys 2009;10(1):129–35.

42. Siochi RA, Pennington EC, Waldron TJ, et al. Radiation therapy plan checks in a paperless clinic. J Appl Clin Med Phys 2009;10(1):43–62.

43. Yang D, Moore KL. Automated radiotherapy treatment plan integrity verification. Med Phys 2012;39(3):1542–51.

44. Kirby TH, Hanson WF, Gastorf RJ, et al. Mailable TLD system for photon and electron therapy beams. Int J Radiat Oncol Biol Phys 1986;12(2):261–5.

45. Ibbott G, Ma CM, Rogers DW, et al. Anniversary paper: Fifty years of AAPM involvement in radiation dosimetry. Med Phys 2008;35(4):1418–27.

46. Ibbott GS, Followill DS, Molineu HA, et al. Challenges in credentialing institutions and participants in advanced technology multi-institutional clinical trials. Int J Radiat Oncol Biol Phys 2008;71(1): S71–5.

47. Broggi S, Cantone MC, Chiara A, et al. Application of failure mode and effects analysis (FMEA) to pretreatment phases in TomoTherapy. J Appl Clin Med Phys 2013;14(5):4329.

48. Cantone MC, Ciocca M, Dionisi F, et al. Application of failure mode and effects analysis to treatment planning in scanned proton beam radiotherapy. Radiat Oncol 2013;8:127.

49. Ciocca M, Cantone MC, Veronese I, et al. Application of failure mode and effects analysis to intraoperative radiation therapy using mobile electron linear accelerators. Int J Radiat Oncol Biol Phys 2012;82(2):e305–11.

50. Perks JR, Stanic S, Stern RL, et al. Failure mode and effect analysis for delivery of lung stereotactic body radiation therapy. Int J Radiat Oncol Biol Phys 2012;83(4):1324–9.

51. Sawant A, Dieterich S, Svatos M, et al. Failure mode and effect analysis-based quality assurance for dynamic MLC tracking systems. Med Phys 2010;37(12):6466–79.

52. Scorsetti M, Signori C, Lattuada P, et al. Applying failure mode effects and criticality analysis in radiotherapy: Lessons learned and perspectives of enhancement. Radiother Oncol 2010;94(3):367–74.

53. Vlayen A. Evaluation of time- and cost-saving modifications of HFMEA: An experimental approach in radiotherapy. J Patient Saf 2011;7(3):165–8.

54. Wilkinson DA, Kolar MD. Failure modes and effects analysis applied to high-dose-rate brachytherapy treatment planning. Brachytherapy 2013;12(4):382–6.

55. Huq MS, et al. Application of risk analysis methods to radiation therapy quality management: Report of AAPM Task Group 100. Med Phys 2015; in review.

56. Ford EC, Smith K, Terezakis S, et al. A streamlined failure mode and effects analysis. Med Phys 2014;41(6):061709.

57. Fraass BA, Lash KL, Matrone GM, et al. The impact of treatment complexity and computer-control delivery technology on treatment delivery errors. Int J Radiat Oncol Biol Phys 1998;42(3):651–9.

58. Mutic S, Brame RS, Oddiraju S, et al. Event (error and near-miss) reporting and learning system for process improvement in Radiation Oncology. Med Phys 2010;37(9):5027–36.

59. Wu AW. The value of close calls in improving patient safety, vol. 1. Oak Brook, IL: Joint Commission Resources; 2011.

60. http://www1.imperial.ac.uk/cpssq/cpssq_publications/resources_tools/the_london_protocol/.

61. Bagian JP, Gosbee J, Lee CZ, et al. The Veterans Affairs root cause analysis system in action. Jt Comm J Qual Improv 2002;28(10):531–45.

62. http://www.jointcommission.org/Framework_for_Conducting_a_Root_Cause_Analysis_and _Action_Plan/.

63. IAEA. Radiation protection and safety of radiation sources: International basic safety standards, in IAEA safety standards, International Atomic Energy Agency. Vienna, Austria: IAEA; 2014.

64. Evans SB, Yu JB, Chagpar A. How radiation oncologists would disclose errors: Results of a survey of radiation oncologists and trainees. Int J Radiat Oncol Biol Phys 2012;84(2):e131–7.

65. Cunningham J, Coffey M, Knöös T, et al. Radiation Oncology Safety Information System (ROSIS): Profiles of participants and the first 1074 incident reports. Radiother Oncol 2010;97(3):601–7.

66. Pawlicki T, Chera B, Ning T, et al. The systematic application of quality measures and process control in clinical Radiation Oncology. Semin Radiat Oncol 2012;22(1):70–6.

67. Pawlicki T, Whitaker M, Boyer AL. Statistical process control for radiotherapy quality assurance. Med Phys 2005;32(9):2777–86.
68. Basran PS, Woo MK. An analysis of tolerance levels in IMRT quality assurance procedures. Med Phys 2008;35(6):2300–7.
69. Breen SL, Moseley DJ, Zhang B, et al. Statistical process control for IMRT dosimetric verification. Med Phys 2008;35(10):4417–25.
70. Gerard K, Grandhaye JP, Marchesi V, et al. A comprehensive analysis of the IMRT dose delivery process using statistical process control (SPC). Med Phys 2009;36(4):1275–85.
71. Palaniswaamy G, Scott Brame R, Yaddanapudi S, et al. A statistical approach to IMRT patient-specific QA. Med Phys 2012;39(12):7560–70.
72. Sanghangthum T, Suriyapee S, Srisatit S, et al. Statistical process control analysis for patient-specific IMRT and VMAT QA. J Radiat Res 2013;54(3):546–52.
73. Kapur A, Potters L. Six sigma tools for a patient safety-oriented, quality-checklist driven radiation medicine department. Pract Radiat Oncol 2012;2(2):86–96.

# PART II

# Clinical Applications

# CHAPTER 13

# Simulation for Radiotherapy Treatment Planning

## 13.1 Introduction

Prior to the early 1990s, "simulation" for an external beam radiotherapy consisted of just that: simulating the treatment with a device that mimicked a linear accelerator (linac) in all aspects except the delivery of a therapeutic beam. These devices (now called "conventional simulators") are equipped with diagnostic x-ray tubes and imaging equipment and are still in use. They have largely given way, however, to computed tomography (CT) simulation whereby a "virtual simulation" is performed on a CT scan acquired with the patient in treatment position. This has enabled the era of 3D conformal radiotherapy (3DCRT, in which targets and normal tissues are delineated on the volumetric CT scan) and image-guided radiation therapy (IGRT) (which uses the CT scan as a reference image). For brachytherapy procedures orthogonal planar imaging is still widely used to locate the applicator and tissue structures, though this is also giving way to volumetric imaging for simulation. A 2010 survey of clinicians performing brachytherapy for gynecologic tumors, for example, showed that the majority of respondents used CT over planar films, though prescription techniques were more often based on 2D definitions.[1]

Technical aspects of CT simulators and QA are considered further in Chapter 7 and in American Association of Physicists in Medicine (AAPM) Task Group (TG)-66, Quality Assurance for Computed-Tomography Simulators and the Computed-Tomography-Simulation Process.[2] Some specific issues to consider here are:

- **Hounsfield units to electron density conversion:** The pixel values in CT scans are in Hounsfield units (HU), and a conversion is required from HU to electron density which is what dose calculations require. Conversion is accomplished with a phantom calibration, and annual checks are required.[2]
- **Metal artifacts:** These can obscure tissue structures and result in inaccurate dose computations. Examples include dental artifacts in the head and neck or a hip prosthesis in the pelvis (see, e.g., AAPM TG-63, Dosimetric considerations for patients with hip prostheses undergoing pelvic irradiation[3]). The density of metal artifacts may need to be overridden in the treatment planning system. Algorithms for metal artifact reduction are now available on some CT scanners. Problems with CT artifacts can also be avoided by using clinical setups which are appropriate for some treatments or by using megavoltage CT (e.g., TomoTherapy).
- **Large-bore CT scanners:** Because it is often necessary to accommodate patients in the treatment position (e.g., on an incline board), large diameter bore scanners are useful. Available models include the Brilliance CT Big Bore (Philips Inc., Eindhoven, Netherlands) with an 85 cm diameter bore, the Somatom (Siemens Inc., Ehrlangen, Germany) with an 80 cm diameter bore, and the Airo intraoperative CT with a 107 cm bore (Brainlab Inc., Feldkirchen, Germany). In addition to the bore size, the size of the field of view (FOV) is also important. If

the scanner has a large bore but a standard FOV, the patient and devices may fit through the bore but the skin surface may not be imaged, rendering the scan useless. Some scanners can reconstruct larger FOVs but these must be checked carefully for HU and geometrical accuracy.

Magnetic resonance imaging (MRI) and positron emission tomography (PET)/CT are being increasingly employed in Radiation Oncology treatment planning. If the goal is to use these studies to define target volumes, then the patient position in the MRI or PET/CT scanner should match the treatment position as closely as possible (e.g., flat table top, same devices, and same pose). MRI-compatible immobilization devices are now available from vendors. One challenge is that MRI or PET/CT scans are often acquired for staging before the radiotherapy simulation has even been performed. The use of MRI in simulation is likely to be an important topic as MRI-enabled treatment devices come into more widespread use.[4]

## 13.2 Immobilization, Setup, and Marking

The technology for patient immobilization is discussed in Chapter 6. Overall, the goal of patient setup is to reduce motion, make daily setup more reproducible, improve comfort, and optimize the avoidance of normal tissue. Reducing motion is especially important given the fact that patients are typically on the treatment table for 15 minutes or more, and even longer for Stereotactic Radiosurgery (SRS)/Stereotactic Body Radiation Therapy (SBRT) treatments. The same immobilization accessories should be used for simulation and treatment. Some options for immobilization include specialized head rests, incline boards and arm holders for breast patients, and prone "belly boards" for some abdominal treatments (see Chapter 6 for a full description of immobilization devices). One widely used device is the thermoplastic shell, typically a perforated plastic that softens when heated. Thermoplastics are available in different thicknesses, with thicker materials offering more rigidity at the cost of decreased skin sparing. Thicker thermo-plastics can double or even triple the skin dose, as described in AAPM TG-176, Dosimetric Effects Caused by Couch Tops and Immobilization Devices.[5] For mildly claustrophobic patients, cutting away the mask above the eyes and, if necessary, above the mouth may increase patient comfort sufficiently to avoid the need for sedatives. Several manufacturers are now offering pre-cut masks for this purpose.

To promote safety, most modern immobilization devices can be "indexed"—that is, affixed to the treatment table at clearly defined locations. Since the patient's position is fixed relative to the treatment table, the X, Y, and Z coordinates of the table can be checked for consistency from day to day. Further description and figures are found in Chapter 6.

### MARKING PATIENTS

A three-point setup is commonly used to align patients. With this technique, three lasers' cross-hairs are visualized on the skin: two lateral points (one on each side) and one anterior point (assuming the patient is supine). Conceptually the three-point setup determines the location of the isocenter and controls for the patient roll (pitch and yaw are somewhat less well constrained). Extra skin marks are sometimes used to aid in positioning. For example, a set of "leveling marks" placed inferiorly can be used to set up a breast cancer patient because the mobility of the breast tissue makes it less suitable for alignment. Prior to CT scanning, a plastic ball bearing (BB) is typically placed on each of the three-point setup marks so that the location can be visualized on the CT scan. Alternative markers are available such as the CT-SPOT plastic crosshair (Beekley Medical Inc., Bristol, CT). The patient is typically given a small permanent ink tattoo at each of the final setup points. In some cases, however, the final isocenter may not be determined at the time of simulation, and so a temporary mark is left on the patient. The necessary shifts are then determined in the treatment planning system, and then final tattoos are made on the patient (e.g., on first imaging day). To verify the correct position of the patient and/or treatment field, radiographs ("port films") are often used on the treatment machine. These images are compared to digitally reconstructed radiographs (DRRs) generated from the simulation CT.

Other markers are sometimes used at the time of simulations for various purposes. For patients receiving postoperative treatment, for example, the surgical scar may be marked for later reference in designing the treatment plan (scars being a site of recurrence in some cases). A radio-opaque plastic "wire" is typically used for this purpose. Metal wire is avoided because it produces artifacts on the CT scan. In postoperative cases it is also common to mark a surgical drain site with wire or a BB. Wires are sometimes used to mark the extent of palpable breast tissue. As a final example, markers are often used to indicate laterality and help ensure that the correct treatment site is identified. An example of this is stereotactic radiosurgery for trigeminal neuralgia. A BB is placed on the patient's head on the involved side, which helps to ensure that the correct fifth cranial nerve is targeted.

There are several pitfalls related to setup and marking: (1) If the isocenter point is moved in the planning system relative to the point set at simulation, this could result in an incorrect patient setup unless the change is clearly communicated to the entire treatment team. (2) Care must be taken to identify the correct BB for the setup point on the CT images. The potential for confusion may exist if extra BBs or other fiducials are present (e.g., a BB on a drain site or plastic wire on a surgical scar). (3) If a patient receives repeat radiation to a similar area care must be taken not to confuse the old tattoo with the new intended location. Good communication is essential. (4) Moles or freckles can sometimes be confused with tattoos. Photos and documentation can help avoid this.

## BOLUS

Tissue-equivalent bolus may be added to photon or electron beams to increase a superficial dose. Although bolus can be added digitally in the treatment planning system, it is sometimes advantageous to place the actual bolus material at the time of simulation to accurately determine its position, shape, and dosimetric effect. An excellent review of bolus material options and effects on dosimetry can be found in Vyas et al.[6] Tissue-equivalent bolus can take a variety of forms, including:

- **Gel sheets such as Superflab or Elastogel:** These are easy to use and thickness is well controlled, but they may not conform well to curved surfaces.
- **Meltable materials such as thermoplastic pellets, bees wax, or paraffin wax (also available in pellet form):** Useful for highly curved surfaces and particularly for electron treatments. For electron treatments bolus material can be formed into shapes to fill air cavities such as the nasal cavity.
- **Superstuff:** Like wax, this material can be molded to shape.
- **Wet gauze or towels:** These are useful for curved surfaces, but the gauze must be consistently saturated with water to achieve its intended dosimetric effect.[7]
- **Brass metal mesh,[8] a beam spoiler, or thick Vaseline:** These are all useful for breast cancer patients.

Whatever bolus material is used, care must be taken to ensure that the material lies flat against the skin and avoid air gaps. Large air gaps produce a lateral spread of electrons, which can lead to a reduced dose on the distal edge of the cavity and even a secondary build-up region. The effect is larger for small field sizes, large air gaps, and higher energies. The effect of air gaps has been studied, but most reports have focused on the accuracy of planning algorithms to predict the dose beyond such air gaps.[9] However, studies in head and neck treatment suggest that the effect of air cavities is on the order of 2% for large field sizes.[10] For air gaps smaller than approximately 1 cm the impact does not appear to be clinically significant.[11]

## SHIELDS

Radiation shields are often constructed or tested at the time of simulation. Examples include:

- **Eye shields used to protect the lens and cornea during electron treatments of the eyelid:** Commercially available devices specifically designed for high energy electrons should be used. An example product is a curved tungsten shield 2 to 3 mm thick covered with acrylic to prevent backscattered electrons. A 2 to 3 mm shield results in an approximately 4% transmission.[12]
- **Lead shields placed on the skin for electron treatments:** The main purpose is to create a sharper penumbra at the field edge. The shield should be made thick enough to attenuate the beam. A typical rule of thumb is: thickness of lead (mm) = Energy (in MV)/2 + 1. A 20% thicker shield should be used if cerrobend is used.
- **Testicular shield or "clamshell":** These are typically constructed from 1.25 cm ($\frac{1}{2}$") thick lead with a slit for access, designed to prevent scatter radiation from reaching the testicles. Clamshells may be useful in a variety of applications because permanent aspermia results at doses >2 Gy.[13] Data from SWOG-8711[14] supports the use of such shields in treatment of testicular cancer. Useful radiation dose data can be found in Mazonakis et al.[15]

# 13.3 Scanning the Patient for CT Simulation

Prior to scanning, the patient should be evaluated for pregnancy status, presence of cardiac or other implanted electronic devices, and possible contraindications for the use of contrast. These are discussed further in Section 13.6. In addition, the patient should have been coached with regard to rectal and/or bladder filling where relevant. The physician should have also noted the goals of simulation and given clear directives as to the technical requirements (e.g., immobilization devices, respiratory control, and anatomic extent of the scan).

After setup and immobilization are complete, the first step is typically to straighten the patient with reference to an anterior-posterior (AP) "scout" image. This aids in later alignment because straight poses are easier to reproduce. An exception is for patients who are for medical reasons more comfortable in a slightly crooked position. It has been noted that forcing such patients into a straight alignment can cause issues with reproducibility during treatment. Of note, the scout images are typically not dimensionally correct in the lateral aspect due to the diverging fan beam. Patients are often positioned head-first supine but other nonstandard poses are possible (e.g., feet-first supine for a lower leg lesion, head-first prone for a patient on a belly board, or even decubitus for other applications). The pose must be noted correctly on the CT scanner console in order for it to correctly populate the DICOM file header. Failure to correctly note the pose can result in orientation problems during treatment planning or image-guided radiation therapy (IGRT) sessions.

Contrast agents are often used during simulation to enhance visualization. These agents have high CT numbers due to their high atomic number. One formulation is a liquid barium sulfate that is swallowed to visualize the lower gastrointestinal (GI) tract or eaten as a paste for the upper GI tract and esophagus. Iodinated contrast agents are injected intravenously (IV) to highlight the vasculature and/or tumors. The timing of IV injection can be correlated with the scan to highlight either arteries (early phase) or veins (late phase). Tumors are also visualized differently in these various phases in a histology-dependent way. The timing of IV injection is typically coordinated through a power injector that remotely administers contrast, through a plastic catheter that is 20 gauge or larger. Detailed information on contrast techniques and medical considerations can be found in the American College of Radiology (ACR) Manual on Contrast Media,[16] and some general safety considerations are discussed in Section 13.6 of this chapter. In theory, the presence of contrast can affect dose calculations since it appears as a high density "bone" to the dose calculation algorithm. Studies have examined this, however, and concluded that the effect is small.[17,18] Contrast can also cause image fusion issues. For example, using barium contrast in patients receiving CyberKnife spine tracking can prevent the imaging algorithm from working correctly. Similar issues are starting to appear as linac-based image-guided setup algorithms are used. To address these issues it is possible to acquire a noncontrast scan first and use that for dose calculations and image guidance while the contrast scan is used as a fusion image set for visualization.

During CT scanning the FOV should be controlled so that the entire patient surface is included in the CT images. Though small FOV scans may be acceptable or even desirable for evaluation in radiology, the external contour of the patient is needed for treatment planning purposes and IGRT alignment. Obese patients represent a challenge since the FOV may not encompass the entire patient. For lateral lesions in obese patients, the patient can be shifted to the contralateral side on the CT couch to catch as much ipsilateral surface as possible. Tissue may also be missed if a patient is positioned away from the scan center. In these situations the CT scan can be modified to incorporate an estimate of the missing tissues, which may be derived from separation measurements.

The measurement and control of respiratory motion are other important aspects of simulation. Respiratory motion can be measured with 4D CT or fluoroscopy as described in AAPM TG-76, The Management of Respiratory Motion in Radiation Oncology.[19] Policies and procedures should be in place for situations in which multiple 4D CT scans might be needed, since the dose is substantially higher for such scans. It is important to remember that respiratory motion affects not only the lung but also the abdomen; large excursions have been measured in the liver and kidneys.[20] Respiratory motion can be controlled by a variety of means, including abdominal compression, respiratory gating, and breath hold. Whatever respiratory management solution is employed, this same system (with the same settings) should be used at simulation and on treatment. Chapter 19 contains a more complete discussion of respiratory motion management in external beam radiotherapy.

A final consideration in CT simulation is the exposure that a patient receives. The "image gently" campaign seeks to reduce exposure in radiology. Though imaging doses are much smaller than the therapeutic doses that the patient will receive, AAPM TG-75, The Management of Imaging Dose During Image-Guided Radiotherapy,[21] suggests that it should be considered and minimized where possible. A further discussion of dose and measurement techniques is found in Chapter 7. CT dose tracking is now being widely used in radiology with several commercial products available as well as an ACR registry (see Talati et al.[22] for a recent review). Some Radiation Oncology departments are adopting the practice as well, and this may become standard practice.

## 13.4 Surface Capture Using Optical Tracking

One system of image guidance relies on aligning and/or tracking the surface of a patient. One technology to accomplish this is the projection and readout of structured light patterns on the patient's surface (e.g., AlignRT, VisionRT Ltd., London, UK). Another technology uses 3D scanning lasers to image the surface (e.g., Sentinel, C-Rad, Uppsala, Sweden). These technologies can use the CT image itself as a reference image, or an optical reference image can be obtained at the time of simulation for later comparison. More information can be found in Chapter 7 and AAPM TG-147, Quality Assurance for Nonradiographic Radiotherapy Localization and Positioning Systems.[23]

## 13.5 Postscan Processing

Following the completion of simulation imaging, quality assurance should be performed. This might include a check of the rectal and/or bladder filling in sites where it is appropriate. It also includes a check of the patient demographics and orientation and the import of these parameters and the images into the planning system. If image fusion is performed (e.g., MRI or PET) the quality of the fusion should also be verified.

The question is sometimes raised as to whether CT scans acquired for radiotherapy planning purposes should be formally evaluated by a radiologist. One recent study[24] examines the incidence of incidental findings and summarizes a handful of other studies that have examined this issue (cf. their Table 3). The authors conclude that although the rate of incidental findings can be substantial (up to 20%) the management is changed in only about 1% of cases. A related question is whether the imaging acquired in Radiation Oncology should be transferred to the radiology picture archiving and communication system (PACS) where available. This is good practice since another physician may then find the images there, and the PACS is an efficient means of archiving data.

## 13.6 Clinical Safety-Related Considerations

### CLINICAL CONSIDERATIONS IN THE USE OF CONTRAST AGENTS

American College of Radiology (ACR)-Society for Pediatric Radiology (SPR) practice guidelines[25] outline general recommendations for the use of contrast and associated policies, procedures, and documentation. A detailed consideration of the clinical issues related to contrast media can be found in the ACR manual on contrast media.[16] One possible adverse event is contrast-induced nephrotoxicity. Patients with risk factors (e.g., age over 60 years, history of renal disease, and other factors) should have kidney function evaluated through a measure of serum creatinine. There is no clear consensus, however, as to safe threshold levels for this test. Other possible adverse events include extravasation of the contrast agent (particularly with a power injector) and allergic-like reactions. Though allergic-like reactions are becoming less common, especially with the switch to nonionic low osmolality contrast media, they are often difficult to predict. Allergies to dairy and shellfish, for example, are not predictive.[16] Staff need to be aware of possible adverse reactions and be trained to react.

### ASSESSING FOR PREGNANCY

The topic of pregnant patients is treated more fully in Chapter 24, but for the purposes of simulation the important consideration is to identify potentially pregnant patients. Simulation is often the first point in the workflow at which a patient would receive radiation exposure and is therefore a point at which the patient's pregnancy status should be evaluated. Radiation dose can be harmful to an embryo or fetus, especially during the first 15 weeks when rapid development occurs in the embryo. A summary of the relevant exposure levels and effects can be found in ACR-SPR's practice guidelines for imaging pregnant or potentially pregnant adolescents and women with ionizing radiation,[26] and AAPM TG-36, Fetal Dose from Radiotherapy with Photon Beams (Table VI),[27] which notes a significant risk of damage above 10 cGy in the first trimester and above 50 cGy in all trimesters. The American Society of Radiologic Technologists (ASRT) radiation therapy clinical performance standards call for the radiation therapist to "verify the patient's pregnancy status."[28] ACR-SPR practice guidelines Appendix D[26] suggests that for substantial risk procedures (of which radiotherapy is one) a urine hCG test should be obtained.

### IMPLANTABLE ELECTRONIC DEVICES

Implantable electronic devices (IEDs) are becoming more common in general and therefore are more commonly encountered in radiation therapy. Examples are pacemakers, insulin pumps, or deep-brain stimulators.

Cardiac implantable electronic devices (CIEDs) take the form of either an implanted cardiac pacemaker (ICP) or an implanted cardiac defibrillator (ICD), both of which are sensitive to radiation. The standard reference has been AAPM TG-34 from 1994,[29] but this is now outdated. A more current review is found in Hurkmans et al.[30] and the forthcoming AAPM TG-203 on the management of radiotherapy patients with implanted cardiac pacemakers and defibrillators.[31] The main concern arises during treatment when permanent circuit damage or soft errors may occur in the memory or logic circuits. This topic is treated more fully in Chapter 24, but for the purposes of simulation the main concern is electromagnetic interference during scanning that may trigger an oversensing event. If the IED will be scanned directly it is recommended that cardiac electrophysiology be consulted.[31] At the time of simulation an IED alert should be put in the chart to direct later planning and management.

## ANESTHESIA AND SEDATION

Any motion of the patient during simulation has a direct effect on the quality of the plan and treatment downstream. It is therefore important to minimize this. Education plays a crucial role for all patients and especially for anxious patients. Anesthesia or conscious sedation are sometimes appropriate. Patients in pain may also find it difficult to remain still. Finally, pediatric patients (especially those under the age of 7 years) often require anesthesia. The experience with anesthesia at St. Jude Children's Research Hospital has been reported recently in the Radiation Oncology literature.[32] Complications were noted in 1.3% of cases (which compares favorably with other series). Simulation was significantly more risk-prone than treatment. Briefer procedures were also less risk-prone. These considerations and complexity make anesthesia and sedation challenging in the nonhospital setting.

# 13.7 Simulation for Brachytherapy

Simulation for brachytherapy procedures has traditionally relied on orthogonal radiographs with x-ray markers to visualize dwell positions or source locations. For some diseases, however, simulation has moved more toward 3D imaging (both CT- and MR-based), which provides for tissue delineation and potentially more accurate localization of the sources. One recent survey of gynecologic procedures, for example, shows that a majority of clinicians use CT-based planning rather than films,[1] although the vast majority still prescribe to point A for gynecological diseases. The use of MRI is particularly useful for visualization of some tumors, and its use continues to evolve and recommendations are appearing.[33] Because metal devices can cause artifacts on CT and MRI, special imaging-compatible applicators should be used. Techniques can also be used to avoid artifacts. In an interstitial implant, for example, a plastic catheter can be used and the metal stylus removed for CT imaging.

**FOR THE PHYSICIAN**

*Technical Considerations*
A variety of technologies are available for simulation, with CT scanners being the modern work horse. For radiotherapy purposes, these scanners are outfitted with large-diameter bores (to accommodate immobilization devices) and flat table tops (versus cushioned surfaces typically used in diagnostic scanners). Regular monthly and annual quality assurance should be performed on these scanners conforming to the recommendations of AAPM TG-66[2] with the appropriate staff time and equipment. A wide variety of immobilization devices are available for simulation (e.g., thermoplastic masks, breast boards, and prone belly boards). Most of these devices can be indexed to the treatment table, which reduces the chance of mispositioning the patient and provides a layer of safety. Immobilization equipment can have an impact on delivered dose (e.g.,

increased skin dose) and should be considered with reference to AAPM TG-176.[5] Other technology relevant for simulation includes bolus material, shields, radiographically visible markers (e.g., plastic wire for scars), and brachytherapy applicators. The impact of contrast material on dose calculation and image fusion should be considered.

### Simulation Process

Prior to scanning, patients should be evaluated for pregnancy status, presence of cardiac implanted electronic devices, possible contraindications for the use of contrast, pain levels, and issues such as claustrophobia and the possible need for anesthesia or sedation. Clear directives should be given as to the technical requirements for the simulation (e.g., immobilization devices, respiratory control, and anatomic extent of the scan). A crucial step in simulation is marking the patient with either a temporary mark or the final isocenter location. Given the importance of this location, it is essential to have a clear policy and procedure for setting and/or moving this point. Good communication and documentation are musts. Quality assurance should be performed post scan to check for such effects as rectal or bladder filling (when clinically indicated) and to assess the quality of any image fusions that might have been performed.

## References

1. Viswanathan AN, Erickson BA. Three-dimensional imaging in gynecologic brachytherapy: A survey of the American Brachytherapy Society. Int J Radiation Oncl Biol Phys 2010;76:104–9.
2. Mutic S, Palta JR, Butker EK, et al. Quality assurance for computed-tomography simulators and the computed-tomography-simulation process: Report of the AAPM Radiation Therapy Committee Task Group No. 66. Med Phys 2003;30:2762–92.
3. Reft C, Alecu R, Das IJ, et al. Dosimetric considerations for patients with HIP prostheses undergoing pelvic irradiation. Report of the AAPM Radiation Therapy Committee Task Group 63. Med Phys 2003;30:1162–82.
4. Raaymakers BW, Lagendijk JJ, Overweg J, et al. Integrating a 1.5 T MRI scanner with a 6 MV accelerator: Proof of concept. Phys Med Biol 2009;54:N229–37.
5. Olch AJ, Gerig L, Li H, et al. Dosimetric effects caused by immobilization devices: Report of AAPM Task Group 176. Med Phys 2014;41(6):061501.
6. Vyas V, Palmer L, Mudge R, et al. On bolus for megavoltage photon and electron radiation therapy. Med Dosim 2013;38:268–73.
7. Benoit J, Pruitt AF, Thrall DE. Effect of wetness level on the suitability of wet gauze as a substitute for Superflab as a bolus material for use with 6 mv photons. Vet Radiol Ultrasound 2009;50:555–9.
8. Healy E, Anderson S, Cui J, et al. Skin dose effects of postmastectomy chest wall radiation therapy using brass mesh as an alternative to tissue equivalent bolus. Pract Radiat Oncol 2013;3:e45–53.
9. Rana S, Rogers K. Dosimetric evaluation of Acuros XB dose calculation algorithm with measurements in predicting doses beyond different air gap thickness for smaller and larger field sizes. J Med Phys 2013;38:9–14.
10. Kan WK, Wu PM, Leung HT, et al. The effect of the nasopharyngeal air cavity on x-ray interface doses. Phys Med Biol 1998;43:529–37.
11. Butson MJ, Cheung T, Yu P, et al. Effects on skin dose from unwanted air gaps under bolus in photon beam radiotherapy. Radiat Measure 2000;32:201–4.
12. Weaver RD, Gerbi BJ, Dusenbery KE. Evaluation of eye shields made of tungsten and aluminum in high-energy electron beams. Int J Radiat Oncol Biol Phys 1998;41:233–7.
13. Ogilvy-Stuart AL, Shalet SM. Effect of radiation on the human reproductive system. Environ Health Perspect 1993;101:109–16.
14. Gordon W Jr, Siegmund K, Stanisic TH, et al. A study of reproductive function in patients with seminoma treated with radiotherapy and orchidectomy: (SWOG-8711). Southwest Oncology Group. Int J Radiat Oncol Biol Phys 1997;38:83–94.
15. Mazonakis M, Kokona G, Varveris H, et al. Data required for testicular dose calculation during radiotherapy of seminoma. Med Phys 2006;33:2391–5.
16. ACR manual on contrast media. Version 9. Reston, VA: American College of Radiology (ACR); 2013.
17. Ramm U, Damrau M, Mose S, et al. Influence of CT contrast agents on dose calculations in a 3D treatment planning system. Phys Med Biol 2001;46:2631–5.

18. Rankine AW, Lanzon PJ, Spry NA. Effect of contrast media on megavoltage photon beam dosimetry. Med Dosim 2008;33:169–74.
19. Keall PJ, Mageras GS, Balter JM, et al. The management of respiratory motion in Radiation Oncology: Report of AAPM Task Group 76. Med Phys 2006;33:3874.
20. Goldstein SD, Ford EC, Duhon M, et al. Use of respiratory-correlated four-dimensional computed tomography to determine acceptable treatment margins for locally advanced pancreatic adenocarcinoma. Int J Radiat Oncol Biol Phys 2010;76:597–602.
21. Murphy MJ, Balter J, Balter S, et al. The management of imaging dose during image-guided radiotherapy: Report of the AAPM Task Group 75. Med Phys 2007;34:4041–63.
22. Talati RK, Dunkin J, Parikh S, et al. Current methods of monitoring radiation exposure from CT. J Am Coll Radiol 2013;10:702–7.
23. Willoughby T, Lehmann J, Bencomo JA, et al. Quality assurance for nonradiographic radiotherapy localization and positioning systems: Report of Task Group 147. Med Phys 2012;39:1728–47.
24. Ye JC, Truong MT, Kachnic LA, et al. Implications of previously undetected incidental findings on 3D CT simulation scans for radiation therapy. Pract Radiat Oncol 2011;1:22–6.
25. ACR-SPR practice guidelines for the use of intravascular contrast media. Vol Resolution 3. Reston, VA: American College of Radiology (ACR); 2012.
26. ACR-SPR practice guideline for imaging pregnant or potentially pregnant adolescents and women with ionizing radiation. Vol Resolution 48. Reston, VA: American College or Radiology; 2013.
27. Stovall M, Balckwell CR, Cundiff J, et al. Fetal dose from radiotherapy with photon beams—Report of AAPM Radiation Therapy Committee Task Group No. 36. Med Phys 1995;22:63–82.
28. ASRT: The practice standards for medical imaging and radiation therapy. Albuquerque, NM: American Society for Radiological Technologists; 2011.
29. Marbach JR, Sontag MR, Van Dyk J, et al. Management of Radiation Oncology patients with implanted cardiac pacemakers: Report of AAPM Task Group No. 34. American Association of Physicists in Medicine. Med Phys 1994;21:85–90.
30. Hurkmans CW, Knegjens JL, Oei BS, et al. Management of Radiation Oncology patients with a pacemaker or ICD: A new comprehensive practical guideline in The Netherlands. Dutch Society of Radiotherapy and Oncology (NVRO). Radiat Oncol 2012;7:198.
31. Miften M, Mihailidis D. Management of radiotherapy patients with implanted cardiac pacemakers and defibrillators: A report of AAPM Task Group 203. Medical Physics in preparation.
32. Anghelescu DL, Burgoyne LL, Liu W, et al. Safe anesthesia for radiotherapy in pediatric oncology: St. Jude Children's Research Hospital experience, 2004-2006. Int J Radiat Oncol Biol Phys 2008;71:491–7.
33. Dimopoulos JC, Petrow P, Tanderup K, et al. Recommendations from Gynaecological (GYN) GEC-ESTRO Working Group (IV): Basic principles and parameters for MR imaging within the frame of image based adaptive cervix cancer brachytherapy. Radiother Oncol 2012;103:113–22.

# CHAPTER 14

# Treatment Planning and Quality Metrics

## 14.1 Introduction

The overall goal of the treatment planning process is to produce the optimal dose distribution for the patient, taking into account the following factors:

1. Treatment intent (curative or palliative)
2. Stage of disease (extent of involvement)
3. Other therapies (chemotherapy, hormones, etc.)
4. Previous treatments
5. Reproducibility (immobilization, patient comfort)
6. Deliverability (collisions, modulation)
7. Safety (sensitivity to changes, robustness)

The process can be very complicated and involves a multidisciplinary approach. A workflow process map for external beam radiation therapy (EBRT) and brachytherapy can be found in the American Association of Physicists in Medicine (AAPM) white paper on incident learning.[1] From the very beginning, the physician, radiation therapist, medical physicist, and dosimetrist must have clear communication regarding the factors mentioned above. As much information as possible should be documented in the medical record so that the sequence of events and current status of the planning process is clear to everyone. This begins with the immobilization and setup ensuring reproducibility and patient comfort. Again, clear communication is important. For instance, if a patient has had shoulder surgery and cannot comfortably raise that arm above the head, other immobilization strategies may need to be employed. Likewise, if a patient becomes agitated during the CT simulation because of claustrophobia, the therapist will need to communicate with the physician and nurse so that steps can be taken to reduce the patient's anxiety. This may involve medication or the use of relaxation techniques. If either method is required, will it be continued during treatments? This should be communicated and well planned. Several references describe the treatment planning process in Radiation Oncology.[2,3] A schematic of the simulation and treatment planning process is shown in Figure 14.1.

The ability to reliably reproduce the treatment over the entire course is the key to successfully delivering radiation therapy. The first step in achieving that goal is a careful setup and immobilization of the patient that maximize comfort while restricting motion. This is discussed in detail in Chapter 6.

After the patient has been positioned, images can be obtained that are used to define the targets and critical structures needed to safely plan the treatment course. In many cases additional imaging studies are used in order to get information about soft tissue definition, functional information, or metabolic information that is unavailable from the primary image set. These image sets must be coregistered to preserve accurate geometric representation of the data.

Accurate contouring of the target(s) and organs at risk (OAR) is critical to developing a high quality treatment plan. If targets are contoured too liberally, the OARs may receive unnecessarily

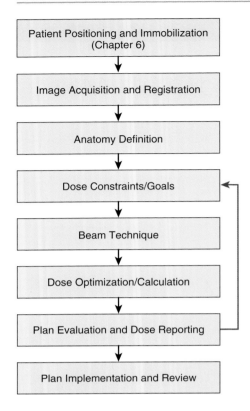

**Figure 14.1** Planning process algorithm.

high doses. Likewise, if OARs are expanded to a degree that is inconsistent with the setup and localization technique being used, the dose to the target may be unnecessarily compromised. The expansion of OARs to account for setup uncertainty and patient motion and the creation of planning volumes is discussed in more detail in Section 14.4.

The physician treatment intent should contain the total planned dose and fractionation and should inform the priorities regarding dose goals and constraints. The stage of the disease will determine the extent of coverage, such as which nodal chains need to be covered. Again, communication is important. For instance, if the physician tells the dosimetrist that it is acceptable to compromise on target coverage to ensure that all OAR goals are met, a note should be made in the medical record so that another dosimetrist taking over the planning or a physicist reviewing the plan will also understand the goals.

A plan must be consistent with the capabilities of the delivery system in order to be delivered safely. For instance, if it was determined that the reproducibility of patient setup and isocenter placement is 3 mm for a given immobilization and imaging technique, the plan margins should reflect this (i.e., do not use 1 mm margins).

After the contouring is complete and the delivery method has been selected, e.g., 3D versus intensity-modulated radiation therapy (IMRT), the plan can be optimized. This can be a manual trial and error process for 3D or an inverse planned IMRT process. In either case, the desired dose goals must be clearly stated. The planner should be aware of the delivery equipment limitations to avoid creating a plan that is undeliverable. Some of these limitations (gantry speed, dose rate, minimum monitor units (MU), maximum MU, etc.) may be input into the treatment planning system (TPS) to prevent creation of plans that exceed limits. Collision detection is not implemented as of this writing. Plans with a high degree of modulation may push systems to their limit and, while possible to deliver, may lead to excessive interlocks.

After the plan has been optimized, the various dose constraints and goals are evaluated to determine if the plan is acceptable. If they are not, beam parameters such as gantry angles or number beams and dose constraints may be modified before another optimization is performed. There may be many iterations before an acceptable plan is achieved. A study by Nelms et al. showed a wide degree of variation of plan quality given the same planning input data.[4] This shows the need for better tools to optimize plans and to provide guidance on what is achievable given a patient's unique anatomy and diagnosis. These will be discussed further in Section 14.4.

By using a multidisciplinary approach, with clear communication and documentation, and taking into account the factors mentioned above, the probability of delivering quality radiation therapy is increased. In the following sections each step in the treatment planning process will be examined. As mentioned, patient positioning and immobilization are covered in Chapter 6, and CT simulation is covered in Chapter 13 and will not be covered in detail in this chapter. In addition, the specifics of IMRT and volumetric modulated arc therapy (VMAT) are discussed in Chapter 16.

## 14.2 Patient Positioning and Immobilization

As described in Chapter 6, the goals for patient immobilization include:

1. Reduce patient motion and improve day-to-day reproducibility of setup.
2. Improve patient comfort.
3. Accommodate the requirements of the physical devices.
4. Avoid normal tissue.

The reader is referred to Chapter 6 for further details.

## 14.3 Image Acquisition and Registration

Computed tomography (CT) is the primary imaging modality in radiation therapy. The CT simulation process is described in Chapter 13. CT does not always yield the best soft tissue contrast for target and organ delineation even with the use of contrast agents. It is currently required for treatment planning to accurately calculate dose because it is the only imaging modality that provides density and therefore attenuation information. High density materials such as hip prostheses and dental implants can cause significant streaking artifacts. These can cause difficulty in the identification of targets and organs at risk. The impact on the dose calculation is minimal in the case of hip prostheses[5] but has been shown to be significant for dental fillings.[6] Magnetic resonance (MR) imaging may be useful in these cases. If available, megavoltage CT (MVCT) can be used to reduce the artifacts due to the decrease in the photoelectric effect at the higher energy. Newer CT scanners have the ability to reconstruct data outside the primary fan beam to create an expanded field of view (FOV). This can aid in contouring the entire external contour of the patient. The density in the expanded areas has been shown to be inaccurate, so care should be taken when used for planning.[7]

Positron emission tomography (PET)/CT scans are often used to obtain metabolic information that would indicate tumor activity. The scans take a relatively long time to acquire, involve the use of radioactive material, have low signal-to-background ratios in some cases, and have poor spatial resolution. The use of PET/CT relies on the use of well-defined protocols for image acquisition, reconstruction, and segmentation.[8]

Investigators are working on methods to correlate MR signals to density.[9,10] If this can be done then MR could be used as the sole modality for planning, which would allow the clinicians to take advantage of the superior soft tissue definition of MR as well as to eliminate the use of ionizing radiation. MR imaging can be used for delineation of soft tissue, obtaining metabolic and functional information, and monitoring the response to treatment. The last use would take advantage of the lack of radiation dose, and thus the scans could be safely done at a higher frequency. Proton spectroscopy can sometimes be used to identify malignancies or necrotic tissue. MR simulation would have the disadvantages of potentially lower geometric accuracy, smaller FOV, much longer acquisition times, and higher cost.

The use of two or three imaging modalities for a single patient is not uncommon because the modalities have different strengths as described above. To accurately combine these images to obtain a complete anatomic, metabolic, and functional picture requires an accurate registration process. This can be particularly challenging if some of the imaging is not done with the patient in treatment position. Image registration algorithms are either rigid or deformable. Rigid registration is a simple geometric translation and rotation of one image set to align with another. It cannot account for differences in patient position or motion. Deformable registration maps one image set to another using a transformation matrix to produce a deformation map. This allows for differences in patient positioning, motion, organ size change, and organ shape change. The validation of deformable registration is very complex. AAPM TG-132, Use of Image Registration and Data Fusion Algorithms and Techniques in Radiotherapy Treatment Planning, is developing a report that will review existing algorithms and discuss issues related to implementation, methods to assess the accuracy of registration, issues related to acceptance testing, and quality assurance (QA). Various publications have looked at the accuracy of different algorithms.[11-13] In general, no algorithm performs with the same accuracy in all situations so they must be evaluated for each clinical application.

## 14.4 Anatomy Definition

The definition of anatomic structures is crucial to achieving high quality radiation therapy delivery. The contouring of targets and OARs can be a time-consuming process in, for example, head and neck IMRT cases or relatively simple in the case of palliative spine treatments.

The issue of standardizing structures and reporting is the topic of two important reports: ICRU-83 on prescribing, recording, and reporting photon-beam IMRT[14] and the American Society for Radiation Therapy (ASTRO) 2009 Recommendations for Documenting IMRT Treatments.[15] Though these reports specifically name IMRT in their titles, they apply to other techniques as well. AAPM in June, 2014, formed AAPM TG-263, Standardizing Nomenclature, which should provide a report in the near future.

The structures outlined in Table 14.1 are a modification and update to ICRU-50 and -62, which defined these concepts.[16,17] ASTRO's 2009 IMRT report recommendations[15] call for the clinician to specify all the volumes in Table 14.1 except for RVR and TV, which are planning structures.

The process sometimes begins with the contouring of the external patient contour, though not all planning systems require this. Some systems do this automatically on the import of the images. The contour should be examined for accuracy because it will determine the depth of treatment and ultimately the MU. Typical areas of concern are around the mouth and nose where the contour can wrap inside the body, wires or markers placed on the skin, and immobilization devices. Most systems do not account for any structure outside the body contour, so the immobilization devices will have to be contoured as part of the body if the dosimetric impact of the devices is to be calculated. Some systems now have the ability to add the treatment couch to the image set to properly account for couch top attenuation. Some planning systems (e.g., TomoTherapy, Pinnacle) account for every structure in the scan FOV and therefore inherently calculate the attenuation of the immobilization devices. One caution when using a system with that capability is that some CT imaging artifacts create a bright ring around the edge of the FOV. This will be seen as a high density region, and the MU will be artificially increased. Careful

**TABLE 14.1** ■ **Treatment Planning Structures Relevant to IMRT/VMAT from ICRU-83[14] and ASTRO 2009 IMRT Report[15]**

| Abbreviation | Definition | Notes and Recommendations |
|---|---|---|
| GTV | Gross Tumor Volume | |
| CTV | Clinical Tumor Volume | A CTV should always be associated with a GTV (ICRU-83) |
| ITV | Internal Target Volume | Determined by evaluating the extent of motion of the target volume throughout the respiratory cycle |
| PTV | Planning Target Volume | Determined by adding a margin to the CTV or ITV to account for motion and setup error |
| OAR | Organ at Risk | Note that some OARs are open or tubular structures. An example is the rectum. ICRU-83 advocates that the inside not be included in such cases. |
| PRV | Planning Organ at Risk Volume | OARs should be expanded to a PRV particularly for serial-like organs (ICRU-83) |
| RVR | Remaining Volume at Risk | Apply DVH constraints to avoid unanticipated hot spots (ICRU-83) |
| TV | Treated Volume | Volume of tissue receiving a "therapeutic dose" of radiation. ICRU-83 suggests this might be defined by $V_{98\%}$, volume receiving at least 98% of the prescription dose. |

evaluation of the image set should be done by zooming out to show the maximum FOV and switching to a lung window to make the ring more obvious. Some TPSs have the capability of filtering out low density artifacts outside the body contour by applying a threshold.

Contouring of targets is done by the physician, who will typically contour a GTV or CTV. The dosimetrist or physicist can then create a PTV using expansion criteria specified by the physician. Margin expansion will be discussed in more detail below. The physician may be aided in target delineation through the use of an atlas-based segmentation algorithm which uses deformable registration from an "expert" case. The final contours must be carefully reviewed and modified as necessary by the physician.

Contouring of OARs is typically done by both dosimetrists and physicians. Dosimetrists often contour bony anatomy, spinal cord, lung, and other easily identifiable structures such as kidney and liver. This can be done using manual techniques, atlas-based segmentation, auto-segmentation, or model-based segmentation. Auto-segmentation relies on following density boundaries and requires the user to place a seed point or bounding volume. These work well for organs with high contrast to surrounding tissue such as the lung. Model-based segmentation algorithms have the typical properties of an organ relating to size, shape, and density that are used to determine the contours. They can also use a seed point or bounding volume. Again, these automated contours must be reviewed and modified as necessary.

Inaccurate contouring can lead to suboptimal plans, delay the planning process by making the achievement of dose goals difficult or impossible, or cause geographic misses. Accurate target and OAR contouring is key to high quality planning. The importance of correct contouring is emphasized in the ASTRO report Safety Is No Accident[2] and the safety white paper on peer-review[18] in which the role of physician peer review of the contours is highlighted. It must be recognized that if contours are not reviewed until after planning (e.g., at new patient rounds or "chart rounds"), the threshold for rejection will be much higher because the planning process will have to be repeated. This has led some groups to explore peer review prior to planning,[19] and this is advocated in Safety Is No Accident. Contouring atlases are available to assist in delineation of volumes. NRG Oncology has contouring atlases available on their website as well as links to atlases for the Radiation Therapy Oncology Group (RTOG), Gynecologic Oncology Group (GOG), and National Surgical Adjuvant Breast and Bowel Project (NSABP) at http://

www.nrgoncology.org/Resources.aspx. There are other atlases that have been described in the literature.[20,21] CTV definitions in atlases, for example, may vary based on staging.

One crucial parameter in treatment planning is the margin that is used to expand from the CTV to PTV. A margin that is too small risks underdosing the CTV. However, if 100% dosimetric coverage of the CTV in all patients were required, a very large CTV-to-PTV margin would be required resulting in higher OAR doses. Clearly some compromise is needed. A solution to this problem comes in the formulation of "margin recipes."

## 14.5 Margins

Margin recipe formulations date back to at least 1995 and are well summarized in ICRU-83[14] Table 4.4. The basic concept is that given information about the setup variability in a population of patients one can calculate the margin needed to ensure dosimetric coverage in, say, 90% of patients. ICRU-83 Table 4.4 lists no fewer than 11 margin formulas for CTV-to-PTV or OAR-to-PRV calculations. Perhaps the most widely used formula is the van Herk et al.[22] margin recipe of $2.5\Sigma + 0.7\sigma$, where $\Sigma$ and $\sigma$ are the systematic and random uncertainties, respectively, in patient setup. $\Sigma$ and $\sigma$ should be measured by each clinic from image-guided radiation therapy (IGRT) or other data. This formula is based on the goal of achieving a minimum CTV dose of 95% for 90% of patients. This population-based margin formula is based on the assumption that the plan is perfectly conformal. It also assumes something about the beam penumbra, though a more generalized formula is available that explicitly accounts for penumbra width.

It is important to recognize that the simplified margin formulas noted above were developed under the assumptions that 3D conformal radiotherapy is being used and that Poisson statistics will be used for standard fractionation. These may not be applicable for IMRT plans, which have different conformality and dose gradients or hypofractionated courses in which the number of fractions is smaller. One study of head and neck cases found margins that were a factor of three smaller than would be suggested by the van Herk et al. formulas.[23] The implication is that margins may need to be different for IMRT. This has been discussed but consensus has not been reached. This topic is discussed further in Section 14.12.

Regardless of the proper formula, it must be recognized that the use of IMRT alone does not generally warrant a reduction in margins. IMRT has more impact on gradients, which can result in less dose to nearby OARs, but does not impact setup variation, which the margin is designed to mitigate. Margin reduction is more properly achieved through the use of IGRT rather than IMRT. In fact, one study has demonstrated increased biochemical failure for prostate patients with inappropriate margin reduction.[24] In this context it is also important to note that a margin formula such as $2.5\Sigma + 0.7\sigma$ suggests that the systematic component of variability ($\Sigma$) is approximately 3 times as important as the random variability ($\sigma$). If margins are to be reduced, it is particularly important to address the systematic component of variability. IGRT is particularly effective at accomplishing this.

The margins to be used to generate the PTV must be specified by the physician in consultation with the medical physicist.[2] This can be done on a case by case basis or as a class solution (e.g., prostate cancer patients receiving 80 Gy in three phases with each phase using a different set of margins). The margins could be determined locally based on analysis of setup variations or based on published recommendations. If using published recommendations, the user should verify the use of an IGRT methodology that is appropriate compared to what was used in the published study.

Another factor to keep in mind is that the treated volume (volume encompassed by the prescription isodose, TV) in general does not match the PTV generated by any margin formula. The TV usually touches the PTV in a few areas and is usually larger than the PTV, although in some cases TV may be smaller than the PTV if OAR constraints are given priority over PTV coverage.

# 14.6 Normal Tissue Dose Constraints and Goals

The aim of the optimization is to maximize the dose to the targets while minimizing the dose to the OARs. In many cases the total dose to the targets is limited by the tolerance doses of the OARs. The establishment of reliable dose constraints has long been a challenge in Radiation Oncology. The seminal paper by Emami et al. outlined tolerance doses for many organs based on a review of the literature and included the concept of a volume effect.[25] More recently an extensive effort was undertaken to update these values. A joint effort of ASTRO and AAPM, the Quantitative Analysis of Normal Tissue Effects in the Clinic (QUANTEC), was published in the *International Journal of Radiation Oncology Biology and Physics* in March 2010[26] and is also available on the AAPM website, http://aapm.org/pubs/QUANTEC.asp. This entire journal issue is devoted to the topic and includes specific articles on 16 organs at risk. Table 14.2 is adapted from the summary table outlining the data for standard fractionation (1.6 to 2.0 Gy/fraction, once or twice daily). Although these numbers are compiled from the QUANTEC reports, there are many factors that affect tolerance doses such as fraction size, total dose, volume of tissue, and combination with chemotherapy. Therefore the reader is cautioned to read the entire QUANTEC report, including the individual organ-specific chapters, before adopting a tolerance dose in the clinic. Tolerances for radiosurgery techniques are given in Chapter 17. Randomized clinical trials often include dose limits and are another good source of data. It should be noted that before adopting a dose constraint for use in your clinic, the complication rate for the constraint must be understood. While a 10% complication rate may be acceptable to some clinicians in some circumstances, it may not be to others.

# 14.7 Treatment Techniques

After the contours have been delineated and reviewed, beams can be placed. This may have been done during the simulation process. There are many possible treatment techniques (e.g., single fields, multiple fixed beams with conformal shapes, field in field, multiple beams with IMRT, arc fields, VMAT fields, or a combination of these). As treatments have evolved from 3D conformal to IMRT to VMAT, there have been distinct changes in the nature of the resulting dose distributions. Each has advantages and disadvantages but the clinical situation will determine which will be used. Communication among team members is crucial. Ultimately the planner will likely try several approaches in order to find the best acceptable plan.

In traditional 3D planning a limited number of fixed beams are used, typically on the order of 3 to 5 beams. The various parameters are manually adjusted to produce an acceptable result. Generally a homogeneous dose across the target is achieved. Beam modulation is achieved using wedges or field-in-field techniques. With the advent of flattening filter free beams (FFF), this can also be achieved by using a half-beam block on the FFF beam, at least in the case of breast tangent fields where a cylindrically symmetric beam is useful.

**TABLE 14.2** ■ **Summary of QUANTEC Tolerance Doses**

| Organ | Tolerance Doses (range) (Gy) or Recommended DVH Constraint | Complication and Estimated Rate |
|---|---|---|
| Brain | 72 Gy, partial volume<br>90 Gy, partial volume<br>V12 <5-10 cc, single fraction | 5% brain necrosis<br>10% brain necrosis<br><20% brain necrosis |
| Optic nerves and chiasm | 55-60 Gy<br>>60 Gy | 3-7% optic neuropathy<br>7-20% optic neuropathy |

*Continued*

TABLE 14.2 ▨ Summary of QUANTEC Tolerance Doses—cont'd

| Organ | Tolerance Doses (range) (Gy) or Recommended DVH Constraint | Complication and Estimated Rate |
|---|---|---|
| Brainstem | <54 Gy entire volume<br>D1-10 cc ≤59 Gy | <5% neuropathy or necrosis<br><5% neuropathy or necrosis |
| Spinal cord | 50 Gy to full thickness cord<br>60 Gy to full thickness cord<br>13 Gy to partial cord, single fraction | 0.2% myelopathy<br>6% myelopathy<br>1% myelopathy |
| Ear (chochlea) | Mean dose <45 Gy | <30% hearing loss |
| Parotid | Mean dose to one gland <20 or <25 for both glands | <20% xerostomia |
| Larynx | V50 <27% and mean dose <44 Gy<br>Mean dose <50 Gy | Reduced risk laryngeal edema<br>Minimize risk of aspiration |
| Lung | V20 ≤30% Gy and mean lung dose (MLD) ≤20 Gy | ≤20% symptomatic pneumonitis |
| Heart | V25 <10%<br><br>Mean pericardium dose ≤26 Gy and V30 ≤46% | <1% probability of cardiac mortality ≈15 years after EBRT<br>Reduced risk of pericarditis (note pericardium volume is different than heart volume) |
| Esophagus | Mean dose <34 Gy<br>V50 <40% | 5-20% Grade 3+ acute esophagitis<br><30% Grade 2+ acute esophagitis |
| Liver | Mean normal liver dose (liver-GTV)<br><28 Gy for primary liver cancer, or those with Child-Pugh A pre-existing liver disease<br><32 Gy for liver mets, excluding patients with pre-existing liver disease | <5% risk of radiation induced liver disease (RILD) |
| Small bowel/ stomach | <45 Gy to whole stomach<br>V15 <120 cc when contouring bowel loops<br>V45 <195 cc when contouring entire volume of peritoneal space | <7% ulceration<br><10% Grade 3+ acute toxicity<br><10% Grade 3+ acute toxicity |
| Kidney | Bilateral kidneys, mean kidney dose <18 Gy<br>Bilateral kidneys, V28 <20%<br>Bilateral kidneys, V23 <30%<br>Bilateral kidneys, V20 <32%<br>Bilateral kidneys, V12 <55% | Estimated risk of kidney damage <5%<br>Estimated risk <5%<br>Estimated risk <5%<br>Estimated risk <5%<br>Estimated risk <5% |
| Bladder | V80 <15%, V75 <25%, V70 <35%, V65 <50%<br>Bladder cancer, whole or partial bladder ≤64-65 Gy in 36 fractions or 40-42 Gy in twice daily fractions | No specific risk given<br><br>RTOG Grade 3 toxicity ≤6% |
| Rectum (segmented from above the anal verge to the turn into sigmoid colon) | Doses up to 78 Gy<br>V50 <50%, V60 <35%, V65 <25%, V70 <20%, V75 <15% | Grade ≥2 <15%<br>Grade ≥3 <10%<br>Reductions in V70 and V75 have greatest impact on reduction of toxicity |
| Penile bulb | Mean dose to 95% of volume <50 Gy D90 <50 Gy | <35% severe erectile dysfunction |

(Adapted from Marks LB, Yorke ED, Jackson A, et al. Use of Normal Tissue Complication Probability Models in the Clinic. Int J Radiat Oncol Biol Phys 2010;76:S10-19.)

The advent of IMRT brought in the concept of inverse planning in which small beam segments are optimized to achieve the desired dose goals. This often results in very heterogeneous target coverage with localized hot spots. IMRT optimization is able to produce steeper gradients in some directions to better spare OARs. In addition, concave distributions can be created, wrapping dose around the spinal cord, for instance. IMRT has been shown to have better OAR sparing at the expense of a larger volume of tissue exposed to low doses.

VMAT has the advantage of optimizing the distribution from all directions in the arc. Though this does give the optimizer more flexibility in some regards, it may be a disadvantage if there are a few discrete angles that have a more optimal geometry. VMAT also spreads out the low doses to an even larger volume. One study showed up to an 11% increase in integral dose using a VMAT approach versus fixed field IMRT.[27]

There is debate as to the significance of the differences in the integral dose between the methods. Will more integral dose lead to more secondary cancers? One study demonstrated an increased risk with higher integral doses.[28] One recent publication reviewed the literature and determined that more long-term studies were needed before any conclusions could be drawn.[29] In general, it is always good practice to minimize the dose outside the irradiated volume to reduce the risk of secondary cancers.

## 14.8 Dose Optimization/Calculation

Dose optimization can be a manual trial and error process of manipulating beam angles, collimator angles, couch angles, beam weights, beam modifiers, and beam energy. Since the mid-1990s automated algorithms utilizing IMRT have been in use. More commonly called inverse planning, the process involves the planner setting desired dose goals for the targets and the OARs. Objective functions and priorities are used by the algorithm to determine which goals to emphasize during the optimization. An objective function describes the cost to exceeding a dose goal for an OAR or not achieving a dose goal for a target. The functions can have thresholds (i.e., cord must not exceed 5000 cGy), linear functions (risk proportional to dose), power functions (as dose exceeds a certain level the risk becomes much greater), or many other possibilities. These are also known as cost functions. Biological models may be used in the optimization process. These models attempt to account for the different biological responses of tissues to physical dose.

It should be noted that dose values and parameters set in the optimization process are not the same as the desired clinical goals, but many TPS systems do not have a way to distinguish between the two. During the optimization process, the dose values for an OAR or target may be set to an artificially low or high value in an attempt to drive the optimization to the desired result. The plan should still be evaluated using the original goals. If the TPS does not have the ability to differentiate between planning goals and optimization values, it should be clearly documented that this is the case.

After a plan has been optimized and it is ready for physician review, it is advisable to have the plan undergo a peer review to confirm its integrity.[2] One study has described an automated method to check plan integrity before it is shown to the physician for approval.[30] Yang et al. developed scripts and software modules that automatically check a wide variety of plan information. A summary of Table I from this report is shown in Table 14.3. The items in this table should be checked using either an automated method as described or a manual method as was done at this institution prior to developing the automated process. Other such studies have also appeared in the literature, though, to date, no vendor solution is available.

## 14.9 Plan Evaluation and Dose Reporting

Both ICRU-83[14] and the ASTRO report[15] strongly advocate for DVH-based dose reporting as opposed to reporting dose to point(s). This is necessary for comparing a particular plan to

TABLE 14.3 ▓ **Summary of Automated Plan Integrity Check**

| Plan Data | Integrity Check |
| --- | --- |
| Patient information and setup | Report patient identification, position, and scan orientation for user verification |
| General plan setup | Outside patient–air density threshold, proper couch removal, proper localization, proper coordinate system |
| Regions of interest (ROI) | Presence of empty contours, density overrides, gaps in axial slices |
| Beams | Named according to institution convention, field ID, consistency of isocenter, machine name, prescription ownership |
| Prescriptions | Empty prescription without beams, invalid prescription definition |
| Dose calculation parameters | Dose calc grid and resolution, heterogeneity corrections, computation algorithm, max dose vs prescription dose, max dose points are inside PTV |
| IMRT optimization | Proper optimization process used, segment MU > institution standard (4 in their case), number of segments per field < institution standard, total number of segments < institution standard, possible conflicts in optimization objectives (i.e., min and max doses for structures that overlap), ROI used for optimization but is partially outside dose grid, empty ROI used in optimization, IMRT objective ranking |

(Adapted from Yang et al. Automated radiotherapy treatment plan integrity verification. Med Phys 2012;39(3): 1542-1551.)

published reports of normal tissue tolerances, for example, the QUANTEC reports.[26,31] It avoids a possible trap in reporting the dose to a specific point, because that point might be low or high dose depending on where in the volume that point happens to be located. The ASTRO 2009 IMRT report notes that if point dose prescription is used the difference between the actual delivered dose and the prescribed dose can vary by upward of 10%. For this reason care should be taken in interpreting treatment records performed at another institution if DVH metrics are not reported.

The most relevant DVH statistic is the $D_{V\%}$ value. For example, the PTV $D_{100\%}$ is the minimum dose received by 100% of the PTV volume. Alternatively this can be stated as a $V_{DGy}$ value (i.e., the percent or absolute volume of an organ receiving a dose of $D$ Gy or more). There is no hard recommendation in ICRU-83 as to which $D_{V\%}$ value should be reported for the target structures. The report notes, though, that PTV $D_{50\%}$ appears to be most consistent across planning systems. ICRU-83 recommends that if $D_{50\%}$ is not used to set the prescription it should at least be reported. The ASTRO 2009 IMRT report goes a little further, recommending that the following doses be reported for both the PTV and CTV: mean dose, $D_{95\%}$, $D_{100\%}$, $V_{100\%}$, and maximum dose. The report recommends that at the very least the prescribed dose (and fractionation) should be noted and the point or volume to which it is prescribed.

For OARs the ASTRO 2009 IMRT report recommends the following doses be reported: maximum, minimum, and mean. ICRU-83 is somewhat more specific and recommends that a "near-maximum" or "near-minimum" dose statistic be used. An example would be $D_{2\%}$ (the dose received by 2% or more of the OAR) and $D_{98\%}$ (the dose received by 98% or more of the OAR). These are more reliable than the minimum or maximum point doses because point doses can be overly sensitive to changes in the dose calculation grid. ICRU-83 recommends that for serial-like organs a near-maximum dose statistic be reported (e.g., $D_{98\%}$) whereas for parallel organs the mean dose should be reported in addition to any relevant statistics for $D_{V\%}$ (or alternatively $V_{DGy}$).

An example might be the lung, where the QUANTEC paper suggests reporting $V_{20Gy}$ and limiting it to ≤30% to 35% to achieve a pneumonitis risk <20%.[32] An open question is whether or not the tumor volume should be subtracted from the organ when reporting dose statistics. In the lung, for example, the normal lung volume is usually defined as the lung excluding the GTV as discussed in the QUANTEC paper on lung.[32] Excluding the PTV would artificially underestimate the dose to the potentially functional lung.

It is important to note that the entire organ must be contoured for the dose statistics to be accurate. In some cases there is an ambiguity as to what extent an OAR should be contoured, an example being the rectum contours in a prostate case. If the rectum is extended far superiorly the result will be an apparently better rectal DVH since the overall volume is larger. In many clinical trials (e.g., RTOG) these details are specified, and it is good practice to develop institutional policies and procedures to standardize dose reporting within an institution. For example, RTOG 0534 specified the rectum should be outlined from the anterior flexion of the rectosigmoid superiorly to the ischial tuberosities inferiorly. The entire bladder should be outlined down to the anastomosis.

There are additional statistics that might be of interest. ICRU-83 refers to these as "level 3" reporting (i.e., optional parameters for research and development). These statistics include:

- Conformity index, *CI*. A measure of how closely the dose conforms to the target region, a value of unity being ideal. A common definition is $CI = \dfrac{V_{pi}}{V_T}$, where $V_{pi}$ is the volume enclosed in the prescription isodose line and $V_T$ is the volume of the target.[15,33]
- Conformity index.[34] CI = c × s where:
  - $c = V_D \cap V_T / V_T$
  - $s = V_D \cap V_T / V_D$
  - $V_D$ = volume receiving prescription dose
  - $V_T$ = target volume
- Homogeneity index, *HI*. A measure of the homogeneity of dose within a target region. There are various formulations of homogeneity index but ICRU-83 advocates the definition $(D_{2\%}-D_{98\%})/D_{50\%}$.
- Dose similarity coefficient, which ICRU-83 defines as $2 \cdot (V_T \cap PTV)/(V_T + PTV)$
- Equivalent uniform dose (EUD), a generalized mean dose[35]
- Biological model parameters. These include tumor control probability (TCP), normal tissue complication probability (NTCP), and probability of uncomplicated control. For further discussion see the QUANTEC papers.[26]

Each plan results in a set of dose–volume parameters, but it must be recognized that each DVH is subject to uncertainties, including the ability of an accelerator to deliver the planned dose and the interfraction and intrafraction variability in patient setup and anatomy. Though the concept of a DVH confidence interval is at least 15 years old,[36] few commercial planning systems have implemented this functionality, with the notable exception of proton radiotherapy planning systems. ICRU-83 recommends that "treatment-planning systems must make an effort to make available new capabilities to report the uncertainty or confidence intervals for their calculated absorbed-dose distributions."[14]

In addition to reviewing the DVH values for the planning goals, the isodose displays should be reviewed to assess for features that could have a clinical impact. For example, where is the location of the PTV hot spot? If it is within an OAR or directly adjacent, an attempt to reoptimize may be warranted. Are there dose "fingers" or peripheral hot spots? These can occur with nonisocentric techniques and noncoplanar beams or arcs. Is the treatment time tolerable for the patient? Are any beams unnecessarily impinging on normal tissue (e.g., exiting through an arm)?

# 14.10 Plan Implementation and Review

Even after the plan has been approved in the TPS many steps remain before the patient can be treated.

1. The plan must be exported to other systems as appropriate (record and verify, MU second check) (see Chapter 5 for details on MU second checks).
2. The information must be imported into those systems and validated.
3. A plan second check is performed by the physicist. This includes the verification of plan parameter transfer to the R&V system, MU verification, consistency of plan with prescription, and overall assessment of plan quality. Patient-specific QA measurements will be performed as needed. It is recommended that these be done before the first treatment.[2]
4. A pretreatment QA is performed by the therapist to confirm the proper transfer of information to the linac control system. Some facilities perform this at the time of plan verification simulation, and others perform it prior to arrival of the patient. If done prior to patient treatment, it may include successful mode-up of all beams and checking for collision issues.
5. Physician peer review. This may not happen prior to the first treatment.

# 14.11 Treatment Interruptions and Changes in Fractionation

It is fairly common for patients to have an interruption in their course of treatment due to a complication such as skin toxicity, low blood counts, or esophagitis. If the break in treatment is prolonged, a significant decrease in tumor control can be expected depending on the type of tumor (lung and head and neck tumors, for example). Models similar to those discussed in Section 14.9 are used to calculate the change in fractionation needed to mitigate the decreased probability of tumor control. The models use a time factor to account for the extension of the treatment course. Typically, an equivalent dose to normal tissue is calculated to determine how much extra dose to give since an increase in complications is undesirable. Two strategies can be employed: keep the dose per fraction the same and increase the number of fractions, or keep the total number of fractions the same and increase the dose per fraction. Another scenario is that a physician may decide to shorten a course of treatment based on response or something unrelated, such as the patient's wish to leave on a planned trip or because the treatment course was delayed due to equipment down time. This can usually be accommodated with weekend treatments but sometimes cannot.

A general methodology to calculate the desired change in fractionation in any of the scenarios discussed above is called the biologically effective dose (BED). Fowler published a review of the BED concept.[37] In it, the reader is cautioned that BED is NOT biologically equivalent dose, but rather biologically effective dose. To get equivalent dose the BED must be divided by a factor that depends on whether the tissue is early or late responding. There is ongoing debate as to whether the BED concept applies to the large fractions used in SRS and SBRT. The BED is calculated with the alpha/beta ratio and time factors as follows:

$$BED = nd(1 + d/[\alpha/\beta]) - \log_e 2(T - T_k)/\alpha T_p$$

where n = number of fractions, d = dose per fraction in Gy, $T_k$ = time factor accounting for the delay in the kickoff of repopulation, and $T_p$ = time factor to account for repopulation. Typical values for $\alpha/\beta$ are 3 for late-reacting tissues, 2 for central nervous system, 10 for early-reacting tissues, and 10 for tumors. A value of 0.35 is generally used for $\alpha$. $T_k$ is approximately 21 days for tumors and 7 days for acute mucosa. $T_p$ is 3 days for tumor and 2.5 days for acute mucosa.[37] Online calculators and smart phone applications are available to perform BED calculations.

# 14.12 Developing Techniques in Treatment Planning

Treatment planning continues to evolve rapidly in an attempt to achieve better optimization, provide better tools for plan evaluation, provide methods to predict probable outcomes, and more accurately describe the actual delivered dose. A few of these emerging techniques are discussed below.

## BIOLOGICAL MODELS

A good introduction to the use of biological models is given in AAPM TG-166, The Use and QA of Biologically Related Models for Treatment Planning.[38] The main idea behind using biological models in treatment planning is to directly correlate the dose distribution to outcomes. In contrast, traditional dose/volume–based planning relies on correlating outcome through a series of empirically determined dose-response relationships. The problem with using these dose/volume metrics is that there may be more than one metric that correlates to the outcome; therefore satisfying one or even several of the metrics does not guarantee the outcome. In addition, the use of more metrics increases the complexity of the optimization problem. With increased complexity comes increased risk of having multiple local minima in the solution space, thus increasing the probability of achieving a suboptimal result. Another confounding issue with dose–volume metrics is that they are dependent on delivery technique (e.g., 3D conformal versus IMRT).[32] The use of biological models directly related to outcomes simplifies the optimization problem, potentially leading to better results. AAPM TG-166 states that because the absolute values of the outcome probabilities may not be reliable, caution should be used with biological models in treatment planning. In addition to using biological models in plan optimization, they can be used for plan evaluation. They may be particularly useful when evaluating several alternative plans when it is unclear as to which is optimal based on dose–volume metrics.

There currently are four common biological models in use.

1. **Generalized Equivalent Uniform Dose (gEUD)** proposed by Niemierko.[35] The gEUD provides a single metric for nonuniform dose distributions. It is defined as the uniform dose that, if delivered over the same number of fractions as the nonuniform dose distribution, yields the same radiobiological effect (AAPM TG-166). It is calculated using the following formula:

$$gEUD = [\Sigma_i v_i D_i^a]^{1/a}$$

where $v_i$ is the fractional organ volume receiving a dose $D_i$ and $a$ is a tissue-specific parameter that describes the volume effect. As $a$ approaches negative infinity, gEUD approaches the minimum dose; thus negative values are used for tumors. As $a$ approaches positive infinity, gEUD approaches the maximum dose (serial organs). For $a = 1$, gEUD is equal to the arithmetic mean dose. For $a = 0$, gEUD is equal to the geometric mean dose.

2. **Tumor Control Probability (TCP).** The TCP is calculated based on the linear quadratic (LQ) model of cell killing which has been linked to DNA damage, specifically double strand breaks. The functions used to calculate TCP typically use the alpha/beta ratio ($\alpha/\beta$) as the sole parameter, and it is usually assumed to be 3 Gy for late-responding normal tissues and 10 Gy for tumors and early-responding normal tissues.

3. **Normal Tissue Complication Probability (NTCP).** These models incorporate volume effects to model dose-response relationships. Parallel organs are those in which function can be retained even if a considerable volume has been damaged. Volume effects are significant in these organs, and the mean dose is often correlated to response. Lung, kidney, and liver are examples of parallel organs. Serial organs are those in which function is impaired if even a small volume is damaged and so the maximum dose is correlated to response. Spinal cord,

intestines, and optic nerves are examples of serial organs. Various models for calculating NTCP are discussed in AAPM TG-166.

4. **Complication Free Cure (P+).** This is an optimization cost function that attempts to maximize the difference between TCP and NTCP.

The general recommendations and precautions from AAPM TG-166 for the use of biologically based models are summarized as follows:

1. Biologically based cost functions for OARs may be preferable to dose–volume constraints because they typically control entire portions of the dose–volume domain whereas dose–volume constraints control only a single point. A single EUD-based cost function can replace multiple constraints if an appropriate volume effect parameter is chosen.
2. Current biological models only control cold spots for targets and therefore can be replaced with simple minimum dose constraints.
3. Current biological models do not effectively control hot spots for targets and therefore should be supplemented by maximum dose constraints.
4. Until the biological models are better understood and validated, treatment plans should be evaluated with traditional dose–volume criteria in addition to biological metrics.
5. A full review of the 3D dose distribution should always be performed.

## PLAN EVALUATION TOOLS

As mentioned previously, the aim of treatment planning optimization is to maximize the dose to the targets while minimizing the dose to the OARs. In many cases the total dose to the targets is limited by the tolerance doses of the OARs. One question that continually comes up is, how do you know when you have achieved the optimal plan? The use of biological models may assist in that regard by directly correlating the plan to outcomes. Strategies such as multicriteria optimization (MCO) have been developed that assist the clinician in the evaluation of many possible solutions quickly.[39] MCO works by creating a database of plans that satisfy different planning goals (i.e., a plan that optimizes target coverage, a plan that optimizes cord sparing, a plan that optimizes left parotid sparing, etc.). The database of plans comprises what is called the Pareto surface. Moving between plans on the Pareto surface results in tradeoffs as one goal is emphasized over another. The database of plans is precalculated so that moving between them can be done in real time, allowing clinicians to quickly optimize the plan to meet their goals. In addition, methods to benchmark the current plan against previous plans of a similar type to determine if further improvement is likely[40] or to predict the achievable DVH based on the distance of a voxel to the target volume have been proposed.[41] These approaches utilize geometric information to estimate what could be achieved in terms of a dose–volume relationship for each OAR.

## ADAPTIVE PLANNING

Adaptive radiotherapy (ART) incorporates changes in anatomy and/or deviations in planned delivered dose due to patient setup deviations or machine delivery deviations to estimate the actual delivered dose to a patient as the treatment progresses. The anatomy changes and setup deviations can be identified using daily 3D IGRT. Transmission detectors mounted on the machine head can detect machine delivery deviations if used on a daily basis. Electronic portal imaging devices (EPIDs) can be used to detect setup and delivery deviations although they cannot differentiate between the two unless used in combination with a transmission detector and/or 3D imaging. Ultimately some or all of this information is used to calculate the daily dose distribution and sum them to generate the estimated delivered dose. If this deviates significantly from the original planned dose, the plan can be reoptimized to bring the final dose back into agreement with the original plan. Recent studies have shown the advantage of ART for pelvis and head and neck treatments.[42,43] Although ART is promising, it should be approached with caution. There is a lack of data concerning what level of deviation is clinically significant and continued replanning will significantly strain resources. To make ART more feasible, automated segmentation of the 3D data sets would be desirable. A recent study performed a risk analysis of ART and found there were significant but manageable risks in the areas of segmentation and planning.[44] It is hoped that these strategies will result in less uncertainty in the final delivered dose, which in turn will enable more accurate determination of dose-response relationships. However, they rely on deformable image registration, which in itself currently has large uncertainties (see upcoming AAPM TG-132). Another issue to consider is that the daily imaging used to calculate the daily doses may have a limited FOV causing the external contour of the patient to be cut off or missing entirely. Approximations must be made in order to calculate the dose.

## ROBUSTNESS

Once a treatment plan has been approved, it is assumed that it will be delivered with an acceptable degree of fidelity over the entire course of treatment. The theory of robustness takes into account possible deviations (random and systematic setup errors, dose delivery errors, organ motion, etc.) during a course and evaluates the sensitivity of a treatment plan to these changes.[45-47] For example, there may be differences in this regard between fixed beam and VMAT approaches. One vendor (RaySearch Labs) has implemented robustness analysis for proton beams, and others are working on it.

The idea of using probability weighted dose distributions and probability weighted objective functions that can produce robust plans rather than margins has been the topic of many studies. Gordon et al.[48] published a description of one such strategy, which has an overview of many of these methods. In these approaches, the planner does not specify a set of margins, but rather a probability function. A common method to account for random setup errors is to convolve the dose distribution with the uncertainty distribution. This basically leads to a blurring of the dose distribution and the creation of dose horns at the edges of the TV. It is unclear if this method provides an adequate solution for systematic errors, which can be more important as discussed above. Gordon has proposed a coverage optimized planning (COP) concept to specifically address systematic errors.[48] One potential advantage of these methods is that they calculate coverage on a per patient basis rather than relying on margins that were calculated on a population basis (e.g., the van Herk margin formulation was designed to ensure that the PTV is covered for 90% of the treatments for a population of patients).

---

### FOR THE PHYSICIAN

Treatment planning can be a very involved and complicated process. As such, clear directives and communication among all team members are very important. Beginning with the first step, patient positioning and immobilization, there should be active involvement by the therapists, dosimetrists, physicists, nurses, and physicians.

Either a single or multiple imaging modalities may be used in the development of the treatment plan. CT is currently the most widely used primary modality, but work is being done to also utilize MR as the primary modality. The primary modality may be supplemented by one or more secondary imaging studies (such as MRI, PET, SPECT) that can provide better target delineation, better visualization of OARs, or functional information. Once these image sets are acquired they must be coregistered so that geometric accuracy is maintained. This can be done in a rigid or deformable manner.

Accurate identification of the target(s) and OARs is critical to developing a high quality treatment plan. There is a lot of ongoing research into methods for automating the contouring process, including auto-segmentation and atlas-based approaches. ICRU and ASTRO recommendations for the naming and definition of certain volumes should be followed. Included in these are expansion volumes used to account for microscopic disease and patient setup deviations. The margins used should be carefully evaluated at each institution to make sure that they are consistent with the technologies being used. Many publications have described "margin recipes" and are reviewed in ICRU-83. Regardless of the method used, it must be recognized that the use of IMRT alone does not generally warrant a reduction in margins. IMRT has more impact on gradients, which can result in less dose to nearby OARs, but does not impact setup variation, which the margin is designed to mitigate. Margin reduction is more properly achieved through the use of IGRT rather than IMRT.

Once the anatomy has been defined, a delivery technique and dose goals for targets and OARs must be identified. The choice of technique (simple single or opposed fields versus 3D conformal versus IMRT versus VMAT, etc.) is determined by the clinical goals. In general, the simplest technique that can achieve the clinical goals should be used. This will lead to shorter treatment times, increasing patient comfort, and by nature of being simpler will lower the risk of errors being introduced.

A treatment plan can be evaluated using many dose–volume metrics. ASTRO and ICRU have published recommendations on what values should be reported. The dose–volume relationships have been determined empirically, and there is a lot of uncertainty in the values due to differences in fractionation, different methods of dose calculation and reporting, and patient biological variability, among other reasons. Widespread use of IMRT and VMAT also calls into question the role of large low dose regions, which were less common in the 3D conformal era. Further, increasing use of hypofractionated or radiosurgery treatments (high dose, few fractions) also calls into question the accuracy of existing dose limits in the high dose region. The QUANTEC reports contain a wealth of information on dose–volume relationships for many organs.

Biological modeling and adaptive planning are two emerging strategies in treatment planning. The goal of biological modeling (such as NTCP, TCP, and gEUD) is to drive better treatment results by directly correlating the dose distribution to outcomes rather than correlating outcome through a series of empirically determined dose-response relationships. In addition, biological models have the potential to improve the optimization process through the use of fewer parameters that affect a greater portion of the dose–volume relationship space. These models are still in active development, and caution should be used when they are implemented. Adaptive radiotherapy (ART) is a process in which the dose is accumulated on a daily basis, accounting for setup deviations, delivery deviations, and changes in anatomy. If this deviates significantly from the original planned dose, the plan can be reoptimized to bring the final dose back into agreement with the original plan. Although ART is promising, it should be approached with caution. There is a lack of data concerning what level of deviation is clinically significant, and in its current form continued replanning will significantly strain resources.

## References

1. Ford EC, Fong de Los Santos L, Pawlicki T, et al. Consensus recommendation for incident learning database structures in Radiation Oncology. Med Phys 2012;39(12):7272–90.
2. Fraass B, Doppke K, Hunt M, et al. American Association of Physicists in Medicine Radiation Therapy Committee Task Group 53: Quality assurance for clinical radiotherapy treatment planning. Med Phys 1998;25(10):1773–829.
3. Safety is no accident: A framework for quality Radiation Oncology and care, American Society for Radiation Oncology (ASTRO), 2012, Available on ASTRO website, https://www.astro.org/uploadedFiles/Main_Site/Clinical_Practice/Patient_Safety/Blue_Book/SafetyisnoAccident.pdf.
4. Nelms BE, Tomé WA, Robinson G, et al. Variation in external beam treatment plan quality: An interinstitutional study of planners and planning systems. Pract Radiat Oncol 2012;2(4):296–305.
5. Keall PJ, Chock LB, Jeraj R, et al. Image reconstruction and the effect on dose calculation for hip prostheses. Med Dosim 2003;28(2):113–17.

6. Mail N, Albarakati Y, Ahmad Khan M, et al. The impacts of dental filling materials on RapidArc treatment planning and dose delivery: Challenges and solution. Med Phys 2013;40(8):081714.

7. Wu V, Podgorsak MB, Tran T-A, et al. Dosimetric impact of image artifact from a wide-bore CT scanner in radiotherapy treatment planning. Med Phys 2011;38(7):4451–63.

8. Gregoire V, Chiti A. PET in radiotherapy planning: Particularly exquisite test or pending and experimental tool? Radiother Oncol 2010;96:275–6.

9. Jonsson JH, Karlsson MG, Karlsson M, et al. Treatment planning using MRI data: An analysis of the dose calculation accuracy for different treatment regions. Radiat Oncol 2010;5:62.

10. Dowling JA, Burdett N, Greer PB, et al. An atlas-based electron density mapping method for magnetic resonance imaging (MRI)-alone treatment planning and adaptive MRI-based prostate radiation therapy. Int J Radiat Oncol Biol Phys 2012;83(1):e5–11.

11. Varadhan R, Karangelis G, Krishnan K, et al. A framework for deformable image registration validation in radiotherapy clinical applications. JACMP 2012;14(1):4066.

12. Kashani R, Hub M, Balter JM, et al. Objective assessment of deformable image registration in radiotherapy: A multi-institutional study. Med Phys 2008;35:5944.

13. Hardcastle N, van Elmpt W, De Ruysscher D, et al. Accuracy of deformable image registration for contour propagation in adaptive lung radiotherapy. Radiat Oncol 2013;8:243.

14. Gregoire V, Mackie TR. ICRU committee on volume and dose specification for prescribing, recording and reporting special techniques in external photon beam therapy: Conformal and IMRT. Radiother Oncol 2005;76:S71. ICRU. Prescribing, Recording, and Reporting Intensity-Modulated Photon-Beam Therapy. ICRU Report 83. Bethesda, MD: International Commission on Radiation Units and Measurements; 2010.

15. Holmes T, Das R, Low D, et al. American Society of Radiation Oncology recommendations for documenting intensity-modulated radiation therapy treatments. Int J Radiat Oncol Biol Phys 2009;74: 1311–18.

16. ICRU. Prescribing, recording and reporting photon beam therapy. ICRU Report 50. Bethesda, MD: International Commission on Radiation Units and Measurements; 1993.

17. ICRU. Prescribing, recording and reporting photon beam therapy (Supplement to ICRU Report 50). ICRU Report 62. Bethesda, MD: International Commission on Radiation Units and Measurements; 1999.

18. Marks LB, Adams RD, Pawlicki T, et al. Enhancing the role of case-oriented peer review to improve quality and safety in Radiation Oncology: Executive summary. Practical Radiat Oncol 2013;3:149–56.

19. Chera BS, Mazur L, Jackson M, et al. Quantification of the impact of multifaceted initiatives intended to improve operational efficiency and the safety culture: A case study from an academic medical center Radiation Oncology department. Practical Radiat Oncol 2014;4(2):e101–8.

20. Ng M, Leong T, Chander S, et al. Australasian Gastrointestinal Trials Group (AGITG) contouring atlas and planning guidelines for intensity-modulated radiotherapy in anal cancer. Int J Radiat Oncol Biol Phys 2012;83(5):1455–62.

21. Nielsen MH, Berg M, Pedersen AN, et al. Delineation of target volumes and organs at risk in adjuvant radiotherapy of early breast cancer: National guidelines and contouring atlas by the Danish Breast Cancer Cooperative Group. Acta Oncol 2013;52(4):703–10.

22. van Herk M, Remeijer P, Rasch C, et al. The probability of correct target dosage: Dose-population histograms for deriving treatment margins in radiotherapy. Int J Radiat Oncol Biol Phys 2000;47:1121–35.

23. Siebers JV, Keall PJ, Wu Q, et al. Effect of patient setup errors on simultaneously integrated boost head and neck IMRT treatment plans. Int J Radiat Oncol Biol Phys 2005;63(2):422–33.

24. Engels B, Soete G, Verellen D, et al. Conformal arc radiotherapy for prostate cancer: Increased biochemical failure in patients with distended rectum on the planning computed tomogram despite image guidance with implanted markers. Int J Radiat Oncol Biol Phys 2009;74:388–91.

25. Emami B, Lyman J, Brown A, et al. Tolerance of normal tissue to therapeutic irradiation. Int J Radiat Oncol Biol Phys 1991;21(1):109–22.

26. Marks LB, Ten Haken RK, Martel MK. Guest editor's introduction to QUANTEC: A users guide. Int J Radiat Oncol Biol Phys 2010;76:S1–2.

27. Lui OY, Li WK, Lock CKM, et al. Dosimetric comparison between RapidArc and conventional fixed-field intensity-modulated radiotherapy for prostate cancer. Biomed Imaging Intervention J 2013; 9(3):e17.

28. Tukenova M, Guibout C, Hawkins M, et al. Radiation therapy and late mortality from second sarcoma, carcinoma, and hematological malignancies after a solid cancer in childhood. Int J Radiat Oncol Biol Phys 2011;80(2):339–46.

29. Zhuang T, Huang L, Qi P, et al. Radiation therapy: Clinical application of volumetric arc therapy. Appl Radiat Oncol 2013;6–11.

30. Yang D, Moore KL. Automated radiotherapy treatment plan integrity verification. Med Phys 2012;39(3):1542–51.

31. Bentzen SM, Constine LS, Deasy JO, et al. Quantitative Analysis of Normal Tissue Effects in the Clinic (QUANTEC). Int J Radiat Oncol Biol Phys 2010;76(Suppl. 3):S3–9.

32. Marks LB, Bentzen SM, Deasy JO, et al. Radiation dose-volume effects in the lung. Int J Radiat Oncol Biol Phys 2010;76:S70–6.

33. Lomax NJ, Scheib SG. Quantifying the degree of conformity in radiosurgery treatment planning. Int J Radiat Oncol Biol Phys 2003;55:1409–19.

34. Paddick I. A simple scoring ratio to index the conformity of radiosurgical treatment plans. Technical note. J Neurosurg 2000;93(Suppl.):219–22.

35. Niemerko A. Reporting and analyzing dose distributions: A concept of equivalent uniform dose. Med Phys 1997;24(1):103–10.

36. Stroom JC, de Boer HC, Huizenga H, et al. Inclusion of geometrical uncertainties in radiotherapy treatment planning by means of coverage probability. Int J Radiat Oncol Biol Phys 1999;43: 905–19.

37. Fowler JF. 21 years of biologically effective dose. Br J Radiol 2010;83(991):554–68.

38. Li XA, Alber M, Deasy JO, et al. The use and QA of biologically related models for treatment planning. Med Phys 2012;39(3):1386–409.

39. Craft DL, Hong TS, Shih HA, et al. Improved planning time and plan quality through multicriteria optimization for intensity-modulated radiotherapy. Int J Radiat Oncol Biol Phys 2012;82(1): e83–90.

40. Moore J, Herman J, Evans K, et al. Clinical deployment of an automatic planning interface for overlap volume histogram based treatment planning. Med Phys 2012;39:3752.

41. Appenzoller L, Tan J, Thorstad W, et al. Predicting dose-volume histograms for organs-at-risk in IMRT planning. Med Phys 2012;39(12):7446–61.

42. Wu QJ, Li T, Wu Q, et al. Adaptive radiation therapy: Technical components and clinical applications. Cancer J 2011;17:182–9.

43. Jaffray DA. Image-guided radiotherapy: From current concept to future perspectives. Nat Rev 2012;9:688–99.

44. Noel CE, Santanam L, Parikh PJ, et al. Process-based quality management for clinical implementation of adaptive radiotherapy. Med Phys 2014;41(8).

45. Chu M, Zinchenko Y, Henderson SG, et al. Robust optimization for intensity modulated radiation therapy treatment planning under uncertainty. Phys Med Biol 2005;50(23):5463–77.

46. Fredriksson A. A characterization of robust radiation therapy treatment planning methods—from expected value to worst case optimization. Med Phys 2012;39(8):5169–81.

47. Chen W, Unkelbach J, Trofimov A, et al. Including robustness in multi-criteria optimization for intensity-modulated proton therapy. Phys Med Biol 2012;57(3):591–608.

48. Gordon JJ, Sayah N, Weiss E, et al. Coverage optimized planning: Probabilistic treatment planning based on dose coverage histogram criteria. Med Phys 2010;37(2):550–63.

# CHAPTER 15

# The Use of Electrons for External Beam Radiotherapy

## 15.1 Introduction

Electron beams have been used in radiotherapy since the 1940s but did not gain widespread use until the 1970s with the commercial development of linear accelerators (linacs). Electrons lose energy as they traverse a medium through various elastic and inelastic collisions with atomic electrons and the nucleus. Inelastic collisions with the nucleus result in a radiative loss of a photon, called bremsstrahlung production. The bremsstrahlung radiation created by electron beam interactions with high atomic number scattering foils and other materials in the beam path is called photon contamination. Electrons are a charged particle with a finite range and are therefore suitable for treatment of superficial or shallow targets.

As charged particles, megavoltage electrons undergo more scattering than megavoltage photons, particularly in air. It is because of this that electron beams use cones with beam trimmers that are close to the patient surface to minimize scatter outside the treatment field. To further customize the shape of the beam, cerrobend cutouts are placed on top of the trimmers.

The electron scatter changes with initial electron energy and depth in the medium. This makes matching of electron fields with other electron fields or photon fields difficult. The many sources of scatter in the electron beam path (scattering foils, linac dose chamber, electron cone) also affect the distance dependence of the beam output. The concept of an effective source position is used to describe this.

Three factors that greatly affect the dose distribution of electron beams are beam obliquity, surface irregularity, and tissue inhomogeneity. Traditional pencil beam algorithms do not accurately calculate dose under these conditions. Monte Carlo calculations for electrons are becoming increasingly common and perform much better in these conditions.

American Association of Physicists in Medicing (AAPM) Task Group (TG)-25, Clinical Electron Beam Dosimetry, provides a good overview of electron beam characteristics.[1] Chapter 8 in the *IAEA Radiation Oncology Physics Handbook* also gives a nice review.[2] Hogstrom and Almond published a review of electron beam therapy physics.[3] AAPM TG-70, Recommendations for Clinical Electron Beam Dosimetry, produced a supplement to AAPM TG-25 that updated the absolute dosimetry sections to reflect the change to absorbed dose in water standards.[4] The discussions in AAPM TG-25 on obliquity, surface dose, effective source position, air gap corrections, and use of diodes remain valid. The AAPM TG-70 report gives a detailed discussion on the use of electrons in many clinical situations. What follows in this chapter is a brief discussion on electron beam characteristics and the impact of the three factors mentioned above, beam obliquity, surface irregularity, and tissue inhomogeneity. This is followed by a discussion of three common clinical situations: bolus, surface shielding, and compensators. Total skin electron therapy is described in Chapter 24, and electron intraoperative therapy is described in Chapter 23.

## 15.2 Beam Characteristics

### DEPTH DOSE

Typical electron beam depth dose curves are shown in Figure 15.1. They show a relatively high surface dose compared to photon beams of the same nominal energy, a build-up to maximum dose, a rapid fall-off in dose, and then a small low dose component called the bremsstrahlung tail or photon contamination. The photon contamination increases with increasing energy as shown in Figure 15.1. There are various depth dose parameters that are used to describe an electron depth dose curve: surface dose, depth of maximum dose (R100 or $D_{max}$), depth of 90% dose (R90), depth of 80% dose (R80), depth of 50% dose (R50), the practical range (Rp), and the photon contamination. Depth dose parameters do change with field size, but the change is small for field sizes larger than the practical range. In fact, the data from Hu et al. demonstrate that for energies less than or equal to 16 MeV, the changes in any of the range parameters are less than 1 mm from 10 cm × 10 cm to 25 cm × 25 cm cone sizes.[5] For energies less than or equal to 12 MeV this extends down to a 6 × 6 cone. Sample data are shown in Table 15.1. For higher energies there can be significant differences, as shown in Figure 15.2. For electrons the surface dose increases with energy, which is the opposite of photons. This is also shown in Figure 15.1.

There are general rules of thumb that can be used to estimate the range parameters, and they are shown in Table 15.2. These are intended to be quick estimates and cannot replace measured data. The values may differ slightly for linacs of different models. In clinical practice, these values should be tabulated in a convenient format similar to the table in Figure 15.1 and made readily available to the clinicians as an aid in selecting beam energy. In clinical practice the energy is often selected so that the R90 depth is at least as deep as the distal-most aspect of the planning target volume (PTV). The energy should also be limited to reduce dose to any normal tissues or organs at risk (OARs) distal to the target.

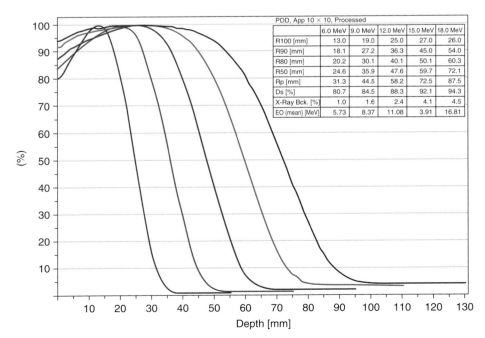

| PDD, App 10 × 10, Processed | | | | | |
|---|---|---|---|---|---|
| | 6.0 MeV | 9.0 MeV | 12.0 MeV | 15.0 MeV | 18.0 MeV |
| R100 [mm] | 13.0 | 19.0 | 25.0 | 27.0 | 26.0 |
| R90 [mm] | 18.1 | 27.2 | 36.3 | 45.0 | 54.0 |
| R80 [mm] | 20.2 | 30.1 | 40.1 | 50.1 | 60.3 |
| R50 [mm] | 24.6 | 35.9 | 47.6 | 59.7 | 72.1 |
| Rp [mm] | 31.3 | 44.5 | 58.2 | 72.5 | 87.5 |
| Ds [%] | 80.7 | 84.5 | 88.3 | 92.1 | 94.3 |
| X-Ray Bck. [%] | 1.0 | 1.6 | 2.4 | 4.1 | 4.5 |
| EO (mean) [MeV] | 5.73 | 8.37 | 11.08 | 3.91 | 16.81 |

**Figure 15.1** Sample electron depth dose curves.

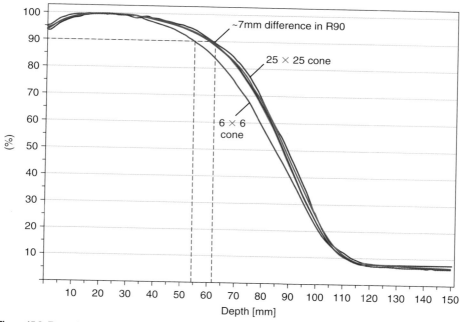

**Figure 15.2** Example of depth dose change with decreasing cone size for a higher energy electron energy (22 MeV).

TABLE 15.1 ▪ **R90 (in mm) by Energy and Cone Size from Hu et al.[5]**

| Energy (MeV) | Cone Size (cm) | | | | |
|---|---|---|---|---|---|
| | **6** | **10** | **15** | **20** | **25** |
| 6 | 18.5 | 18.4 | 18.4 | 18.5 | 18.6 |
| 9 | 28.5 | 28.4 | 28.5 | 28.5 | 28.7 |
| 12 | 39.5 | 39.7 | 39.7 | 39.9 | 40.0 |
| 16 | 49.2 | 51.2 | 51.5 | 51.5 | 51.7 |
| 20 | 54.5 | 59.0 | 60.1 | 60.4 | 61.0 |

TABLE 15.2 ▪ **Electron Beam Range Parameters Rules of Thumb**

| Parameter | Estimation Formula (E is the nominal energy in MeV) |
|---|---|
| R90 in cm | E/(3.2 to 3.3) |
| R80 in cm | E/(2.9 to 3.0) |
| Rp in cm | E/2 |
| Surface dose (%) | E+(70 to 74) |

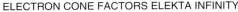

ELECTRON CONE FACTORS ELEKTA INFINITY

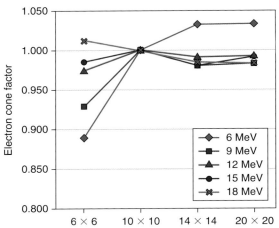

**Figure 15.3** Sample electron cone output factors by cone size and energy.

## OUTPUT AND CUTOUTS

The output trend of the electron cones will vary by energy. The Radiological Physics Center (RPC), now IROC Houston, has published benchmark data for many linac models.[6] There are also other benchmark data sets as described in Chapter 5. A sample set of data is shown in Figure 15.3. As mentioned above, the depth dose is unchanged for field sizes greater than the practical range. Similarly, there is little change in the output of an electron beam down to cutout sizes equal to the practical range. Given that Rp can be estimated by E/2, this implies that only fields less than 3 cm for a 6 MeV beam will have significant changes. This is only an estimate, and the validity for a particular linac should be established at the time of commissioning. AAPM TG-70 describes a method to estimate the depth dose and output of rectangular cutouts of dimension X × Y via the geometric mean:

$$OF_{X,Y} = (OF_X \times OF_Y)^{1/2}$$

$$PDD_{X,Y} = (PDD_X \times PDD_Y)^{1/2}$$

This requires that a series of cutouts be measured at the time of commissioning. Although it does work for rectangular cutouts, it is not particularly accurate for small or irregularly shaped cutouts. Khan described a method based on the lateral buildup ratio (LBR) concept that more accurately describes changes in output and depth dose.[7] The LBR is derived from the ratio of the percent depth dose (PDD) for a 2 cm diameter cutout to that for the open cone. For irregular cutouts, a method of sector integration is used to calculate the PDD and output. This is easily implemented in computer code but is difficult to use in a manual calculation. Kehwar and Huq have proposed an improvement in this method.[8] In practice, small or irregular cutouts should be measured to confirm the output and depth dose.

For small cutouts, the depth dose curve will shift toward the surface as shown in Figure 15.4. Therefore both the output and depth dose should be verified because this may change the choice of energy. Figure 15.4 also shows that the effect is more pronounced at higher energies, as expected.

The shape of the isodose lines for electron beams is also energy and depth dependent. Table 15.3 shows the 90% width, proximal depth, and distal depth of 2 cm × 9 cm, 4 cm × 9 cm, and 9 cm × 9 cm cutouts in a 10 cm × 10 cm cone for various energies. The 90% width is measured

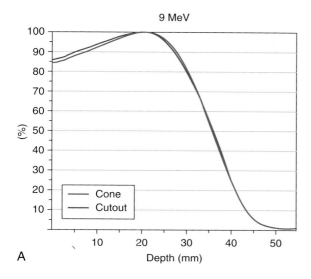

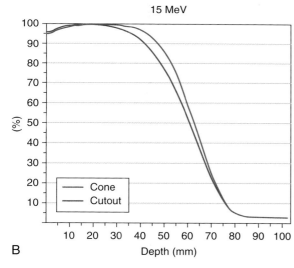

**Figure 15.4** The change in depth dose with smaller cutout size (4 cm).

TABLE 15.3  ▓ **90% Coverage for Different Cutout Sizes**

| Cutout Size (cm) | 90% Width at $D_{max}$ Depth for the Smallest Dimension/ Proximal 90% Depth/Distal 90% Depth (cm) | | | |
|---|---|---|---|---|
| | **6 MeV** | **9 MeV** | **12 MeV** | **15 MeV** |
| 9 × 9 | 8.0/0.5/1.8 | 8.1/0.7/2.9 | 8.1/0.4/3.8 | 8.5/0.2/4.6 |
| 4 × 9 | 2.8/0.5/1.8 | 2.9/0.6/2.8 | 3.1/0.3/3.6 | 3.3/0.2/4.2 |
| 2 × 9 | 1.1/0.3/1.7 | 1.3/0.2/2.4 | 1.4/0.1/2.8 | 1.4/0.1/3.1 |

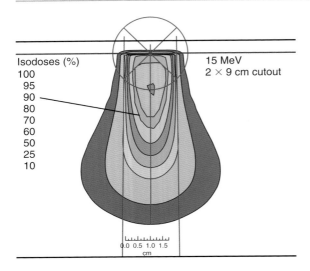

Isodoses (%)
100
95
90
80
70
60
50
25
10

15 MeV
2 × 9 cm cutout

0.0 0.5 1.0 1.5
cm

**Figure 15.5** Isodose lines for a narrow cutout for a high energy electron beam.

TABLE 15.4 ▦ **Measured Penumbra in mm from Hu et al.[5] for a Varian Linac**

| Depth | 6 MeV | 9 MeV | 12 MeV | 16 MeV | 20 MeV |
|-------|-------|-------|--------|--------|--------|
| R100 | 22.1 | 24 | 25.7 | 20.6 | 12.3 |
| R90 | 25.9 | 30.7 | 37.9 | 44 | 46.6 |
| R50 | 25.9 | 32.3 | 41 | 50.8 | 60.6 |

at the depth of maximum dose. The data show that the margin needed for the cutout is about 1 cm. It should be noted that the 90% width narrows significantly with depth and the distal 90% depth becomes much shallower as the cutout size decreases for higher energies, so computerized treatment planning is recommended to ensure coverage (see Figure 15.5). Lead collimation resting on the skin is sometimes used for small fields since the penumbra is relatively wide compared to the tumor. Skin collimation can also achieve better shielding for superficial nearby structures.

The thickness of the cutouts should be sufficient to reduce the transmission to less than 5%. If lead is used, a good rule of thumb is the thickness required in mm is E/2; if cerrobend is used, multiply by a factor of 1.2 (TG-25).

## PENUMBRA

The penumbra of an electron beam is a function of beam energy and depth. The International Commission on Radiation Units and Measurements (ICRU) recommends that penumbra be reported as the distance from the 80% point to the 20% point on a beam profile.[9] They also recommend that the penumbra be reported at the depth of R85/2. The penumbra increases with depth for all energies, with higher energies showing the most dramatic increases. Table 15.4 shows the measured penumbra from Hu et al.[5] The dramatic changes of the penumbra with depth make matching of adjacent beams difficult.

## EXTENDED DISTANCE

Because scatter increases with distance between the cone and the surface of the patient, the output and penumbra will change for extended source to surface distance (SSDs). One study showed an

8 mm to 10 mm increase in the penumbra for a 6 MeV beam at an SSD of 110 cm.[10] The multiple scatter sources in an electron beam cause a cone/cutout and energy dependent relationship between output and SSD. By plotting the change in output versus SSD the effective SSD (f) can be calculated. The effective SSD can then be used to calculate the output at an arbitrary SSD. Measurements could be made at 100 cm, 110 cm, and 120 cm SSD, for example. If $I_0$ is the reading at $d_{max}$ depth with an air gap = 0 (nominal SSD of 100 cm) and $I_g$ is the reading at $d_{max}$ for an air gap distance of g cm, a plot of $(I_0/I_g)^{1/2}$ versus g will yield a straight line with a slope of $(1/f + d_{max})$. Therefore $f = (1/\text{slope}) - d_{max}$. The inverse square law can then be used with f as the nominal SSD instead of 100 cm. The dose at an air gap of g ($D_g$) is then calculated from the dose at air gap of 0 ($D_0$) as follows:

$$D_g = D_0 \, (f + d_{max})2/(f + g + d_{max})$$

The plot of of $(I_0/I_g)^{1/2}$ versus g will be linear only up to about 115 cm. At greater distances the change in output should be confirmed with measurements. Alternatively, a series of measurements can be taken during commissioning for future reference. AAPM TG-25 states that the effective SSD correction does not vary with depth and the entire depth dose curve can be corrected using the same factor, meaning the PDD does not change significantly with SSD at least up to 115 cm SSD.

## 15.3 Obliquity and Surface Irregularity

Beam obliquity and surface irregularity are closely related in that they both involve beam incidence at non-normal angles. Since standard dosimetry data are measured at normal incidence, corrections for oblique beams must be made. For angles of incidence less than 30 degrees the corrections are small. The isodose curves are merely shifted parallel to the surface. For angles equal to or greater than 30 degrees, three changes are seen as shown in Figure 15.6:

1. An increase in dose near $d_{max}$
2. Shift in the therapeutic depth ($\approx$90%) toward the surface
3. Increase in dose at oblique depths near the practical range

Rounded surfaces have the effect of pulling the isodoses closer to the surface as the obliquity gradually changes. This is shown in Figure 15.7.

Tissue protrusions (i.e., the nose) or deficits (i.e., surgical deficits) have an effect like that of an inhomogeneity. As will be discussed in the following section, hot spots are created on the lower density side of an interface, as is shown in Figure 15.8. Section 15.5 discusses the use of bolus material to minimize these hot spots. Examples of these are shown in AAPM TG-25.[4]

## 15.4 Inhomogeneity

There are two concerns with tissue inhomogeneity: attenuation and scatter. The attenuation beyond a slab inhomogeneity can be estimated by calculating the coefficient of equivalent thickness (CET). The CET is approximately equal to the ratio of the stopping power for the inhomogeneity to that of water and can be estimated by the ratio of electron densities. The dose beyond an inhomogeneity is then determined by calculating the effective depth in water ($d_{eff}$) as follows:[1]

$$d_{eff} = d - t(1 - CET)$$

The CET for bone is $\approx$ 1.65 and for lung is $\approx$ 0.33. For depth (d) = 5 cm and inhomogeneity thickness (t) = 2 cm, $d_{eff}$ is 6.3 for bone and 3.66 for lung. To estimate the dose at the depth d, the PDD for $d_{eff}$ is used. It should be emphasized that this is only an estimate and a properly commissioned TPS is highly recommended to accurately calculate the doses for inhomogeneities.

6 MeV electrons, PDD vs. obliquity angle 14 cm cone,
110 cm SSD dose normalized to 0 degree max dose

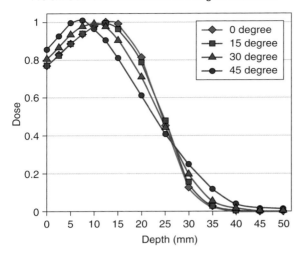

15 MeV electrons, PDD vs. obliquity angle 14 cm cone,
110 cm SSD dose normalized to 0 degree max dose

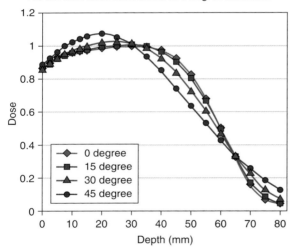

**Figure 15.6** Effect of obliquity on electron beams.

As mentioned in the previous section, hot spots form lateral to an inhomogeneity interface on the lower density side. This is due to increased scatter out from the higher density material that is not compensated by scatter from the low density material. Figure 15.9 and Figure 15.10 demonstrate this.

## 15.5 Bolus and Compensators

Bolus can be used with electron beams for three reasons: (1) to increase the surface dose, (2) to compensate for surface irregularities, and (3) to shape the distal isodose to conform to the PTV.

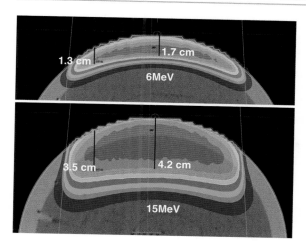

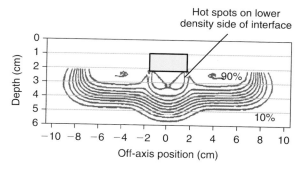

**Figure 15.7** Effect of rounded surfaces on electron beams.

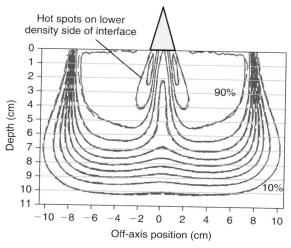

**Figure 15.8** Demonstration of hot spots on the low density side of tissue interfaces. Top figure shows a low density cavity inside a water phantom. Lower figure shows a water density protrusion creating lower density region adjacent to it. *(Adapted from Boyd et al, A measured data set for evaluating electron-beam dose algorithms, Med Phys 2001;28:950-958.)*

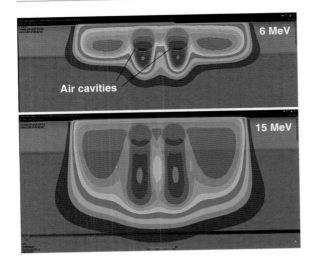

**Figure 15.9** Effect of air inhomogeneity on electron beams.

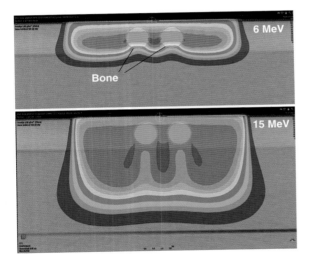

**Figure 15.10** Effect of bone inhomogeneity on electron beams.

Surface doses range from 70% to 90% depending on the linac model and beam energy. To achieve the recommended 90% dose to the PTV most energies will require some bolus if there is a surface component to the PTV. Many materials are available for use as bolus. AAPM TG-70 describes paraffin wax, polystyrene, acrylic, Super Stuff, Superflab, Superflex, and thermoplastic sheets. Paraffin wax, polystyrene, and acrylic are labor intensive to construct. The Super- products are flexible and can mold to the skin surface but can be difficult to use in covering large curved areas without bulging. If covered with plastic wrap daily, they can be reused. Thermoplastic sheets have the advantage of being able to cover large areas without bulging. Unless the patient sets up exactly the same each day it can sometimes be difficult to achieve the same conformity to the skin. Air gaps of up to 10 mm are unlikely to significantly affect the surface dose,[11] but if it is suspected that there are sizable air gaps, the patient should be scanned with the bolus in place to confirm the extent of the gap or a new bolus should be constructed. A more recent review of bolus

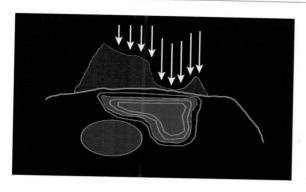

**Figure 15.11** Use of a compensator to shape the distal isodose lines.

materials was published by Vyas et al.[12] They discuss additional bolus materials such as Play-Doh, wet gauze, and petroleum jelly, among others.

Bolus material may also be used to fill voids to eliminate potential hot and cold spots due to air cavities such as the external auditory canal or the nasal passages. Paraffin wax is normally used in these cases. Water has been proposed for the auditory canal but can be uncomfortable for the patient.

Compensators can be used to fill in tissue deficits, build up a surface to make it more uniform, or shape the distal isodose line to cover a PTV. Tissue deficits can be filled with wax molds, petroleum jelly, or strips of oil gel sheets. In the example of treating the nose, a wax mold can be created to level the surface and eliminate the types of hot spots demonstrated in Figure 15.8.

If the PTV is not at a uniform depth, a given electron energy will either compromise coverage or treat excessive normal tissue. A custom bolus compensator can be created by adding material over the shallower depth areas of the PTV to pull the isodose toward the surface as shown in Figure 15.11. This can be done manually through a trial and error process as described by Low.[13] The patient should be scanned with the final bolus in place and computerized planning performed to confirm PTV coverage. Sharp surface gradients on the compensator should be avoided so as not to produce hot spots. One company (.decimal) has developed a process to custom mill the compensator based on the patient surface, PTV shape, and electron beam energy. This is much less time intensive and more accurate.

# 15.6 Shielding Adjacent Structures

If an OAR is adjacent to the treatment field, shielding may need to be placed directly on the patient to sharpen the field edge and to shield the structure. This is particularly important at extended distances where out-of-field scatter increases. Examples are the lens of the eye, lacrimal glands, or the inside of the mouth. While 3 to 5 mm of lead may be sufficient to shield the underlying tissues,[14] an internal shield can cause a significant increase in dose to tissues upstream due to backscatter. The backscatter increases with increasing atomic number of the shield and decreases with increasing electron energy. According to the formula given in AAPM TG-25 to estimate the backscatter, it can be up to 60%. A more modern calculation by Chow and Grigorov has shown that the effect is in the range of 20% to 50% depending on electron energy.[15] This study shows depth dose curves with a 2 mm lead shield placed at depths ranging from 0.5 to 2 cm for energies 4 MeV to 16 MeV. To minimize this backscatter a laminated shield with increasing atomic number should be used. For example, the proximal layer could be wax, followed by an aluminum layer, and then a lead layer could be used. The design of any shield should be verified with measurements.

## 15.7 General Clinical Considerations

AAPM TG-70 has a series of sections on clinical situations ranging from intact breast, chest wall, nose, eye, scalp, and parotids.[4] Some general similarities run through these sections and are worth consideration.

1. Computerized treatment planning is highly recommended, particularly for abutting fields, oblique beams, surface irregularities, and inhomogeneity. A pencil beam algorithm may have significant limitations in these areas, and a more modern algorithm such as Monte Carlo is preferable.
2. Cutout margins should account for penumbra and breathing motion. For small cutouts, the margins may need to be increased, particularly for higher energies.
3. If fields are abutted, it is recommended that the junction be moved at least once during the course of treatment to minimize hot and cold spots.
4. In-vivo and in-phantom dosimetry should be performed to validate complicated setups.
5. Good immobilization is required for complicated setups.
6. Custom bolus is recommended for irregular surfaces, for tissue deficits, and for shaping the distal isodose lines to conform to the PTV. Because electron beam surface doses range from 70% to 90%, bolus will almost always be needed if there is a surface component to the PTV. Bolus should be at least 2 cm wide to avoid a cold spot under the bolus.
7. Eye shields designed for photon treatments should not be used for electrons.

## 15.8 Emerging Trends in Electron Beam Radiotherapy

Though the basics of electron beam treatments have remained unchanged since the 1970s, there are several emerging techniques, including arcs, electron multi-leaf collimators (eMLC), energy modulation, and electon/photon intensity modulated radiation therapy (IMRT).

Electron arcs have been used by a few centers for a long time but have not been widely implemented due to their complexity. Because the standard cones with a typical 95 cm distance to the trimmers would cause a collision during an arc, either a custom cone is needed or the photon jaws can be used. The width should be 4 cm to 8 cm. If the surface curvature changes in the superior-inferior direction, a tapered width can be used. Surface shielding is needed for two reasons: to sharpen beam edge because the trimmers from the standard cone are not used and to allow for uniformity at the beginning and end of the arc. The surface dose is less for arc treatments because areas closer to the isocenter are exposed to larger arc segments. The photon contamination component will also increase at depth since it is focused on the isocenter.[4] A recent study demonstrated that electron arcs may become more feasible with the advent of advanced features on newer linacs.[16]

Several studies have examined the development of electron MLCs.[17,18] They propose that this will eliminate the fabrication time for cutouts, eliminate the exposure of staff to a hazardous material (cerrobend), and allow for electron IMRT. It remains to be seen if the cost and complexity of commissioning such systems will make them widely accepted into clinical practice.

Electron IMRT through the use of energy modulation also has been investigated.[19,20] There is a commercial product available (Trumpet eIMRT, Standard Imaging) that will determine a mix of beam energies based on desired dose homogeneity over the PTV and the bolus to be used.

A recent report has described the use of photon beam IMRT fields in combination with electron beams to reduce the penumbra, improve dose uniformity over the PTV, and reduce doses to OARs.[21]

**FOR THE PHYSICIAN**

With the advent of IMRT the use of electrons has declined, particularly in pelvic and head and neck cancers. Electrons, however, remain a useful tool for the treatment of superficial and shallow (less than 7 cm deep) targets. Typical energies used are 4 MeV to 22 MeV. Because electrons scatter more easily than photons, collimation close to the patient's surface is required to minimize penumbra. In fact, if critical structures are adjacent to the field, shielding placed directly on the patient surface may be required. The backscatter off high atomic number shields such as lead can be in the range of 20% to 50%, with higher values for lower energies. Therefore, if shields are placed internally (behind the lip, for example) the shield should be coated with increasingly lower atomic number materials such that the lowest atomic number material is next to the tissue.

The characteristics of electron beams can be estimated by several rules of thumb. The depth of 90% dose in cm is approximately E/3.2 where E is the nominal energy of the beam. Likewise, the depth of 80% dose and the practical range (Rp) are E/2.9 and E/2 respectively. Surface dose (%) can be estimated by E+72. The amount of lead in mm required to shield to less than 5% transmission is estimated by E/2. The thickness is about 20% larger for cerrobend. Another key characteristic of electron beams is the widening of the penumbra as the depth increases, making it difficult to match adjacent electron fields. The wide penumbra also requires that a margin of about 1 cm be added to the target size when creating the cutout.

Output and depth dose are significantly affected by small cutouts, particularly for higher energies. Small cutouts reduce the dose per MU and move the $d_{max}$ depth closer to the surface. The dosimetry for small cutouts should be validated individually or by comparing to a library of previously measured values. This includes an analysis of the 90% isodose width, which can be severely constricted. A rule of thumb is that the output and depth dose will be affected if the minimum cutout dimension is less than Rp.

Electron beam depth dose is largely unaffected by changes in SSD up to about 115 cm. Because of the multiple scattering materials in the path of the electron beam (scattering foils, dose chamber, collimator jaws, electron cone) the effective source position is different from the nominal 100 cm distance. By measuring the output at varying distances, an effective source position can be determined. This depends on the energy, cone, and cutout and should be measured for each combination.

Beam obliquity, surface irregularity, and inhomogeneities can cause complex changes in the dose distribution. Hot spots can be created laterally to an inhomogeneity interface on the lower density side. Tissue protrusions (nose) and deficits (surgical deficits) can produce the same effect as the adjacent air acts as an inhomogeneity. Bolus material can be used to build up around a protrusion or to fill in a deficit. Bolus also can be used as a compensator to shape the distal isodose line to better conform to the PTV by placing material over the shallower parts of the PTV. Sharp edges in the compensator should be avoided because they will produce hot spots similar to a tissue protrusion.

AAPM TG-70 describes a series of clinical issues that should be considered. See Section 15.7 for details.

## References

1. Khan FM, Doppke KP, Hogstrom KR, et al. Clinical electron beam dosimetry. Med Phys 1991;18(1):73–107.
2. Radiation Oncology Physics: A Handbook for Teachers and Students. International Atomic Energy Agency. 2005. Available at: http://www-pub.iaea.org/books/IAEABooks/7086/Radiation-Oncology-Physics-A-Handbook-for-Teachers-and-Students.
3. Hogstrom K, Almond P. Review of electron beam therapy physics. Phys Med Biol 2006;51:R455–89.
4. Gerbi BJ, Antolak JA, Deibel FC, et al. Recommendations for clinical electron beam dosimetry: Supplement to the recommendations of Task Group 25. Med Phys 2009;36(7):3239–79.
5. Hu YA, Song H, Chen Z, et al. Evaluation of an electron Monte Carlo dose calculation algorithm for electron beams. J Appl Clin Med Phys 2009;9(3):2720.

6. Tailor RC, Followill DS, Hernandez N, et al. Predictability of electron cone ratios with respect to linac make and model. J Appl Clin Med Phys 2003;4(2):172–8.

7. Khan FM, Higgins PD, Gerbi BJ, et al. Calculation of depth dose and dose per monitor unit for irregularly shaped electron fields. Phys Med Biol 1998;43:2741–54.

8. Kehwar TS, Huq MS. The nth root percent depth dose method for calculating monitor units for irregularly shaped electron fields. Med Phys 2008;35(4):1214–22.

9. Prescribing, recording, and reporting electron beam therapy. J ICRU 2004;4(1):39–48.

10. Steel J, Stewart A, Satory P. Matching extended-SSD electron beams to multileaf collimated photon beams in the treatment of head and neck cancer. Med Phys 2009;36(9):4244–9.

11. Kong M, Holloway L. An investigation of central axis depth dose distribution perturbation due to an air gap between patient and bolus for electron beams. Australas Phys Eng Sci Med 2007;30(2):111–19.

12. Vyas V, Palmer L, Mudge R, et al. On bolus for megavoltage photon and electron radiation therapy. Med Dosim 2013;38:268–73.

13. Low DA, Starkschall G, Bujnowski SW, et al. Electron bolus design for radiotherapy treatment planning: Bolus design algorithms. Med Phys 1992;19:115–24.

14. Chow CL, Grigorov GN. Dosimetric dependence of the dimensional characteristics on a lead shield in electron radiotherapy: A Monte Carlo study. J Appl Clin Med Phys 2009;10(2):75–91.

15. Chow CL, Grigorov GN. Monte Carlo simulation of backscatter from lead for clinical electron beam using EGSnrc. Med Phys 2008;35(4):1241–50.

16. Rodrigues A, Yin F, Wu Q. Dynamic electron arc radiotherapy (DEAR): A feasibility study. Phys Med Biol 2014;59(2):327–45.

17. Eldib A, Jin L, Li J, et al. Feasibility of replacing patient specific cutouts with a computer-controlled electron multileaf collimator. Phys Med Biol 2013;58(16):5653–72.

18. O'Shea TP, Ge Y, Foley MJ, et al. Characterization of an extendable multi-leaf collimator for clinical electron beams. Phys Med Biol 2011;56(23):7621–38.

19. Gentry JR, Steeves R, Paliwal BA. Inverse planning of energy-modulated electron beams in radiotherapy. Med Dosim 2006;31(4):259–68.

20. Olofsson L, Mu X, Nill S, et al. Intensity modulated radiation therapy with electrons using algorithm based energy/range selection methods. Radiother Oncol 2004;73(2):223–31.

21. Mosalaei H, Karnas S, Shah S, et al. The use of intensity-modulated radiation therapy photon beams for improving the dose uniformity of electron beams shaped with MLC. Med Dosim 2012;37(1):76–83.

# CHAPTER 16

# IMRT and VMAT

## 16.1 Introduction

Intensity-modulated radiotherapy (IMRT) provides exceptional control over the delivery of dose. Figure 16.1 shows an example of a 7-field IMRT plan for a patient with T3 oropharyngeal carcinoma of the head and neck.[1] This case illustrates the ability to sculpt dose around nearby organs at risk (in this case the cord and parotid) while irradiating the gross tumor volume and at-risk nodal regions to a high dose. This case also demonstrates the technique of "dose painting" or "simultaneous integrated boost" in which a single plan is used to deliver a total of 70 Gy to the gross disease while nodal regions simultaneously receive a dose of either 59.4 Gy or 54 Gy. Similar dose sculpting capabilities are available with volumetric modulated arc therapy (VMAT).

Examination of the clinical evidence behind IMRT can be found in the 2008 meta-analysis from Veldeman et al.,[2] which identified 49 published studies with well-defined clinical endpoints. A similar analysis for the UK health system was published in 2010.[3] Though only six randomized controlled trials were identified (three for breast cancer and three for head and neck), overall the case studies showed a benefit to IMRT in terms of toxicity and quality-of-life endpoints. Specific benefits were noted for the following endpoints: xerostomia in head and neck cases, rectal toxicity in prostate cases, gastrointestinal/genitourinary (GI/GU) toxicity in uterine cancer, and cosmesis in breast cancer.

### Further Reading

Technical reviews of IMRT/VMAT can be found in several review papers.[4,5] Several IMRT/VMAT textbooks are available including clinically oriented presentations,[6,7] more technically oriented presentations,[8] and the proceedings of the 2003 American Association of Physicists in Medicine (AAPM) Summer School.[9] It is worth noting that these texts date back some 10 years and fewer reference books are being written about IMRT/VMAT as the technology matures. Another source for reference materials are the sections in various standard textbooks (e.g., Chapters 6 through 8 in *Principles and Practice of Radiation Oncology*).[10]

### HISTORY OF TECHNICAL DEVELOPMENTS IN IMRT AND VMAT

Prior to 1994 optimal treatment plans were developed using beam aperture, collimator angle, gantry angle, beam energy, beam weighting, and modifiers such as wedges or compensators. Some basic modulation may have been accomplished using a field-in-field approach. The planner would manually adjust the various parameters until an acceptable, not necessarily optimal, result was achieved. With the development of the multi-leaf collimator (MLC) and inverse planning, the adjustments moved from mechanical parameters to target and organ-at-risk (OAR) parameters. The objectives and dose constraints are modified to produce an acceptable, but still not necessarily optimal, result. This is achieved through the automatic adjustment of the various mechanical

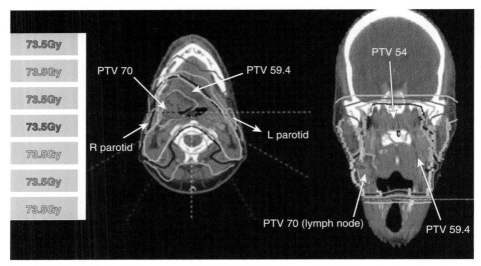

**Figure 16.1** Dose distribution for an example 7-field IMRT plan for a patient with head and neck carcinoma. *(From de Arruda FF, Puri DR, Zhung J, et al. Intensity-modulated radiation therapy for the treatment of oropharyngeal carcinoma: the Memorial Sloan-Kettering Cancer Center experience. Int J Radiat Oncol Biol Phys 2006;64:363-373.)*

parameters by the optimization algorithm in sequential trials to meet the specified goals and constraints. The first versions only modified the beam intensity throughout a beam aperture. This was called intensity-modulated radiation therapy. More modern systems can optimize gantry angle and collimator angle as well.

The first commercially available IMRT system (Peacock, NOMOS Corp.) became available in 1994 and used a binary collimator as an add-on device for a standard linear accelerator (linac) in an arc delivery. The beam intensity was modulated throughout the arc by the opening and closing of the collimator leaves. Since the binary collimator leaves are either open or closed the intensity of a given arc segment was determined by the amount of time the leaf was open during that segment. Once an arc was completed, the couch was indexed a precise amount to treat the next volume or "slice" of the target. This was repeated until the entire target was covered. Because of this slice-by-slice approach, it is referred to as serial or axial TomoTherapy. This original system led to the development of helical TomoTherapy as implemented in the TomoTherapy Hi-Art system (Accuray Systems Inc.). The implementations that followed on traditional linacs used the standard MLC to modulate the beam at fixed gantry and collimator angles as mentioned above. This can be done by delivering the dose at multiple fixed segments where the beam is turned off while the MLC is changing shape, called step and shoot, or by having the MLC continuously change shape as the beam is constantly on, called sliding window delivery or dynamic MLC (dMLC). For sliding window delivery the dose rate may be fixed or variable. The next development was to use the conventional linac and MLC and to perform the dynamic delivery throughout an arc, which is called VMAT. This is sometimes referred to by its original development name of intensity-modulated arc radiotherapy (IMAT) or by vendor-specific names such as RapidArc (Varian Inc.) or SmartArc (Philips Inc.).

In terms of the usage of IMRT and VMAT, a 2004 survey of U.S. practices found that IMRT was used by 73% of respondents.[11] Given that 91% of nonusers at the time planned to adopt IMRT, the availability in U.S. clinics is now likely close to 100%. Studies of Medicare billing patterns show that IMRT was used in 54% of cases in 2010.[12] A 2010 Canadian survey demonstrated that IMRT was available in 87% of centers, up from 37% in 2006.[13]

## 16.2 Nomenclature for Structures

Because of the complexity of IMRT/VMAT treatments, it is essential to have a well-defined schema for specifying structures and doses. This issue is the central topic of two important reports: ICRU-83, Volume and Dose Specification for Prescribing, Recording, and Reporting Photon-Beam IMRT,[14] and the American Society for Radiation Oncology (ASTRO) 2009 Recommendations for Documenting IMRT Treatments.[15] Though these reports specifically name IMRT in their titles, they are clearly intended to apply to VMAT as well. These reports advocate the use of a standard nomenclature for planning structures: gross tumor volume (GTV), clinical tumor volume (CTV), internal target volume (ITV), planning target volume (PTV), OAR, and planning OAR volume (PRV) (see Chapter 14 for a further discussion). These nomenclatures are a modification and update to ICRU-50 and -62, which defined these concepts).[16,17] The ASTRO 2009 IMRT report recommendations[15] call for the clinician to specify the regions of interest listed above.

## 16.3 Margins in IMRT/VMAT Planning

Another important planning concept is margins (see Chapter 14 for further discussion). Especially crucial for IMRT/VMAT is the margin used to expand CTV to PTV. This directly impacts tumor coverage. Population-based margin recipes have been developed and are well summarized in ICRU-83 Table 4.4. One widely used margin formula is from van Herk et al.:[18] $2.5\Sigma + 0.7\sigma$, where $\Sigma$ and $\sigma$ are the systematic and random uncertainties respectively in patient setup. It should be noted, however, that this margin formula was developed for 3D conformal radiotherapy and may not be applicable for IMRT plans, which have different conformality and dose gradients. One study of head and neck cases[19] found that the required margins were substantially smaller than those suggested by the van Herk et al. formula.

Regardless of the proper formula, it must be recognized that the use of IMRT alone does not generally warrant a reduction in margins. IMRT has more impact on gradients, which can result in less dose to nearby OARs, but does not impact setup variation, which the margin is designed to mitigate. Margin reduction is more properly achieved through the use of IGRT rather than IMRT. In this context it is also important to note that a margin formula such as $2.5\Sigma + 0.7\sigma$ suggests that the systematic component of variability ($\Sigma$) is approximately 3 times as important as the random variability ($\sigma$). If margins are to be reduced, it is particularly important to address the systematic component of variability. IGRT is particularly effective at accomplishing this.

## 16.4 Dose Reporting and Record Keeping

Both ICRU-83 and the ASTRO report strongly advocate for dose volume histogram (DVH)-based dose reporting as opposed to reporting dose to point(s). Point dose specifications are no longer adequate because IMRT/VMAT plans often have a more heterogeneous dose distribution within the target. If a point dose prescription is used, the overall target may get more or less dose depending on which point happened to be selected for defining the prescription. DVH-based reporting is also necessary for comparing a particular plan to published reports of normal tissue tolerances, for example, the QUANTEC reports.[20,21] DVH statistics are considered in further detail in Chapter 14, which includes such parameters as $D_{V\%}$ and $V_{DGy}$ value (i.e., the percent volume of organ receiving a dose of $D$ Gy or more) as well as homogeneity index and conformality index.

The ASTRO 2009 IMRT report recommends that IMRT treatment documentation should include the following: IMRT treatment planning directive, a treatment goal summary, an image guidance summary, and a motion management summary. The report lists in detail what information should be included in each of these components. The following should also be included:

MD treatment summary note, daily treatment record, and treatment plan printout. The details of what should be in this last component are also given. The records should also include the make, model, and software version of the treatment planning system that was used. The ASTRO 2009 IMRT report recommends that treatment records be kept for at least 5 years, while ICRU-83 uses the more stringent, but reasonable, recommendation of "five years or the life of the patient, whichever is longer."[14]

## 16.5 IMRT/VMAT Treatment Planning

### INVERSE PLANNING

There is a vast literature on IMRT/VMAT inverse treatment planning. Though it is not possible to summarize here, ICRU-83 Chapter 2 has a helpful presentation of the basic concepts in inverse planning, objective functions, and gradient-search optimization. A more recent development in inverse planning is the technique of multicriteria optimization (MCO).[22-24] The basic concept behind MCO is that one does not know, *a priori*, which objective function should be employed. In other words, the relative importance of various target and OAR objectives is itself a free variable. In practice, the treatment planner changes objective functions in an iterative fashion until a clinically acceptable plan is achieved. With MCO, multiple objective functions are evaluated, allowing a more complete exploration of the space of possible treatment plans.

### TECHNIQUES AND ISSUES IN IMRT/VMAT TREATMENT PLANNING

There is a wide array of planning techniques in use to achieve a good IMRT plan. Some practical techniques include:

1. Use a large number of equally spaced beams (e.g., 7 to 9 coplanar beams for head and neck). This obviates the need to optimize beam angle.
2. Avoid parallel-opposed beams, since the beamlet or apertures of opposing beams are directly competing in terms of the objective function.
3. Use "rings" or donuts around the target volume to increase dose conformality around the target volume.
4. Evaluate possible collision problems between the patient and the beam delivery hardware. This is especially important with VMAT deliveries when couch kicks are used or the isocenter is located in a lateral lesion.

In some cases the PTV will overlap with a PRV or even an OAR. The classic example is the prostate, which, when extended to a PTV, overlaps the rectum. One way to handle this overlap is to define a subregion of the PTV (e.g., PTV ∩ rectum for a prostate case). A DVH objective is applied to this subregion in order to drive the inverse planning to provide less coverage in the subregion. ICRU-83 suggests this as a reasonable approach but advocates that when the plan is complete the dose to the whole PTV still be reported and not just the DVH for the modified PTV. ICRU-83 also strongly advocates that the coverage of the PTV not be compromised in favor of OAR sparing, though this is a clinical decision and it may not be possible to achieve both objectives in some cases.

Compared to 3D conformal radiotherapy (CRT), IMRT and VMAT tend to spread the low dose region around the patient in ways that are not always predictable. Figure 16.2 illustrates the case of a patient being treated for cervical cancer. The sparing of bowel and bladder is apparent, but a high dose "finger" also is observed in the IMRT plan. It is important to evaluate plans for such unintended high dose regions, and this is especially important for plans involving couch kicks or nonisocentric delivery.

In some cases the PTV can extend near the skin or even into air (see ICRU-83 Section 5.3.1 for a discussion). This presents a problem for inverse planning since the algorithm can attempt

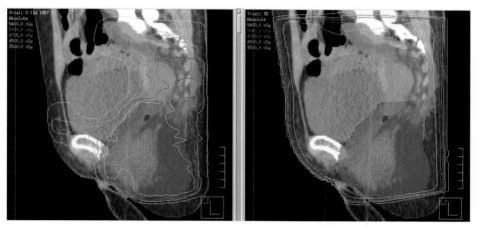

**Figure 16.2** Dose distributions for a patient receiving treatment for cervical cancer using a 9-field IMRT plan (left) and a 3D CRT plan (right).

to artificially enhance the beam fluence in the apparently low dose region near the skin or in the air. This situation can be avoided by creating a modified PTV volume that is truncated at the skin or even pulled back. This modified PTV is used for inverse planning objectives. This approach may have the negative effect of underdosing the superficial regions of the PTV and/or eliminating "flash" outside the skin. One solution is to make a subvolume of the PTV near the skin and assign a low weight to the objective function for that volume (ICRU-83). Another way to drive MLC leaves out near the skin and provide flash is to construct a "PTV air" or "fake bolus," which is a region that extends outside the skin in which density is overridden to a value of 1 g/cm$^3$. This region is assigned a very low objective weight. This serves to drive the MLC leaves out during optimization. After the final optimization is complete, the "PTV air" is removed and the dose is recalculated. Care must be taken with this method, however, since the "PTV air" does not represent a true anatomic structure.

On a more general note, the question arises as to what makes a "good" treatment plan. This is an area of active investigation to identify a meaningful metric for plan quality. For example, the McNutt et al. group[25] has developed the "overlap volume histogram" metric, which provides a method of quantifying the OAR sparing that is achievable on a population basis. Other metrics have been defined for the purposes of the "plan challenge," an annual contest administered by Radiation Oncology Resources Inc. (now owned by Sun Nuclear Inc.) in which a single treatment planning case is provided to multiple dosimetrists and physicists. Though these results are not yet widely available, the quality scores appear not to correlate with the planners' experience, education, or certification status.[26]

Another practical question is: How long does it (or should it) take to complete an IMRT or VMAT plan? This question has been partially addressed in a 2009 multi-institutional survey of IMRT practices.[27] The authors found that the answer depended on which planning system was being used but concluded that head and neck cases required an average of 30 hours total (11 hours for planning), lung cases 15 hours (8 hours' planning), and prostate cases 14 hours (6 hours' planning).

## 16.6 IMRT and VMAT Delivery and QA

As mentioned above, there are many different methods for delivering IMRT and VMAT treatments and each has special considerations. These include delivery time, beam on-time, minimum and maximum gantry speeds, minimum and maximum dose rates, collision issues, imaging policy, interrupted delivery procedure, and motion management. Because many of the segments used in IMRT are very small, small changes in aperture size can significantly affect the dose delivered. Because of these issues, more rigorous commissioning and QA of equipment are required where IMRT/VMAT are concerned. For example, the QA tolerances in AAPM TG-142 are different for a machine performing IMRT versus one that does not. Chapters 4 and 5 consider the issue of commissioning and QA in more detail. This includes a discussion of patient-specific QA for IMRT/VMAT plans, which is an evolving topic. Some important information and tools for validating the performance of IMRT can be found in AAPM TG-119[28] (including verification test plans that may be downloaded). Anthropomorphic test phantoms from IROC (formerly RPC) are also a valuable verification tool. A description can be found in Molineu et al.[29]

### FOR THE PHYSICIAN

IMRT and VMAT are now widely available in industrialized countries and are used by nearly every clinic. Like any technology, the pros and cons must be weighed, and it must be recognized that IMRT and VMAT are not appropriate for all cases. On the positive side, these delivery techniques provide unparalleled control of dose in three-dimensional space. In a head and neck case, for example, the dose to the spinal cord can be kept very low while still providing 59.4 Gy to a nodal target volume that surrounds the cord on three sides. This capability comes at a cost, however. Operationally, these techniques are more complex than conventional plans (head and neck IMRT planning can require 30 hours of work, for example). With this complexity, it is essential to have a schema for specifying structures and doses, which have guidelines from ICRU and ASTRO. IMRT and VMAT require special care in prescribing and reporting doses, especially since plans can be more heterogeneous. "Deliver 6000 cGy in 30 fractions to the isocenter" is no longer an appropriate prescription because the isocenter is just one point and may not be representative of the target volume as a whole. Rather, dose volume statistics should be used to prescribe and report dose as recommended in ICRU-83 on IMRT.

Extra patient-specific quality assurance tests are required with IMRT and VMAT. IMRT and VMAT are also more sensitive to errors and uncertainties in the treatment delivery hardware, and therefore more rigorous regular quality assurance is required of the equipment.

At a more conceptual level, IMRT and VMAT tend to spread dose out into a "low dose bath" as compared to 3D or 2D planning. This is especially true of VMAT. The clinical effect of this must be weighed, and it may be more appropriate in some cases to deliver higher doses to a smaller volume of normal tissue than lower doses to a larger volume. There are several noted advantages of VMAT over IMRT, one being the shorter treatment delivery times and fewer MU (leading to less leakage dose), but again this must be weighed against the complexity. One final issue is plan quality. What constitutes a "good" plan? This is an open question for any treatment plan, but especially for IMRT and VMAT because the skill of the planner and the performance of the inverse planning algorithm have such a crucial impact. Metrics that measure plan quality are under development, and this represents an active area of advancement in the coming years.

### References

1. de Arruda FF, Puri DR, Zhung J, et al. Intensity-modulated radiation therapy for the treatment of oropharyngeal carcinoma: The Memorial Sloan-Kettering Cancer Center experience. Int J Radiat Oncol Biol Phys 2006;64:363–73.
2. Veldeman L, Madani I, Hulstaert I, et al. Evidence behind use of intensity modulated radiotherapy: A systematic review of comparative clinical studies (vol 9, pg 367, 2008). Lancet Oncol 2008;9:513.
3. Staffurth J, Board RD. A review of the clinical evidence for intensity-modulated radiotherapy. Clin Oncol 2010;22:643–57.
4. Bortfeld T. IMRT: A review and preview. Phys Med Biol 2006;51:R363–79.
5. Yu CX, Amies CJ, Svatos M. Planning and delivery of intensity-modulated radiation therapy. Med Phys 2008;35:5233–41.

6. Chao KSC, Apisarnthanarax S, Ozyigit G, editors. Practical essentials of intensity modulated radiation therapy. 2nd ed. Philadelphia: Lippincott, Williams and Wilkins; 2005.

7. Mundt A, Roeske JC, editors. Intensity modulated radiation therapy: A clinical perspective. Hamilton, Ontario: BC Decker Inc.; 2005.

8. Staff MS-KCC. A practical guide to intensity modulated radiation therapy. Madison, WI: Medical Physics Publishing; 2003.

9. Palta J, Mackie TR, editors. Intensity-modulated radiation therapy: The state of the art. Madison, WI: Medical Physics Publishing; 2003.

10. Halperin EC, Wazer DE, Perez CA, et al., editors. Perez and Bradys principles and practice of Radiation Oncology. 6th ed. Philadelphia, PA: Lippincot Williams and Wilkins; 2013.

11. Mell LK, Mehrotra AK, Mundt AJ. Intensity-modulated radiation therapy use in the U.S., 2004. Cancer 2005;104:1296–303.

12. Shen X, Showalter TN, Mishra MV, et al. Radiation Oncology services in the modern era: evolving patterns of usage and payments in the office setting for medicare patients from 2000 to 2010. J Oncol Pract 2014;10(4):e201–7.

13. AlDuhaiby EZ, Breen S, Bissonnette JP, et al. A national survey of the availability of intensity-modulated radiation therapy and stereotactic radiosurgery in Canada. Radiat Oncol 2012;7:18.

14. Gregoire V, Mackie TR. ICRU committee on volume and dose specification for prescribing, recording and reporting special techniques in external photon beam therapy: Conformal and IMRT. Radiother Oncol 2005;76:S71.

15. Holmes T, Das R, Low D, et al. American Society of Radiation Oncology recommendations for documenting intensity-modulated radiation therapy treatments. Int J Radiat Oncol Biol Phys 2009;74:1311–18.

16. ICRU. Prescribing, recording and reporting photon beam therapy. ICRU Report 50. Bethesda, MD: International Commission on Radiation Units and Measurements; 1993.

17. ICRU. Prescribing, recording and reporting photon beam therapy (supplement to ICRU Report 50). ICRU Report 62. Bethesda, MD: International Commission on Radiation Units and Measurements; 1999.

18. van Herk M, Remeijer P, Rasch C, et al. The probability of correct target dosage: Dose-population histograms for deriving treatment margins in radiotherapy. Int J Radiat Oncol Biol Phys 2000;47:1121–35.

19. Siebers JV, Keall PJ, Wu QW, et al. Effect of patient setup errors on simultaneously integrated boost head and neck IMRT treatment plans. Int J Radiat Oncol Biol Phys 2005;63:422–33.

20. Marks LB, Ten Haken RK, Martel MK. Guest editor's introduction to QUANTEC: A users guide. Int J Radiat Oncol Biol Phys 2010;76:S1–2.

21. Quantitative Analysis of Normal Tissue Effects in the Clinic (QUANTEC). Int J Radiat Oncol Biol Phys 2010;76(3):S1–160.

22. Cotrutz C, Lahanas M, Kappas C, et al. A multiobjective gradient-based dose optimization algorithm for external beam conformal radiotherapy. Phys Med Biol 2001;46:2161–75.

23. Craft D, Halabi T, Bortfeld T. Exploration of tradeoffs in intensity-modulated radiotherapy. Phys Med Biol 2005;50:5857–68.

24. Holdsworth C, Kim M, Liao J, et al. The use of a multiobjective evolutionary algorithm to increase flexibility in the search for better IMRT plans. Med Phys 2012;39:2261–74.

25. Wu BB, Ricchetti F, Sanguineti G, et al. Data-driven approach to generating achievable dose-volume histogram objectives in intensity-modulated radiotherapy planning. Int J Radiat Oncol Biol Phys 2011;79:1241–7.

26. Nelms BE, Robinson G, Markham J, et al. Variation in external beam treatment plan quality: An inter-institutional study of planners and planning systems. Pract Radiat Oncol 2012;2:296–305.

27. Das IJ, Moskvin V, Johnstone PA. Analysis of treatment planning time among systems and planners for intensity-modulated radiation therapy. J Am Coll Radiol 2009;6:514–17.

28. Ezzell GA, Burmeister JW, Dogan N, et al. IMRT commissioning: Multiple institution planning and dosimetry comparisons, a report from AAPM Task Group 119. Med Phys 2009;36(11):5359–73.

29. Molineu A, Followill DS, Balter PA, et al. Design and implementation of an anthropomorphic quality assurance phantom for intensity-modulated radiation therapy for the radiation therapy oncology group. Int J Radiat Oncol Biol Phys 2005;63:577–83.

# CHAPTER 17

# SRS and SBRT

## 17.1 Introduction

Stereotactic radiosurgery (SRS) was originally defined as fulfilling all of the following conditions:

1. Single-fraction treatment
2. High dose per fraction (>5 Gy)
3. Target with diameter of <3.5 cm in the brain
4. Delivery accuracy of <1 mm as defined by the Winston-Lutz test[1]
5. No planning target volume (PTV) or internal target volume (ITV) margins are used; clinical target volume (CTV) margins may be used

SRS was later expanded to also include single-fraction treatments of spinal lesions and then also to include fractionated treatments. The current definition includes:

1. 1 to 5 fraction treatment
2. High dose per fraction (>5 Gy)
3. Target with diameter of <3.5 cm in the central nervous system (CNS) (brain or spine)
4. Delivery accuracy of <1 mm as defined by an end-to-end test

Stereotactic body radiation therapy (SBRT), also sometimes called SABR (stereotactic ablative radiation therapy), is defined by the following conditions:

1. 1 to 5 fraction treatment (up to 8 in Canada)
2. High dose per fraction (>5 Gy)
3. Target size up to 4 cm diameter in the lung or 5 cm to 7 cm for target locations in the thoracic and abdomino-pelvic cavity
4. Technical delivery accuracy of <1.5 mm to 2 mm as defined by an end-to-end test
5. ITV and PTV margins are used to compensate interfraction and intrafraction motion and deformation. Most targets except prostate require respiratory motion management.

## 17.2 Technical Requirements

The high doses and steep dose gradients of SRS/SBRT delivered in very few fractions result in a much smaller margin of error than for conventionally fractionated radiation therapy. A machine being used for the delivery of SRS/SBRT must therefore at minimum fulfill the following stringent technical requirements outlined in Part I of this book:

1. Chapter 4: The machine must meet the mechanical tolerances outlined in American Association of Physicists in Medicine Task Group (AAPM TG)-142

2. Chapters 1/2: Small field beam commissioning
3. Chapter 7: Image guidance capabilities (or frame for SRS)
4. Chapter 16: End-to-end (E2E) test results <1 mm and delivery quality assurance (DQA) results <3%/2 mm
5. Chapter 19: Respiratory motion management techniques

The E2E test is an adaptation of the Winston-Lutz test[1] for the era of image-guided, frameless SRS/SBRT. Ideally, each of the steps would be performed by the treatment team member(s) who will perform the same function for a patient treatment. Performing an E2E test in this way as part of the commissioning process can help clarify the workflow and information flow and serve as a tool to develop the initial set of policies and procedures:

1. An appropriate anthropomorphic phantom for the treatment site, equipped with fiducials for localization similar to what will be used in a patient, is loaded with in-vivo dosimetry tools such as thermoluminescent dosimeter (TLD), optically stimulated luminescent detector (OSLD), metal-oxide semiconductor field-effect transistors (MOSFETs), gel, or film (physicist).
2. The phantom is immobilized and scanned, using the same immobilization devices and scan protocols that would be used for the patient (radiation therapist).
3. The images are imported into the treatment planning system, and the hidden target is contoured (physician).
4. A treatment plan is developed fulfilling the prescribed dose constraints (dosimetrist).
5. The plan is signed and reviewed (physician).
6. The plan documentation is processed and the plan exported to the treatment unit (dosimetrist).
7. A second check, secondary monitor unit (MU) calculation, and patient-specific QA measurements if applicable are performed (physicist).
8. The treatment is delivered (radiation therapist).
9. The dose measurement result is analyzed (physicist).

## 17.3 Policies and Procedures

Before starting an SRS/SBRT program, a set of policies and procedures (P&Ps) must be developed in a multidisciplinary setting of all care providers involved. To determine which P&Ps are needed, a patient flowchart can serve as a useful tool. This flowchart will also serve as a quality control tool to make sure all members of the patient treatment team understand their role in the care process, the order of care steps, and the information flow.

Table 17.1 outlines a sample set of P&Ps to meet the American College of Radiology (ACR) practice accreditation guidelines and the Canadian Association of Radiation Oncologists (CARO) scope of practice guidelines for lung, liver, and spine SBRT[2] recommendations. The ASTRO white paper on quality and safety considerations in SBRT[3] emphasizes that SRS/SBRT is not

TABLE 17.1 ■ **Sample SBRT Policies and Procedures**

| Treatment Step | Nursing | Dosimetry | Physician | Physicist | RTT |
|---|---|---|---|---|---|
| Simulation | x | | x | | x |
| Planning | | x | x | x | |
| Treatment Delivery | | | x | x | x |
| Final Treatment Chart Review | | | x | x | x |

one technique/modality and that expertise in one anatomic target area does not constitute expertise for other sites. It is therefore necessary to develop procedures that are specific to the technology in use at the institution, as well as specific to disease site(s).

The P&Ps should be tested using a mock patient treatment scenario, preferably including the image acquisition, treatment planning, and treatment delivery of a patient care plan to a phantom. After the initial patients have been treated, the P&Ps should be revised. After the initial revision, the P&Ps should be reviewed and, if applicable, updated on an annual basis.

In lieu of binders at multiple locations, which are difficult to keep current, an electronic system should be used to centrally store the P&P manual. The P&P should be accessible to all members of the Radiation Oncology department, be reachable from the majority of clinical workstations, and offer version tracking and sign-off capabilities to easily identify the most up-to-date iteration of the P&P.

## 17.4 Staffing

The implementation and maintenance of an SRS/SBRT program require adequate staffing to achieve safe, high-quality treatments. The 2008 Abt study[4] provides median work estimates for SRS/SBRT procedures once they are established into the clinical routine. The American Society for Radiation Oncology (ASTRO) white paper on quality and safety considerations in SBRT states that "Adequate levels of specialty staff is closely related to a reduction in medical errors." Furthermore, it recommends providing adequately trained personnel, opportunities for continuing education, and "ample time for staff to perform their required tasks, without undue stress or fatigue ...."[3]

The ACR practice guidelines on SBRT[5] and SRS,[6] as well as the ASTRO white paper on quality and safety considerations in SBRT, recommend that a qualified medical physicist (QMP) with specific training in SBRT should be responsible for the technical aspects of SRS/SBRT. A QMP for the purpose of overseeing SRS/SBRT is defined as an individual who has received board certification in therapeutic medical physics or the equivalent subspecialty by the American Board of Radiology (ABR), Canadian College of Medical Physics (CCMP), or American Board of Medical Physics (ABMP). This recommendation has been strengthened compared to now-retired practice guidelines in which all subspecialties of medical physics were listed as appropriate to perform SRS/SBRT. The responsibilities of the QMP include all technical aspects of SRS/SBRT, establishing a quality control (QC) checklist for the entire treatment process, supervising treatment planning, second MU check and patient-specific delivery QA, and communication with the radiation oncologist.

The CARO scope of practice guideline for lung, liver, and spine SBRT[2] expects the QMP to communicate to the radiation oncologist when limitations and assumptions made at each step of the treatment process are reached. This requires an in-depth understanding by the QMP of limitations and assumptions used in the process. Furthermore, the QMP is expected to review all SBRT treatment plans before delivery. The QMP is expected to have specific training in SBRT through either an educational course or mentoring. The QMP also should be versed in published guidelines (e.g., applicable AAPM TGs) that guide the implementation of rigorous QA for SRS/SBRT.

## 17.5 Patient Selection and Development of Treatment Protocols

AAPM TG-101, Stereotactic Body Radiation Therapy,[7] recommends enrolling SRS/SBRT patients in a clinical trial. If this is not feasible, it is recommended to treat patients per trial or peer-reviewed published guidelines. Any significant deviation from clinical trial protocols or published guidelines should be structured as a prospective study under IRB review. These recommendations are confirmed by the CARO scope of practice guideline for lung, liver, and spine

SBRT.[2] The ASTRO white paper on quality and safety considerations in SBRT[3] recommends collecting a library of peer-reviewed published studies relevant to specific SBRT sites and that the institution clearly document plans for patient selection, treatment planning, and treatment delivery prior to starting an SRS/SBRT program.

## 17.6 Simulation Imaging

In frame-based SRS or spine SBRT procedures it is assumed that the target structure does not move relative to the stereotactic coordinate system. If potential changes in the tumor location or changes in the frame position (e.g., slippage) are suspected, frame-based methods can and should be supplemented with pretreatment imaging. In frameless SRS/SBRT if fiducials are used to localize the tumor, the fiducials should be appropriately placed in or around the tumor to achieve the necessary accuracy. Anatomic landmarks such as bony structures or, in the case of lung tumors, the tumor itself can also be directly used as fiducials.

For spine SRS, the CARO scope of practice guidelines for lung, liver, and spine SBRT[2] recommends using a near-rigid body immobilization system to minimize intrafraction motion. For delivery systems able to image and correct for patient intrafraction motion, the requirements for the immobilization system may be less stringent. For all frameless SRS/SBRT procedures, the ACR practice guideline on SBRT recommends that the patient position be comfortable enough for the patient to hold still throughout the whole procedure.

High resolution simulation imaging is the basis for gross target volume (GTV) identification and hence accuracy of contouring. For image-guided SRS/SBRT delivery, the resolution of the simulation scan will influence the accuracy of image guidance during treatment. For SRS, an axial slice thickness of <1.25 mm is required. In SBRT, where tumors and organs at risk (OARs) are generally larger, a slice thickness of <3 mm is recommended by AAPM TG-101.[7] The CARO scope of practice guidelines for lung, liver, and spine SBRT[2] recommends a computed tomography (CT) slice thickness of <2.5 mm for spine and <3 mm for liver. Generally, a CT scan will be used as the baseline imaging modality for SRS/SBRT treatment planning. It provides accurate information on electron density, although the influence of using contrast during simulation on the dose calculation accuracy should be investigated. CT images generally have very low spatial distortion. In addition, 4D imaging is readily available to match the planned respiratory motion management during treatment.

AAPM TG-101 recommends a scan length extending 5 to 10 cm superior and inferior beyond the borders of the treatment or 15 cm if non-coplanar beams are to be used. All OARs should be included and evaluated using dose-volume histograms (DVH). If the target or OAR cannot be identified accurately due to imaging artifacts, SRS/SBRT should not be considered a safe treatment option. The CARO scope of practice guidelines for lung, liver, and spine SBRT[2] suggests magnetic resonance imaging (MRI) (axial volumetric T1 and T2) extending to one vertebral body above and below the target region for spine SRS. ACR practice guidelines on SBRT recommend investigating all digital images for spatial distortions that may arise in the imaging chain. The following are further considerations for simulation and imaging:

- **Contrast:** The CARO scope of practice guidelines for lung, liver, and spine SBRT[2] recommend using multiphase MRI imaging with intravenous gadolinium contrast for liver cancer. For primary liver cancer, late arterial phase imaging is recommended, whereas liver metastases are best visualized in the venous phase. For lung, the recommendation is to use contrast for medial lesions or lesions near atelectasis, but contrast can mostly be avoided for more peripheral lesions.
- **Image fusion:** For many SBRT targets, CT imaging is not the optimum diagnostic tool to define a lesion. For brain lesions, MRI is the image modality of choice. In the lung and abdomen, positron emission tomography (PET) is used, often as a PET/CT scan. If secondary image sets to the simulation CT are used for target definition, correct transfer of these image

TABLE 17.2 ■ **List of Commonly Used PTV Margins from the Major SRS/SBRT Trials**

| Site | Study | Margin |
| --- | --- | --- |
| Liver | RTOG-1112 | >4 mm minimum<br><20 mm maximum<br><10 mm goal<br>Asymmetric margins permitted |
| Lung | RTOG-0236 | 5 mm axial<br>10 mm longitudinal |
|  | RTOG-0915 | Conventional CT (non-4D):<br>5 mm axial<br>10 mm longitudinal<br>4D CT:<br>ITV + 5 mm |

RTOG, Radiation Therapy Oncology Group.

sets into the treatment planning system must be verified. In addition, the fusion algorithms—including their strengths and weaknesses—must be well understood and tested. Especially when using deformable image registration, it is necessary for the physicist and physician to have a clear understanding of the potentially large uncertainties involved in the fusion process. AAPM TG-132, Use of Image Registration and Data Fusion Algorithms and Techniques in Radiotherapy Treatment Planning, is currently under review for publication at the time of writing. This publication will provide more detailed guidance on image fusion.

■ **Respiratory motion management:** Must be considered for lesions in the lung and abdominal cavity. Chapter 19 discusses the clinical process in detail.

## 17.7 Margins

Traditionally, no explicit CTV margins are used in SRS with the exception of the treatment of resection cavities in the brain, where some institutions add a 2 mm CTV margin.[8] For SRS treatment of spinal metastases, the International Spine Radiosurgery Consortium has published detailed consensus contouring guidelines for common scenarios in spine radiosurgery.[9]

The van Herk[10] margin formula is often used for determining PTV margins in traditionally fractionated treatment regimens. However, it is based on the assumption of a sufficiently high number of fractions for a Poisson statistic of the random error to be valid. It also assumes the use of 3D conformal radiotherapy. There have been efforts to adapt the van Herk formula for SRS/SBRT, and more recently, Monte Carlo–based studies have been published on margin size specifically for SRS/SBRT.[11] Because frameless SRS/SBRT is still a relatively new modality, it is recommended to use margins based on recommendations from clinical trial groups or, if those are not available, to refer to published prospective clinical studies using similar processes and equipment (see Table 17.2).

In lung, the CARO scope of practice guidelines for lung, liver, and spine SBRT[2] recommends using a maximum intensity projection (MIP) image for the delineation of the ITV but not for dose calculation. Some groups, however, have noted that MIP images do not provide adequate image quality in the presence of respiratory motion and so employ 4D-CT scans for delineation of the GTV.

## 17.8 Dose Constraints and Treatment Planning

This section discusses the clinical aspects of treatment planning for SRS/SBRT. Technical QA of treatment planning systems, including image import, image fusion, and treatment export, is

TABLE 17.3 ▮ **Target Dose from Society Recommendations and Phase II/III Clinical Trials**

| | Target | Source | Dose Rx |
|---|---|---|---|
| Lung | Medically inoperable T1/T2 N0M0 non-small cell | CARO | 60 Gy/8 Fx |
| | Lung mets | | 50 Gy/5 Fx |
| | Tumors <5 cm | | 48 Gy/4 Fx |
| | | | 54-60 Gy/3 Fx |
| | | | 34 Gy/1 Fx |
| | Inoperable Stage I/II NSCLC, peripheral lesions | RTOG-0236 (Phase II) RTOG-0618 (Phase II) | 60 Gy/3 Fx over 1.5-2 weeks |
| | Inoperable Stage I/II NSCLC, peripheral lesions | RTOG-0915 (Phase II) | 34 Gy/1 Fx or 48 Gy/4 Fx (consecutive days) |
| Liver | Hepatocellular CA <8 cm | CARO | 42-60 Gy/5 Fx |
| | Liver mets <6 cm and/or ≤5 lesions | | 50 Gy/5 Fx |
| | | | 48 Gy/5 Fx |
| | | | 45 Gy/3 Fx |
| | Hepatocellular CA | RTOG-1112 (Phase III) | 27.5-50 Gy/5 Fx, 24-72 hr between Fx |
| Spine | Previously irradiated spine mets | CARO | 35 Gy/5 Fx |
| | Spine mets with no prior radiation | | 30 Gy/4 Fx |
| | Post-op patients (±prior radiation) | | 24-26 Gy/3 Fx |
| | Selected primary spine tumors | | 24-26 Gy/2 Fx |
| | No more than 3 consecutive vertebrae | | 16-24 Gy/1 Fx |

covered in Chapter 5. The ASTRO white paper on quality and safety considerations in SBRT recommends that the planning system must be able to support multimodality and multidimensional image data from CT, MRI, and PET (Tables 17.3 and 17.4).

## RTOG AND OTHER PROTOCOLS

The RTOG has come forward with a compactness constraint of PTV + 2 cm to limit the volume of intermediate dose to OARs. Indirectly, the use of the compactness constraint forces the use of multiple beams, lowering the risk for skin toxicity caused by beam entry hot spots far away from the target. Hot spots within the target are not only acceptable, but often desirable; for example, some lung SBRT treatment protocols specify a 25% to 30% hot spot within the GTV. The dose gradient outside the target should be steep (e.g., from 1 Gy/mm in spine SRS up to 16 Gy/mm for trigeminal neuralgia SRS). To accurately calculate dose given the steep dose gradients, the dose calculation grid of the treatment planning system should be set to the highest resolution that keeps the calculation time clinically reasonable. At this time, it is ≤2 mm for most treatment planning systems and 2% for most MC-based treatment planning systems.

Underdosing the PTV may be necessary to protect critical organs abutting the target. A typical example would be in spine SRS, where the dose limit to the cord combined with the currently achievable dose gradient for photon beams will almost always require a small area of the posterior vertebral body to be underdosed.

Lung tumors, but also tumors in the head and neck and brain, are located near large tissue inhomogeneities. The ability of the treatment planning system to accurately calculate dose and dose gradients for a small treatment field should be evaluated and documented. AAPM TG-65, Tissue Inhomogeneity Corrections for Megavoltage Photon Beams,[12] gives site-specific recommendations on the use of inhomogeneity calculations. ASTRO's white paper on quality and safety considerations in SBRT recommends that the treatment planning system should correct for tissue inhomogeneity with sufficient accuracy, although it does not state a specific limit other than

TABLE 17.4 ▪ Organ-at-Risk Dose Limits

| Organ at Risk | Source | Max Volume Above TH (cm³) | 1 Fx DVH (Gy) | 1 Fx Max (Gy) | 3 Fx DVH (Gy) | 3 Fx Max (Gy) | 4 Fx DVH (Gy) | 4 Fx Max (Gy) | 5 (6) Fx DVH (Gy) | 5 (6) Fx Max (Gy) | Endpoint (≥Grade 3) |
|---|---|---|---|---|---|---|---|---|---|---|---|
| Optic apparatus | TG-101 | 0.2 | 8 | 10 | 15.3 | 17.4 | | | 23 | 25 | Neuritis |
| Cochlea | TG-101 / QUANTEC | | — / 9.1* | 9 / 6.9 | | 17.1 | | | | 25 | Hearing loss / Serviceable hearing |
| Brain | QUANTEC | 5-10 | 12 | | | | | | | | |
| Brainstem | TG-101 / QUANTEC | 0.5 | 10 | 15 / 12.5 | 18 | 23.1 | | | 23 | 31 | Cranial neuropathy |
| Spinal cord/medulla | TG-101 & RTOG-0915 / RTOG-0236 / RTOG-0618 | 0.35 / 1.2 / Point | 10 / 7 | 14 / — | 18 / 12.3 | 21.9 / — / 18 | 20.8 / 13.6 | 26 | 23 / 14.5 | 30 / — | Myelitis |
| Cauda equina | TG-101 | 5 | 14 | 16 | 21.9 | 24 | | | 30 | 32 | Neuritis |
| Sacral plexus | TG-101 | 5 | 14.4 | 16 | 22.5 | 24 | | | 30 | 32 | Neuropathy |
| Esophagus | TG-101 & RTOG-0915 / RTOG-0236 / RTOG-0618 | 5 / Point | 11.9 | 15.4 | 17.7 | 25.2 / 27 | 18.8 | 30 | 19.5 | 35 | Stenosis/fistula |
| Brachial plexus | TG-101 & RTOG-0915 / RTOG-0236 / RTOG-0618 | 3 / Point | 14 | 17.5 | 20.4 | 24 / 24 | 23.6 | 27.2 | 27 | 30.5 | Neuropathy |
| Heart/pericardium | TG-101 & RTOG-0915 / RTOG-0236 / RTOG-0618 | 15 / Point | 16 | 22 | 24 | 30 / 30 | 28 | 34 | 32 | 38 | Pericarditis |
| Great vessels | TG-101 & RTOG-0915 | 10 | 31 | 37 | 39 | 45 | 43 | 49 | 47 | 53 | Aneurysm |
| Trachea and large bronchus | TG-101 & RTOG-0915 / RTOG-0236 / RTOG-0618 | 4 / Point | 10.5 | 20.2 | 15 | 30 / 30 | 15.6 | 34.8 | 16.5 | 40 | Stenosis/fistula |
| Bronchus/smaller airways | TG-101 | 0.5 | 12.4 | 13.3 | 18.9 | 23.1 | | | 21 | 33 | Stenosis with atelectasis |

| Organ | Reference | | | | | | | | | | Complication |
|---|---|---|---|---|---|---|---|---|---|---|---|
| Rib | TG-101 & RTOG-0915 | 1 | 22 | 30 | 28.8 | 36.9 | 32 | 40 | 35 | 43 | Pain or fracture |
| | | 30 | — | — | 30 | — | 33.2 | 36 | 36.5 | 39.5 | |
| Skin | TG-101 & RTOG-0915 | 10 | 23 | 26 | 30 | 33 | | | 18 | 32 | Ulceration |
| Stomach | TG-101 & RTOG-0915 | 10 | 11.2 | 12.4 | 16.5 | 22.2 | 17.6 | 27.2 | 18 | 32 | Ulceration/fistula |
| Duodenum | TG-101 | 5 | 11.2 | 12.4 | 16.5 | 22.2 | 17.6 | 27.2 | 18 | 32 | Ulceration |
| | | 10 | 9 | — | 11.4 | — | | | 12.5 | | |
| Jejunum/Ileum | TG-101 | 5 | 11.9 | 15.4 | 17.7 | 25.2 | | | 19.5 | 35 | Enteritis/obstruction |
| Colon | TG-101 | 20 | 14.3 | 18.4 | 24 | 28.2 | | | 25 | 38 | Colitis/fistula |
| Rectum | TG-101 | 20 | 14.3 | 18.4 | 24 | 28.2 | | | 25 | 38 | Proctitis/fistula |
| Bladder wall | TG-101 / QUANTEC | 15 | 11.4 | 18.4 | 16.8 | 28.2 | | | 18.3 | 38 | Cystitis/fistula |
| Penile bulb | TG-101 | 3 | 14 | 34 | 21.9 | 42 | | | 30 | 50 | Impotence |
| Femoral heads | TG-101 | 10 | 14 | — | 21.9 | — | | | 30 | — | Necrosis |
| **PARALLEL TISSUE** | | | | | | | | | | | |
| Renal | TG-101 | <2/3 | 10.6 | | 18.6 | | | | 23 | | Malignant hypertension |
| Lung | TG-101 & RTOG-0915 | <1500 | 7 | | 11.6 | 11.6 | | | 12.5 | | Basic lung function |
| | | <1000 | 7.4 | | 12.4 | 12.4 | | | 13.5 | | Pneumonitis |
| | RTOG-0236 | Comment: see end of table for dose conformality and gradient values | | | | | | | | | |
| | RTOG-0618 | | | | | | | | | | |
| | RTOG-0915 | Comment: see end of table for dose conformality and gradient values | | | | | | | | | |
| Liver | TG-101 | <700 | 9.1 | | 19.2 | | | | 21 | | Basic liver function |
| | RTOG-1112 | | | | | Liver mean dose | | | Rx dose (max = 150% of Rx) | | |
| | | | | | | 13 | | | 50 | | |
| | | | | | | 15 | | | 45 | | |
| | | | | | | 15 | | | 40 | | |
| | | | | | | 15.5 | | | 35 | | |
| | | | | | | 16 | | | 30 | | |
| | | | | | | 17 | | | 27.5 | | |

All dose limits are in Gy.

*mean dose

*Continued*

**TABLE 17.4** ▓ **Organ-at-Risk Dose Limits—cont'd**

**RTOG-0236 Lung Dose Constraint Table**

| Maximum PTV Dimension (cm) | Ratio of Prescription Isodose Volume to the PTV | | Ratio of 50% Prescription Isodose Volume to the PTV, $R_{50\%}$ | | Maximum Dose 2 cm from PTV in Any Direction, $D_{2\,cm}$ (Gy) | | Percent of Lung Receiving 20 Gy Total or More, $V_{20}$ (%) | | PTV Volume (cc) |
|---|---|---|---|---|---|---|---|---|---|
| | Deviation | | Deviation | | Deviation | | Deviation | | |
| | None | Minor | None | Minor | None | Minor | None | Minor | |
| 2.0 | <1.2 | 1.2-1.4 | <3.9 | 3.9-4.1 | <28.1 | 28.1-30.1 | <10 | 10-15 | 1.8 |
| 2.5 | <1.2 | 1.2-1.4 | <3.9 | 3.9-4.1 | <28.1 | 28.1-30.1 | <10 | 10-15 | 3.8 |
| 3.0 | <1.2 | 1.2-1.4 | <3.9 | 3.9-4.1 | <28.1 | 28.1-30.1 | <10 | 10-15 | 7.4 |
| 3.5 | <1.2 | 1.2-1.4 | <3.9 | 3.9-4.1 | <28.1 | 28.1-30.1 | <10 | 10-15 | 13.2 |
| 4.0 | <1.2 | 1.2-1.4 | <3.8 | 3.8-4.0 | <30.4 | 30.4-32.4 | <10 | 10-15 | 21.9 |
| 4.5 | <1.2 | 1.2-1.4 | <3.7 | 3.7-3.9 | <32.7 | 32.7-34.7 | <10 | 10-15 | 33.8 |
| 5.0 | <1.2 | 1.2-1.4 | <3.6 | 3.6-3.8 | <35.1 | 35.1-37.1 | <10 | 10-15 | 49.6 |
| 5.5 | <1.2 | 1.2-1.4 | <3.5 | 3.5-3.7 | <37.4 | 37.4-41.7 | <10 | 10-15 | 69.9 |
| 6.0 | <1.2 | 1.2-1.4 | <3.3 | 3.3-3.5 | <39.7 | 39.7-41.7 | <10 | 10-15 | 95.1 |
| 6.5 | <1.2 | 1.2-1.4 | <3.1 | 3.1-3.3 | <42.0 | 42.0-44.0 | <10 | 10-15 | 125.8 |
| 7.0 | <1.2 | 1.2-1.4 | <2.9 | 2.9-3.1 | <44.3 | 44.3-46.3 | <10 | 10-15 | 162.6 |

Note 1: For values of PTV dimension or volume not specified, linear interpolation between table entries is required.
Note 2: Protocol deviations greater than listed here as "minor" will be classified as "major" for protocol compliance (see Section 6.7).

TABLE 17.5 ■ **Hardware and Delivery Techniques for SRS/SBRT**

| SRS (cranial) | Cones | GK | Isocentric shots |
| | | Linac | Non-coplanar arcs |
| | | CK | Isocentric & nonisocentric shots |
| | MLC | Linac | Isocentric non-coplanar conformal beams, IMRT, VMAT |
| | | CK | Isocentric & nonisocentric conformal |
| SRS (body) | Cones | CK | Isocentric & nonisocentric shots |
| and SBRT | MLC | Linac | Isocentric non-coplanar conformal beams, IMRT, VMAT |
| | | CK | Isocentric & nonisocentric conformal |

GK = Gamma Knife, CK = Cyber Knife

excluding most pencil beam algorithms for this purpose. The white paper also recommends QA of the heterogeneity correction during the commissioning process using an appropriate phantom.

Several treatment planning options are available, depending on the use of collimation (cones or MLC) as well as delivery system. Table 17.5 lists treatment beam configurations used in SBRT planning. When using non-coplanar beams, performing a delivery dry run to identify potential collision risks is advised. The CARO scope of practice guidelines for lung, liver, and spine SBRT[2] recommends using conformity indices, as they are helpful when evaluating the overall plan quality. The ACR practice guideline on SBRT recommends having a documented process for commissioning a treatment planning system into clinical use for SRS/SBRT and ongoing monitoring of the treatment planning system's performance. Chapter 5 in Part 1 provides guidelines on how to put such a process in place.

## 17.9 Treatment Delivery

For frameless SRS/SBRT treatments, accurate image guidance systems must be used for patient setup and intrafraction motion monitoring. Image guidance options include 2D-3D registration using orthogonal x-rays, kV-MV image registration, and kV or MV cone-beam computed tomography (CBCT). More recently, nonionizing technologies using visible light (VisionRT), electromagnetic tracking (Calypso), or ultrasound (Clarity) have become available for routine clinical use. AAPM TG-101[7] recommends defining action levels for translation and rotations above which the patient setup position should be corrected. The ACR practice guideline on SBRT and SRS[6] recommends testing both the image guidance system and treatment delivery system in an integrated manner to verify that they accurately work together during the treatment delivery process. The systems should demonstrate the capability to localize and position a hidden target and subsequently irradiate the target to a specified accuracy. This type of test is an integral part of an E2E test. Furthermore, AAPM TG-142, Quality Assurance of Medical Accelerators,[13] recommends daily verification of the agreement between imaging and treatment delivery system.

Respiratory motion management must be applied to stereotactic targets in the thoracic and abdominal cavities. The techniques are identical to respiratory motion management in intensity-modulated radiation therapy (IMRT) and 3D conformal treatments, which are covered in Chapter 19.

The CARO scope of practice guidelines for lung, liver, and spine SBRT[2] recommend that the treatment should be delivered within a short timeframe from simulation, although "short" is not explicitly defined in the document. For longer SRS/SBRT procedures on linacs where intra-fraction motion monitoring is not available, the treatment can be interrupted halfway to image and confirm target position.

Before the start of any SRS/SBRT treatment, a procedural pause should be used to confirm patient identity, target location, dose per fraction, and fraction number and verify accurate setup

Medical Record Number

Patient Name

Addressograph or Label - Patient Name, Medical Record Number

PROCEDURE • CYBERKNIFE RADIOSURGERY PATIENT
SAFETY CHECKLIST

Allergies _____

Plan Name _____   Start Date _____   Number of fractions _____ *  CK1 or CK2 ____
*cross out rows of unused fractions*

**Section I - Before First Fraction**

| Safety Check | Completed | Radiation Therapist Signature | Print Name | Date | Time |
|---|---|---|---|---|---|
| 1.  Correct patient (name/DOB/photo) | | | | | |
| 2.  History and physical in chart | | | | | |
| 3.  Signed consent in chart | | | | | |
| 4.  Physics double check signed | | | | | |
| 5.  Site and side correspond to Rx Plan | | | | | |
| 6.  Trigeminal neuralgia checklist done | ❏ Yes ❏ NA | | | | |
| 7.  Functional disorder checklist done | ❏ Yes ❏ NA | | | | |
| 8.  Prone position checklist done | ❏ Yes ❏ NA | | | | |

**Section II - Immediately Before Each Fraction**

| Fraction | Radiation Therapy Technologist | Radiation Physicist | Physician |
|---|---|---|---|
| **Fraction 1** | ☐ Correct Patient (name/DOB/photo)<br>☐ Correct Procedure on consent (first Tx)<br>☐ Correct Position (supine/prone)<br>☐ Correct Collimator(s)<br>☐ Plan Corresponds to Prescription<br>☐ Monitor Units Correct<br>☐ Patient Voided<br>Date: _____ Time: _____<br>Signature: _____<br>Print Name: _____ | ☐ Correct Patient (name/DOB/photo)<br>☐ Correct Position (supine/prone)<br>☐ Correct Collimator(s)<br>☐ Plan Corresponds to Prescription<br>☐ Monitor Units Correct<br><br><br>Date: _____ Time: _____<br>Signature: _____<br>Print Name: _____ | ☐ Correct Patient (name/DOB/photo)<br>☐ Plan Corresponds to Prescription<br>☐ Medication Needs Evaluated<br>☐ Image tracking verified<br><br><br><br>Date: _____ Time: _____<br>Signature: _____<br>Print Name: _____ |
| **Fraction 2**<br>*cross out if single fraction* | ☐ Correct Patient (name/DOB/photo)<br>☐ Correct Position (supine/prone)<br>☐ Correct Collimator(s)<br>☐ Plan Corresponds to Prescription<br>☐ Monitor Units Correct<br>☐ Patient Voided<br>Date: _____ Time: _____<br>Signature: _____<br>Print Name: _____ | ☐ Correct Patient (name/DOB/photo)<br>☐ Correct Position (supine/prone)<br>☐ Correct Collimator(s)<br>☐ Plan Corresponds to Prescription<br>☐ Monitor Units Correct<br><br>Date: _____ Time: _____<br>Signature: _____<br>Print Name: _____ | ☐ Correct Patient (name/DOB/photo)<br>☐ Plan Corresponds to Prescription<br>☐ Medication Needs Evaluated<br>☐ Image tracking verified<br><br><br>Date: _____ Time: _____<br>Signature: _____<br>Print Name: _____ |
| **Fraction 3**<br>*cross out if < 3 fractions* | ☐ Correct Patient (name/DOB/photo)<br>☐ Correct Position (supine/prone)<br>☐ Correct Collimator(s)<br>☐ Plan Corresponds to Prescription<br>☐ Monitor Units Correct<br>☐ Patient Voided<br>Date: _____ Time: _____<br>Signature: _____<br>Print Name: _____ | ☐ Correct Patient (name/DOB/photo)<br>☐ Correct Position (supine/prone)<br>☐ Correct Collimator(s)<br>☐ Plan Corresponds to Prescription<br>☐ Monitor Units Correct<br><br>Date: _____ Time: _____<br>Signature: _____<br>Print Name: _____ | ☐ Correct Patient (name/DOB/photo)<br>☐ Plan Corresponds to Prescription<br>☐ Medication Needs Evaluated<br>☐ Image tracking verified<br><br><br>Date: _____ Time: _____<br>Signature: _____<br>Print Name: _____ |
| **Fraction 4**<br>*cross out if < 4 fractions* | ☐ Correct Patient (name/DOB/photo)<br>☐ Correct Position (supine/prone)<br>☐ Correct Collimator(s)<br>☐ Plan Corresponds to Prescription<br>☐ Monitor Units Correct<br>☐ Patient Voided<br>Date: _____ Time: _____<br>Signature: _____<br>Print Name: _____ | ☐ Correct Patient (name/DOB/photo)<br>☐ Correct Position (supine/prone)<br>☐ Correct Collimator(s)<br>☐ Plan Corresponds to Prescription<br>☐ Monitor Units Correct<br><br>Date: _____ Time: _____<br>Signature: _____<br>Print Name: _____ | ☐ Correct Patient (name/DOB/photo)<br>☐ Plan Corresponds to Prescription<br>☐ Medication Needs Evaluated<br>☐ Image tracking verified<br><br><br>Date: _____ Time: _____<br>Signature: _____<br>Print Name: _____ |
| **Fraction 5**<br>*cross out if < 5 fractions* | ☐ Correct Patient (name/DOB/photo)<br>☐ Correct Position (supine/prone)<br>☐ Correct Collimator(s)<br>☐ Plan Corresponds to Prescription<br>☐ Monitor Units Correct<br>☐ Patient Voided<br>Date: _____ Time: _____<br>Signature: _____<br>Print Name: _____ | ☐ Correct Patient (name/DOB/photo)<br>☐ Correct Position (supine/prone)<br>☐ Correct Collimator(s)<br>☐ Plan Corresponds to Prescription<br>☐ Monitor Units Correct<br><br>Date: _____ Time: _____<br>Signature: _____<br>Print Name: _____ | ☐ Correct Patient (name/DOB/photo)<br>☐ Plan Corresponds to Prescription<br>☐ Medication Needs Evaluated<br>☐ Image tracking verified<br><br><br>Date: _____ Time: _____<br>Signature: _____<br>Print Name: _____ |

15-2767 (09/10)

**Figure 17.1** Sample pretreatment procedural pause checklist for a multifraction SRS/SBRT treatment.

and other parameters. The use of a standardized checklist, initialed as applicable by the round-trip time (RTT), physicist, and physician, is highly recommended. The checklist can either reside in the electronic medical record (EMR) system or be a paper checklist scanned into the EMR system as documentation for this critical clinical safety step. A sample checklist is provided in Figure 17.1 as a starting point for developing a customized checklist.

AAPM TG-101[7] recommends the documentation of treatment interruptions or deviations from the intended fractionation time interval and also recommends that the physicist be present throughout the first treatment procedure for supervision and to provide direct supervision for subsequent fractions. Billing codes published by Centers for Medicare & Medicaid Services (CMS) for stereotactic procedures may contain differing provisions for physicist presence, which should be evaluated with a medical billing specialist to ensure compliance with current Medicare rules.

There is currently no uniform guideline for supervision by physicians and physicists during treatment delivery. Supervision requirements can be separated into three levels:

1. Legal requirements set by federal or state regulations, requirements specified in billing codes
2. Requirements by accrediting bodies (if applicable)
3. Best practice recommendations as specified in society recommendations and institutional policies and procedures

After the patient treatment is completed, a formal final chart review should be conducted by the therapist, physicist, and physician to verify that treatment was delivered as intended, any deviations from the treatment protocol were documented, and follow-up instructions/appointments are in place.

## FOR THE PHYSICIAN

Due to the high risk nature of high dose, hypofractionated radiosurgical treatment, machines used to deliver these treatments must meet the most stringent technical requirements, including mechanical tolerances and commissioning. A multidisciplinary approach is needed during the design and setup of the radiosurgery program to ensure all policies and procedures are present to ensure safe and efficient treatment. Prior to treatment, mock patient treatment scenarios and phantoms should be used in end-to-end testing of the workflow. The ACR practice guideline on SBRT and SRS and the ASTRO white paper on quality and safety considerations both provide guidance on best practices. There is more emphasis recently on having qualified medical physicists with specific SBRT training be responsible for technical aspects of a radiosurgical program.

With the high dose per fraction and sharp penumbra in radiosurgical treatments, patient immobilization is even more critical than it is in conventionally fractionated radiation. Many immobilization systems are available for this purpose, and needs vary based on body site. Patient comfort must be factored into the setup position because treatment times are often long. Respiratory motion management must be considered for lung and abdominal cavity treatment. The concept of margins is different for radiosurgery versus conventional radiation, and CTV is rarely used. In clinical practice PTV margins are typically based on published or ongoing clinical trials.

To accurately target the tumor with high dose radiation, high resolution simulation imaging is needed for tumor and normal tissue definition. If imaging modalities other than CT are used for contouring (e.g., MRI, PET), there must be a rigorous fusion algorithm to ensure accuracy. Physicians and physicists need an understanding of the uncertainties involved in the fusion process, and can refer to the forthcoming AAPM TG-132 for more information.

In treatment planning for radiosurgery, the sharp dose gradients require that treatment planning systems calculate at the highest resolution possible while still keeping the calculation time clinically reasonable. Hot spots are often expected and desired inside the target volume. When reviewing plans, attention must be paid to the intermediate dose region, and most clinical protocols have dose conformality constraints to limit the size of this region. Tissue inhomogeneity needs to be accounted for by the treatment planning system, especially for small field sizes.

Prior to radiosurgery treatment delivery, there must be confirmation of patient setup and immobilization. Various imaging modalities can be used, and AAPM TG-101 provides recommendations for translation and rotations above which the patient setup position should be corrected. Part of the quality assurance process for radiosurgery equipment should ensure that the image guidance system and treatment delivery system work in an integrated manner during the treatment delivery process.

### References

1. Lutz W, Winston KR, Maleki N. A system for stereotactic radiosurgery with a linear accelerator. Int J Radiat Oncol Biol Phys 1988;14:373–81. doi:10.1016/0360-3016(88)90446-4.
2. Sahgal A, Roberge D, Schellenberg D, et al. The Canadian Association of Radiation Oncology scope of practice guidelines for lung, liver and spine stereotactic body radiotherapy. Clin Oncol 2012;24:629–39. doi:10.1016/j.clon.2012.04.006.
3. Solberg TD, Balter JM, Benedict SH, et al. Quality and safety considerations in stereotactic radiosurgery and stereotactic body radiation therapy: Executive summary. Prac Radiat Oncol 2012;2(1):2–9.
4. Mills MD. Analysis and practical use: The Abt study of medical physicist work values for Radiation Oncology physics services—Round II. J Am College Radiol 2005;2:782–9. doi:10.1016/j.jacr.2005.02.009.
5. Potters L, Steinberg M, Rose C, et al. American Society for Therapeutic Radiology and Oncology (ASTRO) and American College of Radiology (ACR) practice guideline for the performance of stereotactic body radiation therapy. Int J Radiat Oncol Biology Phys 2004;60(4):1026–32.
6. Seung SK, Larson DA, Galvin JM, et al. American College of Radiology (ACR) and American Society for Radiation Oncology (ASTRO) practice guideline for the performance of stereotactic radiosurgery (SRS). Am J Clin Oncol 2013;36(3):310–15. doi:10.1097/COC.0b013e31826e053d.
7. Benedict SH, Schlesinger DJ, Goetsch SJ, et al. Stereotactic body radiation therapy: The report of AAPM Task Group 101. Med Phys 2012;37:4078–101.
8. Soltys SG, Adler JR, Lipani JD, et al. Stereotactic radiosurgery of the postoperative resection cavity for brain metastases. Int J Radiat Oncol Biology Phys 2008;70(1):187–93. doi:10.1016/j.ijrobp.2007.06.068.
9. Cox BW, Spratt DE, Lovelock M, et al. International Spine Radiosurgery Consortium consensus guidelines for target volume definition in spinal stereotactic radiosurgery. Int J Radiat Oncol Biol Phys 2012; 83(5):e597–605.
10. van Herk M. Errors and margins in radiotherapy. Semin Radiat Oncol 2004;14:52–64. doi:10.1053/j.semradonc.2003.10.003.
11. Herschtal A, Foroudi F, Silva L, et al. Calculating geometrical margins for hypofractionated radiotherapy. Phys Med Biol 2013;58(2):319–33. doi:10.1088/0031-9155/58/2/319.
12. Papanikolaou N, Battista JJ, Boyer AL, et al. Report of the AAPM Task Group No. 65: Tissue inhomogeneity corrections for megavoltage photon beams. Madison, WI: Medical Physics Publishing; 2004.
13. Klein EE, Hanley J, Bayouth J, et al. Task Group 142 report: Quality assurance of medical accelerators. Med Phys 2009;36(9):4197–212.

# Clinical Aspects of Image Guidance and Localization in Radiotherapy

## 18.1 Introduction

Image-guided radiotherapy (IGRT) is well established; however it is important to note that there has never been a prospective randomized trial to examine its value. There are, however, a number of retrospective series examining the impact of IGRT as outlined in recent papers.[1,2] The potential impact of IGRT can be appreciated by considering a recent study that linked biochemical failures in prostate cancer patients to mislocalization of the target caused by rectal distention at the time of simulation.[3] This issue can be corrected with IGRT.[4]

IGRT becomes crucial when considering high dose-per-fraction treatments, the most extreme example of which is stereotactic body radiotherapy (SBRT). The American Society for Radiation Oncology (ASTRO) white paper Quality and Safety Considerations in Stereotactic Radiosurgery (SRS) and SBRT notes that image guidance is "a prerequisite for all SBRT applications."[5] IGRT is also important when lower, nonablative doses are used, for example, in the hypofractionated treatment of early stage prostate cancer, which is being pursued based on the advantageous biology of a low $\alpha/\beta$ ratio[6] in early trials[7] and now in cooperative group trials (e.g., Radiation Therapy Oncology Group (RTOG) 0938).

While further outcomes-based research on IGRT will be welcome, it is clear that the technology is beneficial in many settings and essential in some. This chapter explores the physics-related aspects of IGRT in clinical use.

## 18.2 Overview of Image Guidance Definitions and Procedures

Image-guided radiotherapy can come in any of several flavors as defined in International Electrotechnical Commission (IEC) and also American Association of Physicists in Medicine Task Group (AAPM TG)-104:[8]

- "Online" correction (i.e., immediately prior to or during the therapeutic irradiation session and requiring operator-initiated adjustments)
- "Offline" correction (i.e., to be applied in subsequent treatment delivery)
- "Real-time" IGRT is similar to online, but means imaging throughout treatment allowing for automatic adjustment without the intervention of an operator.

The type of image guidance depends on the clinical needs. In SBRT, for example, the ASTRO white paper on stereotactic safety[5] calls for image guidance to be applied "ideally … at the start of each treatment fraction," i.e., online. Offline corrections are valuable for reducing systematic errors but do not address random day-to-day variations. While online corrections can greatly reduce random variations, they come at the cost of technical complexity. Online CT systems typically require 2 to 3 extra minutes for image acquisition plus the time for interpretation. They also deliver extra dose, which deserves consideration. AAPM TG-75, The Management of Imaging Dose During IGRT,[9] notes that "management of imaging dose during radiotherapy is a different problem than its management during routine diagnostic or image-guided surgical procedures." Although this application may not call for a diagnostic radiology program like Image Gently (http://www.pedrad.org/associations/5364/ig/) or Image Wisely (http://www.imagewisely .org/), clearly a balanced cost/benefit consideration is required. The report notes that it is "no longer safe to … assume that the cumulative imaging dose is negligible compared to the therapeutic dose."

There are a wide variety of technologies to accomplish the various flavors of IGRT as outlined in Table 18.1. Note that with the possible exception of on-treatment MR technologies, no one platform can accomplish all IGRT clinical goals. A technical review of IGRT system capabilities is found in Chapter 7.

It is necessary to have a clear understanding of the IGRT process and workflow. Here we consider two examples that encapsulate most of the features of IGRT: (1) computed tomography (CT)-based IGRT and (2) real-time IGRT during treatment. Obvious parallels can be drawn to other forms of IGRT.

## WORKFLOW EXAMPLE 1: CT-BASED IGRT

A first step in IGRT and a key foundation is the reference image used for treatment planning (in this case the simulation CT, Figure 18.1A). An isocenter and region-of-interest structure sets are defined in the treatment planning system. These are transferred (if necessary) to the image guidance system. When the patient is ready for treatment and positioned at the intended isocenter, a CT is acquired (Figure 18.1B). This CT is aligned with the reference data set using an interactive image fusion software interface (Figure 18.1C). Registration uses rigid body alignment with 3D translations and (optionally) rotations around three axes. Registration can be accomplished manually or automatically via various algorithms that can be set to focus on particular regions of the image (e.g., a 3D box) or on different threshold values of the CT number (e.g., bony features or soft tissue gray values). The registration results in a calculated shift correction. The patient is moved according to these shift calculations, a process that is often accomplished automatically via a command to the linac table. Some patient support systems (e.g., HexaPod) allow for "six-degree-of-freedom" positioning (i.e., translational movements in three directions as well as rotations of up to 3 degrees about the three principle axes). One issue is that the rotation may correctly describe the anatomic alignment near the isocenter but may be less accurate away from the isocenter. A rotation of 1 degree corresponds to a shift of approximately

TABLE 18.1    **Flavors of IGRT Enabled by Various Technologies and the Associated Imaging Capabilities (Visualization of Soft Tissue and/or Fiducials) as Well as IGRT Correction Strategies**

| Technology Platform | Soft-Tissue | Fiducials | Online Correction | Offline Correction | Real-Time IGRT |
|---|---|---|---|---|---|
| kV-CBCT & planar | ✓ | ✓ | ✓ | ✓ | ✗ |
| MV-CT | ✓ | ✓ | ✓ | ✓ | ✗ |
| CyberKnife | ✓(lung) | ✓ | ✓ | ✓ | ✓ |
| Calypso | ✗ | ✓ | ✓ | ✗ | ✓ |
| MR-guided RT | ✓ | ✓ | ✓ | ✓ | ✓ |

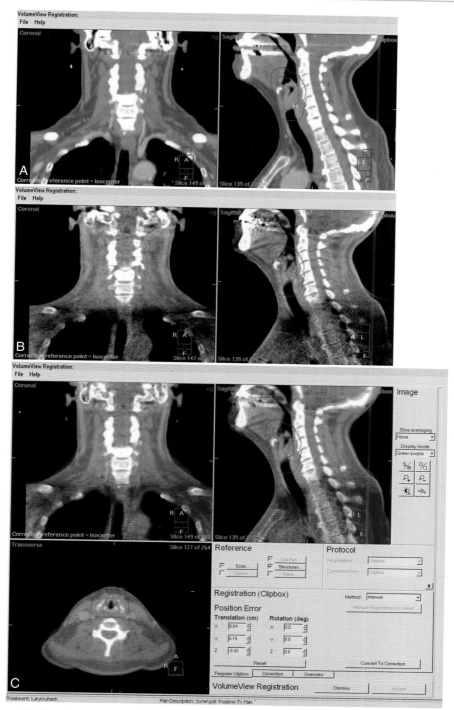

**Figure 18.1** Cone-beam CT (CBCT)-based alignment of a patient being treated for head and neck cancer. Prior to treatment a CBCT scan is acquired (**B**) and fused with the reference CT from simulation (**A**). Note that some regions align well but others do not (**C**).

TABLE 18.2  ■  **Example IGRT Protocol and Professional Responsibilities**

| IGRT Protocol. Memorial Harbor Hospital. Site: Abdominal Tumors. Conventional Fractionation | |
| --- | --- |
| **Professional Group** | **Role and Protocol** |
| Radiation Therapy Technologist | Perform scan and initial alignment; consult physician if shift >10 mm in any dimension. |
| Radiation Oncologist | Consult with RTT prior to treatment on expected alignment; be present at first treatment. |
| Medical Physicist | System quality assurance (QA); analyze shift data to determine random and systematic errors; be present at first treatment. |

2 mm at 10 cm from the isocenter. Such inaccurate alignments off-axis can have implications for doses to organs at risk.

Whatever the correction strategy, it is valuable to have a predefined protocol for IGRT that includes the roles and responsibilities for each professional group and the associated protocols (see ASTRO safety white paper on IGRT[2]). An example protocol from a fictional hospital is presented in Table 18.2. The protocol spells out who is responsible for IGRT alignment (therapists in this case). It also lists threshold limits for shifts (10 mm in this case) after which they must consult a radiation oncologist. Such thresholds are a specific recommendation of the ACR/ASTRO practice guidelines for IGRT[10] and ideally should be site-specific and based on an analysis of the random and systematic errors. The example protocol also spells out professional roles. Here the physician and physicist are expected to be present for the alignment procedure on the first day but not thereafter. This would vary for other treatment protocols. In SBRT cases, for example, the physician would typically be present for each treatment.

To this idealized IGRT process are added the many issues and challenges that can arise in actual practice. One well-worn error pathway is related to isocenter placement. The image guidance system must have the correct reference point defined, typically the isocenter from the treatment planning computer. If an incorrect reference point is transferred the patient alignment will be incorrect. This error is particularly insidious because it is not visible to the operator. Similarly, on a TomoTherapy system the reference or red lasers must be set to the reference point in the planning system. Not doing so will lead to systematic errors.

Other, less gross errors are possible. For example, the bladder filling for a pelvis case might be different at the time of treatment compared to simulation. In such a situation it would not be possible to align all the pelvic anatomy without intervening with the patient and rescanning. Figure 18.1B shows an example from a patient with head and neck cancer where part of the anatomy is well aligned (cervical vertebrae) but another part is not (mandible and skull). Such region misalignments represent a significant challenge where extensive regions are being treated and underscore the importance of the physician being involved in defining the alignment objectives for IGRT cases.

Another question is how well the CT planning scan (acquired prior to treatment) represents the anatomy during the actual treatment. Several issues come into play here: patient movement, nonideal immobilization, long wait times between scanning and treatment, changes in tumor size or position during the course of therapy, and changes in patient body habitus (e.g., weight loss). A few publications have addressed this issue, but there is relatively little peer-reviewed literature given the wealth of IGRT data that have been collected. In the future more reports will hopefully appear, providing practical guidance on IGRT setup issues. To evaluate movement on individual cases it may be useful to perform a repeat CT just after treatment to assess movement (perhaps for several fractions). For longer treatments (e.g., SRS/SBRT) repeat imaging may be performed mid-treatment.

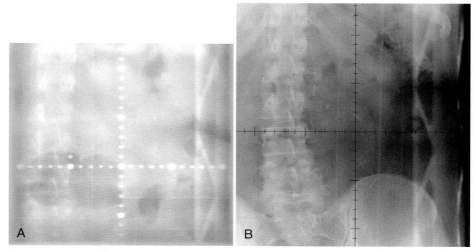

**Figure 18.2** Planar images acquired for alignment using the MV linac beam (**A**) and the kV beam (**B**).

## WORKFLOW EXAMPLE 2: REAL-TIME IGRT

Workflow scenarios for real-time IGRT share many similarities with the preceding discussion about CT-based IGRT. The details are technology dependent, but one simple example is planar images on a linac-based system. Again a reference image (digitally reconstructed radiograph (DRR)) is required. Modern IGRT systems allow one to overlay or fuse the DRR with the online image and also to draw regions on the DRR (e.g., a bony landmark or implanted fiducial), which are then overlaid with the online image. The online images can be megavoltage (MV) electronic portal imaging device (EPID) images, but kV planar imaging typically results in better image quality and lower doses (Figure 18.2). In the example in Figure 18.2B, the alignment of surgical clips is being monitored during treatment. Another example of real-time guidance is the use of implanted radiofrequency beacons, currently approved for use in the prostate. Each beacon is identified on the reference CT scan and has a unique frequency. The beacon positions are then monitored in real time during treatment. When real-time image guidance is used, action levels should be established for the interruption of treatment. In the setting of respiratory motion, these action levels may depend on the method used for respiratory compensation. More details on this can be found in Chapter 19.

# 18.3 Imaging Protocols and Issues in Clinical Use

There are numerous parameters controlling image acquisition. The technical details can be found in Chapter 7, while here we consider the clinical context more fully. One important setting for CT is the extent of anatomy imaged. This can be controlled by collimation as shown in Table 18.3. Settings can be used in various combinations with associated trade-offs between image quality and extent of visible anatomy. A large setting (e.g., L20 or half-fan, see Table 18.3) yields extensive anatomy, perhaps even the outer contour of the patient. However, compared to a smaller setting (e.g., S10 or full-fan) it results in increased noise due to scatter and cupping artifacts as well as increased exposure to the patient.

The number of projection images acquired is also controllable. On one system (Elekta Inc.) the acquisition can be either from an entire gantry rotation ("full-scan") or can be limited to 200° of a rotation ("half-scan"). A half-scan is faster (70 sec versus 1.5 min) but is subject to streaks

TABLE 18.3 ■ System Settings and Nominal Parameters for CT-Based IGRT Systems

| System | Lateral Field of View | | Superior-Inferior | | Clearance |
| | Setting | FOV Diameter | Setting | Extent | |
| --- | --- | --- | --- | --- | --- |
| Elekta XVI | S | 28 cm | 2 | 3.5 cm | 53.6 cm |
| | M | 43 cm | 10 | 12.5 cm | |
| | L | 52 cm | 15 | 18 cm | |
| | | | 20 | 26 cm | |
| Varian OBI | Full-fan | 24 cm | | 15 cm | 50 cm |
| | Half-fan | 45 cm | | 14 cm | |
| TomoTherapy | | 40 cm | | Variable | 85 cm bore |

Note that the "S" setting is used for kV planar imaging and fluoroscopy. Geometric distance between the isocenter and the panel is listed, which is an indicator of the clearance.

on axial cuts. The size of the voxels used in reconstruction can also be controlled. This system uses isotropic voxels (low res: 2 mm, med res: 1 mm, and high res: 0.5 mm) with slice averaging selectable in the longitudinal dimension. The On-Board Imaging (OBI) system from Varian uses other protocols (full-fan: $0.47 \times 0.47 \times 2.5$ mm or half-fan: $0.88 \times 0.88 \times 2.5$ mm). TomoTherapy uses preprogrammed pitch values of 1, 2, and 3 (fine, normal, and coarse) with a 4 mm collimator (i.e., nominal slice thicknesses of 2, 4, and 6 mm). As reviewed in AAPM TG-148,[11] the TomoTherapy rotational period during the image acquisition is fixed at 10 sec, which translates to an acquisition rate of one slice per 5 sec for a half-scan reconstruction technique. The axial field of view is set at 40 cm with a voxel size of 0.78 mm. The superior-inferior extend depends on how many slices are acquired.

Beyond these technical considerations, image quality and guidance are affected in more complex ways by various clinical situations. Figure 18.1B shows a CBCT scan where the image quality is good in one region (the thinner head and neck area) but worse in another region (the thicker region near the shoulders). In some cases this is acceptable, but in other cases the technique would need to be modified (e.g., higher mAs settings, higher kVp, or use of full-scan (instead of half-scan) technique).

Another issue affecting image quality is patient motion, which is common given the long scan acquisition times (>1 minute). Motion results in blurring, which is sometimes difficult to appreciate. Respiratory motion is a special case of this. New developments allow for 4D CBCT by which respiratory motion can be visualized, albeit with a long acquisition time (3 to 4 minutes). If a patient is being treated with respiratory motion management (e.g., gating or breath hold), then CBCT should be acquired with this management in place. In this case motion is of course minimal, but scan times can be long (e.g., five or more breath-hold acquisitions for a single CT).

## 18.4 Anatomic Changes and Adaptive Radiation Therapy

Anatomic changes represent one of the key advantages of IGRT and also one of the most significant challenges. On the positive side, IGRT allows one to correct for systematic changes on treatment versus at the time of simulation. The 2005 study of de Crevoisier et al. from MD Anderson[3] found that increased rectal filling at the time of simulation resulted in increased biochemical failure. This was thought to be due to the systematic posterior displacement of the prostate during treatment relative to the treatment plan. Similar effects of rectal distention were noted in a Dutch dose-escalation prostate trial.[12] IGRT provides an opportunity to correct this.

Anatomic changes can also present significant challenges for IGRT. One particularly difficult situation is the on-treatment changes in patients with non–small cell lung cancer undergoing standard treatment (e.g., 60 Gy delivered in 33 fractions). Some of these tumors will shrink during treatment to less than half of their original size. If the centroid of the tumor is aligned each day, the surrounding anatomy will be greatly offset by the end of the treatment. Furthermore, the shrinkage is often directionally asymmetric. Alignment can be further complicated by the resolution of atelectasis during treatment. To reduce the impact of these effects some physicians will resimulate and plan such patients midway through treatment. Other examples of anatomic changes are noted in the following applications section.

Adaptive radiation therapy (ART) is one approach to addressing anatomic changes during treatment. The basic concept is to reoptimize a patient's plan using a CT scan acquired at the time of treatment. This can either be done online with fast planning or offline whereby a replan is developed to be applied the following day. At the time of this writing, only one vendor-supplied ART system is currently cleared by the Food and Drug Administration (FDA) (an MR-based system from ViewRay Inc.). No task-group level recommendations exist yet on the use of ART, though there is clearly a need for guidance given the important workflow, delivery, and safety considerations. However, there is an extensive body of literature on this topic (see Ghilezan et al.,[13] for example, for a review for prostate cancer). At least one prospective trial employing ART has appeared.[14] In the absence of widespread commercial tools, some clinics are employing ART "by hand" by rescanning and replanning patients in cases with large enough anatomic changes to have a clinically significant dosimetric impact as judged by the physician.[15] In the presence of anatomic changes, however, such a composite dose distribution is approximate at best. It may not be possible to recalculate dose, in which case the system would have to deform the dose rather than recalculate, a process that does not account for changes in density or external contours. Even in fully ART-capable systems there may be situations in which dose cannot be recomputed (e.g., truncated online CT).

# 18.5 Organizing and Managing an Image Guidance Program

The safety and effectiveness of an IGRT program arguably depend at least as much on organizational and management aspects as on the technical and clinical features discussed above. Useful discussions of this issue can be found in the ASTRO white paper on IGRT safety[2] and the ACR/ASTRO guidelines on IGRT.[10] The ASTRO white paper on IGRT safety Table 2 lists "ten foundational elements for good IGRT," some of which also appear in the ACR/ASTRO guidelines.

1. Establish a multiprofessional team responsible for IGRT activities.
2. Establish and monitor a program of daily, monthly, and annual QA.
3. Provide device- and process-specific training for all staff operating IGRT systems or responsible for IGRT delivery. IGRT requires a set of skills beyond that traditionally required. Radiation therapists, for example, require expertise in cross-sectional anatomy and reading ultrasound images.
4. Perform "end-to-end" testing for all new IGRT procedures.
5. Establish process-specific documentation and procedures for IGRT.
6. Clearly identify who is responsible for approval of IGRT correction decisions and the process whereby these decisions are made and documented.
7. Establish and document site-specific planning procedures, including the procedure for defining planning target volume (PTV) margins.
8. Perform multiprofessional peer review of PTV volumes and peer review of gross tumor volume/clinical target volume (GTV/CTV) volumes by radiation oncologists.
9. Verify proper creation and transfer of IGRT reference data (PTV, OARs, DRRs, etc.) to the IGRT system.
10. Establish a reporting mechanism for IGRT-related variances in the radiation treatment process.

# 18.6 Image Guidance Applications

This section presents example case studies of IGRT as applied to various specific disease sites.

## PROSTATE

The sharp dose gradients typically used on the posterior edge of the prostate make IGRT particularly useful, especially since it allows one to move beyond bony anatomy and localize the prostate gland itself. Various technologies have been used: ultrasound (see American Association of Physicists in Medicine Task Group (AAPM TG)-154[16]), on-treatment computed tomography (CT), and implanted markers or radiofrequency beacons (Calypso Inc.). Soon magnetic resonance (MR)-guided radiotherapy will undoubtedly be used for this disease site. IGRT provides direct localization of the gland as well as visualization of rectal and bladder filling when volumetric imaging is used.

Though IGRT is indisputably valuable for this disease site, special challenges must be recognized. First, in terms of visualization, the prostate gland can be difficult to distinguish from surrounding soft tissue, especially on megavoltage CT (MVCT). Several recent studies have explored the use of long-lasting hydrogels inserted between the prostate and rectum mainly to create space but also to assist in visualization.[17,18]

Another challenge in prostate IGRT concerns the target structures, which are sometimes complex. In treating a multiple phase course, for example, the initial phase may include the seminal vesicles and/or regional nodes, and these anatomic regions cannot all be aligned simultaneously. In the absence of adaptive radiotherapy (or creating a set of plans in advance) a strategy of aligning bony anatomy may be chosen. For the boost or "conedown" phase, the alignment would focus on the prostate itself, looking at the prostate/bladder/rectum interfaces in particular. Even in this case, however, the gland can undergo pitch rotations, particularly if bladder or rectal filling changes. These rotations may not be fully corrected for even with a six-degree-of-freedom patient positioning system (typically limited to <3 degree rotation). Some groups have observed substantial interfractional variations in rectal volume, leading them to advocate planning and treatment with an empty rectum, which appears to reduce this variability.[19]

A final challenge concerns the movement of the prostate during treatment due to peristalsis and relaxation of the pelvic muscles, resulting in a slow posterior drift over the course of a treatment. This motivates real-time imaging, which, for the time being, is accomplished with implanted markers or radiofrequency beacons (Calypso Inc.). These carry their own set of challenges, however. One early concern was migration of markers within the prostate tissue, but this appears to not be a problem. It is crucial, however, to implant the markers accurately. Typically three markers are implanted, and if these markers are too close to each other the 3D localization accuracy is reduced. Of course these issues are particularly important for systems that do not rely on volumetric imaging.

A final warning about IGRT relates to margins. Though IGRT provides increased confidence in tumor localization, margins that are too tight may negatively affect outcomes. Just such an effect was noted in a 2009 study from a European center.[20] Freedom from biochemical failure was significantly reduced in the patients who received marker-based IGRT. This was attributed to a reduction in margins that was too aggressive (3 mm LR, 4 mm CC, and 5 mm AP where 6 mm may have been more appropriate).[20]

## HEAD AND NECK

Radiotherapy of the head and neck (H&N) is a prime candidate for IGRT because tumor regions lie close to organs at risk (e.g., cord and parotid gland). Treatment plans often have sharp dose gradients. H&N is challenging, however, due to the fact that extensive treatment fields are often used to treat gross disease or at-risk nodal regions in the neck. Large tumor volumes, combined with the flexible neck anatomy, make IGRT alignment challenging. Some centers simply use a rigid alignment technique and ignore daily anatomic deformation due to nonrigid movement (e.g., neck flexion, mandible position). Studies suggest, however, that this is not appropriate.[21] One early study of volumetric imaging for H&N aligned one part of the vertebral anatomy and then measured residual errors in other parts and noted a 2 to 6 mm residual error.[22] Later studies have confirmed this[21] and suggest an approach whereby multiple regions are simultaneously aligned.

A second challenge in H&N is the notable change in tissue volume over the course of treatment. One early study reported that GTVs shrink to roughly half their size over the course of treatment.[23] Lymph nodes and parotid glands also shrink and shift medially. These effects are due to the resolution of tumor, postsurgical changes, and/or weight loss in the patient. If these changes are not accounted for, tumors can be significantly underdosed and normal structures significantly overdosed.[15] The ultimate solution to this issue likely lies in adaptive radiotherapy using deformable image registration, a technique that is in development and represents a future direction for the field.[24]

## LUNG

IGRT of lung tumors is unique in several respects. Tumors are well visualized especially in the peripheral lung, which is not the case in other sites such as liver where fiducial markers are often necessary to localize tumors. Gross tumor can even be visualized on planar radiographs (and/or tomosynthesis), which allows one to perform intrafraction alignment. This is routine on CyberKnife treatments but can also be performed on linear accelerator platforms.

One significant challenge for IGRT in lung is respiratory motion as discussed further in Chapter 19 and AAPM TG-76, The Management of Respiratory Motion in Radiation Oncology report.[25] Motion can be measured at the time of simulation using 4D CT, which allows one to visualize movement and also addresses the various artifacts and systematic offset inherent in "snapshots" taken with standard CT (see AAPM TG-76 section III). 4D CT data can be included in treatment planning to generate an internal target volume (ITV). The data can also be processed to produce a maximum intensity projection (MIP, the maximum in pixels over all respiratory phases) or an average CT (the average in each pixel). Recently 4D CT has also become available on some treatment units, which is useful for confirming alignment and motion.[26] The above techniques are useful mainly for free-breathing treatments, but respiratory motion can be controlled by various means including compression devices, respiratory gating, or breath hold. Whatever the approach, on-treatment IGRT techniques must be consistent with those used at the time of simulation.

Like H&N, another significant challenge in lung IGRT is the resolution of tumors and atelectasis during standard fractionation treatments. Volumes of non-small cell lung cancer tumors shrink by approximately 1% per day,[27-29] and this shrinkage is asymmetric. As with H&N, the ultimate solution to this problem may lie in adaptive radiotherapy.

### FOR THE PHYSICIAN

IGRT plays a central role in modern Radiation Oncology, especially for hypofractionated or stereotactic treatments. IGRT can increase confidence that treatments are targeting the desired site and help decrease treatment volume margins when appropriate. IGRT also underlies the emerging technique of ART, which addresses anatomic changes during treatment by reoptimizing a patient's plan using new imaging information. A wide variety of technology is available for IGRT (Table 18.1), with the goal of improving treatment precision through one or more of the following strategies: online correction (immediately prior to treatment), offline correction (applied prior to the next fraction), or real-time monitoring (during treatment). Benefits of IGRT must be weighed against potential downsides. Online CT systems typically require 2 to 3 extra minutes for image acquisition plus the time for interpretation. They also deliver extra dose, which deserves consideration and can become significant if using IGRT daily for several weeks of treatment. On the technical end, IGRT acquisition protocols can be controlled to some extent to optimize the various dependent variables such as image quality, scan time, and extent of anatomy visualized. These factors often have tradeoffs against each other, and physician guidance is needed to find the optimal scanning protocol (i.e., more images acquired might lead to better resolution but take longer and give more dose to the patient).

Several application case studies are outlined here (Section 18.6) that illustrate the advantages and challenges of IGRT. Large tumor volumes in the head and neck, for example, make IGRT alignment challenging, especially given the flexible anatomy of the neck. In the lung, a major challenge is respiratory motion, and techniques for alignment must take this into account. More generally, normal tissue dose can sometimes be *higher* with IGRT, which is somewhat counterintuitive. An example is the rectum in a prostate cancer treatment. Due to daily setup variations, the rectum is sometimes positioned in a low dose region. If IGRT is used, however, the rectum may be positioned more consistently in the high dose region compared to a case in which no IGRT is used.

The safety and effectiveness of an IGRT program arguably depend at least as much on organizational and management aspects as on the technical and clinical features. Guidelines are available from professional organizations to assist with this, including the importance of training, a multiprofessional team approach, and a structured quality management program.

## References

1. Bujold A, Craig T, Jaffray D, et al. Image-guided radiotherapy: Has it influenced patient outcomes? Semin Radiat Oncol 2012;22:50–61.
2. Jaffray D, Langen KM, Mageras G, et al. Safety considerations for IGRT: Executive summary. Pract Radiat Oncol 2013;3:167–70.
3. de Crevoisier R, Tucker SL, Dong L, et al. Increased risk of biochemical and local failure in patients with distended rectum on the planning CT for prostate cancer radiotherapy. Int J Radiat Oncol Biol Phys 2005;62:965–73.
4. Kupelian PA, Willoughby TR, Reddy CA, et al. Impact of image guidance on outcomes after external beam radiotherapy for localized prostate cancer. Int J Radiat Oncol Biol Phys 2008;70:1146–50.
5. Solberg T, Balter J, Benedict S, et al. Quality and safety considerations in stereotactic radiosurgery and stereotactic body radiotherapy: Executive summary. Pract Radiat Oncol 2012;2:2–9.
6. Fowler J, Chappell R, Ritter M. Is alpha/beta for prostate tumors really low? Int J Radiat Oncol Biol Phys 2001;50:1021–31.
7. Pollack A, Walker G, Horwitz EM, et al. Randomized trial of hypofractionated external-beam radiotherapy for prostate cancer. J Clin Oncol 2013;31:3860–8.
8. Yin F, Wong J. The role of in-room kv x-ray imaging for patient setup and target localization: Report of Task Group 104. College Park, MD: AAPM; 2009.
9. Murphy MJ, Balter J, Balter S, et al. The management of imaging dose during image-guided radiotherapy: Report of the AAPM Task Group 75. Med Phys 2007;34:4041–63.
10. ACR–ASTRO practice guidelines for image-guided radiation therapy (IGRT). Reston, VA: American College of Radiology; 2009.
11. Langen KM, Papanikolaou N, Balog J, et al. QA for helical TomoTherapy: Report of the AAPM Task Group 148. Med Phys 2010;37:4817–53.
12. Heemsbergen WD, Hoogeman MS, Witte MG, et al. Increased risk of biochemical and clinical failure for prostate patients with a large rectum at radiotherapy planning: Results from the Dutch trial of 68 GY versus 78 Gy. Int J Radiat Oncol Biol Phys 2007;67:1418–24.
13. Ghilezan M, Yan D, Martinez A. Adaptive radiation therapy for prostate cancer. Sem Radiat Oncol 2010;20:130–7.
14. Schwartz DL, Garden AS, Thomas J, et al. Adaptive radiotherapy for head-and-neck cancer: Initial clinical outcomes from a prospective trial. Int J Radiat Oncol Biol Phys 2012;83:986–93.

15. Hansen EK, Bucci MK, Quivey JM, et al. Repeat CT imaging and replanning during the course of IMRT for head-and-neck cancer. Int J Radiat Oncol Biol Phys 2006;64:355–62.
16. Molloy JA, Chan G, Markovic A, et al. Quality assurance of US-guided external beam radiotherapy for prostate cancer: Report of AAPM Task Group 154. Med Phys 2011;38:857–71.
17. Susil RC, McNutt TR, DeWeese TL, et al. Effects of prostate-rectum separation on rectal dose from external beam radiotherapy. Int J Radiat Oncol Biol Phys 2010;76:1251–8.
18. Song DY, Herfarth KK, Uhl M, et al. A multi-institutional clinical trial of rectal dose reduction via injected polyethylene-glycol hydrogel during intensity modulated radiation therapy for prostate cancer: Analysis of dosimetric outcomes. Int J Radiat Oncol Biol Phys 2013;87:81–7.
19. Chen L, Paskalev K, Xu X, et al. Rectal dose variation during the course of image-guided radiation therapy of prostate cancer. Radiother Oncol 2010;95:198–202.
20. Engels B, Soete G, Verellen D, et al. Conformal arc radiotherapy for prostate cancer: Increased biochemical failure in patients with distended rectum on the planning computed tomogram despite image guidance by implanted markers. Int J Radiat Oncol Biol Phys 2009;74:388–91.
21. van Kranen S, van Beek S, Rasch C, et al. Setup uncertainties of anatomical sub-regions in head-and-neck cancer patients after offline CBCT guidance. Int J Radiat Oncol Biol Phys 2009;73:1566–73.
22. Zhang LF, Garden AS, Lo J, et al. Multiple regions-of-interest analysis of setup uncertainties for head-and-neck cancer radiotherapy. Int J Radiat Oncol Biol Phys 2006;64:1559–69.
23. Barker JL, Garden AS, Ang KK, et al. Quantification of volumetric and geometric changes occurring during fractionated radiotherapy for head-and-neck cancer using an integrated CT/linear accelerator system. Int J Radiat Oncol Biol Phys 2004;59:960–70.
24. Jaffray DA, Lindsay PE, Brock KK, et al. Accurate accumulation of dose for improved understanding of radiation effects in normal tissue. Int J Radiat Oncol Biol Phys 2010;76:S135–9.
25. Keall PJ, Mageras GS, Balter JM, et al. The management of respiratory motion in Radiation Oncology report of AAPM Task Group 76. Med Phys 2006;33:3874.
26. Sonke JJ, Zijp L, Remeijer P, et al. Respiratory correlated cone beam CT. Med Phys 2005;32:1176–86.
27. Kupelian PA, Ramsey C, Meeks SL, et al. Serial megavoltage CT imaging during external beam radiotherapy for non-small-cell lung cancer: Observations on tumor regression during treatment. Int J Radiat Oncol Biol Phys 2005;63:1024–8.
28. Siker ML, Tome WA, Mehta MP. Tumor volume changes on serial imaging with megavoltage CT for non-small-cell lung cancer during intensity-modulated radiotherapy: How reliable, consistent, and meaningful is the effect? Int J Radiat Oncol Biol Phys 2006;66:135–41.
29. Fox J, Ford E, Redmond K, et al. Quantification of tumor volume changes during radiotherapy for non-small-cell lung cancer. Int J Radiat Oncol Biol Phys 2009;74:341–8.

# CHAPTER 19

# Respiratory Motion Management for External Beam Radiotherapy

## 19.1 Introduction

One of the primary goals in radiation therapy is to maximize the dose to the target while minimizing the dose to healthy tissue. For targets that exhibit significant motion (>5 to 10 mm) during the respiratory cycle this creates a challenge. If a target is 3 cm in diameter (volume = 14.1 $cm^3$) and moves ±10 mm in one direction and ±5 mm in the other directions, the volume encompassing the motion becomes an ellipsoid of about 42 $cm^3$, which would be the volume needed to ensure that the target is covered throughout the respiratory cycle. This means that approximately 28 $cm^3$ of normal tissue (200% of the target volume) is irradiated just to account for the target motion.

The motion of organs and tissue also leads to artifacts during the acquisition of treatment planning images. Respiratory-induced blurring can make the delineation of targets and critical structures difficult. In addition to blurring, the interplay of the respiratory cycle and the temporal aspect of the image acquisition can lead to discontinuities in structures or to a complete failure to detect small tumors. If a simulation computed tomography (CT) with such artifacts is used as a reference image during image-guided radiation therapy (IGRT) treatments, major misalignments can occur.

While the preceding discussion certainly applies to the lung, it must be remembered that other treatment sites are affected as well. The liver is strongly affected by respiratory-induced motion and deformation, especially at the dome of the liver. Other organs in the abdomen have been shown to move substantially with respiration (e.g., approximately 7 mm superior-inferior (SI) excursion of the kidneys in an average patient[1]). This has implications for margins and motion control in sites such as pancreas or Wilms tumor.

Thus the driving forces behind respiratory motion management are to more accurately delineate targets and critical structure and to reduce the volume of normal tissue if possible and thereby reduce complications and/or increase the dose that can be delivered. Therefore methods must be developed to control (or at least account for) respiratory motion. The methods are summarized in Table 19.1.

Each of these methods has strengths and weaknesses and varying degrees of complexity. Regardless of the method selected, there are some common issues.

1. The method must undergo rigorous commissioning and ongoing quality assurance (QA).
2. The respiratory motion must be accounted for during simulation.
3. The planning margins must be identified.
4. The respiratory motion during simulation must accurately reflect the respiratory motion during treatment (e.g., if motion control devices are used these must be identical and have the same settings during treatment).
5. The patient must be able to comply with the motion management strategy.

TABLE 19.1 ■ **Methods to Account for or Control Respiratory Motion**

| Method | Implementations |
| --- | --- |
| Motion encompassing | Slow CT |
|  | Inhale and exhale breath-hold CT |
|  | 4D CT (respiration-correlated CT) |
| Respiratory gating | Respiratory gated simulation and treatment delivery |
| Breath hold | Deep inspiration breath hold |
|  | Assisted breath hold |
|  | Self-held breath hold without respiratory monitoring |
|  | Self-held breath hold with respiratory monitoring |
| Forced shallow breathing | Abdominal compression |
| Respiratory synchronization | Real-time tumor tracking |

6. There may be an additional interplay with respect to intensity-modulated radiation therapy (IMRT) delivery.
7. Motion management will require more resources and may result in longer treatment times.
8. Target and normal tissue motion is not limited to the lung. Abdominal structures are also affected.
9. All imaging modalities are affected by respiratory motion.
10. Tumor motion is not the only source of uncertainty and may not even be the largest.

The American Association of Physicists in Medicine (AAPM) Task Group (TG)-76, The Management of Respiratory Motion in Radiation Oncology, has produced a comprehensive report detailing each of these strategies.[2] The report is freely available on the AAPM website, and the reader is encouraged to obtain it.

## 19.2 Measuring Respiratory Motion

The respiratory cycle is initiated by an inhalation caused by the contraction of the diaphragm and the intercostal muscles, which pull the diaphragm down and the ribs anteriorly and superiorly. This increases the size of the thoracic cavity, drawing air into the lungs. At exhale the muscles relax and the thoracic cavity returns to its pre-inhale position. The motion of the diaphragm causes the abdomen to shift inferiorly and anteriorly. The respiration can be characterized as shallow, normal, or deep. During normal inspiration the lung volume can increase by 10% to 25%.

Respiratory motion can be measured by direct observation of the structure of interest, by the use of an implanted fiducial marker, or by a surrogate structure such as the diaphragm or chest wall. Breathing patterns vary from patient to patient, indicating the need for any motion management strategy to be patient specific. Even for the same patient the cycle can vary during a single session or from day to day. Figure 19.1 shows an example of breathing patterns for one patient over a span of minutes. The patient's breathing is regular in the first session (panel A) but becomes more irregular in the second session (panel B). For some patients, audiovisual feedback and respiratory training can be used to help regularize the breathing cycle. This involves displaying the detected respiratory cycle to the patient as the patient breathes, along with visual cues as to the desired amplitudes to "train" the patient to breathe in a regular pattern.

Many imaging modalities have been used to measure organ motion during the respiratory cycle. Table 1 in AAPM TG-76 gives modality-specific references for various organs circa 2006. Table 2 in AAPM TG-76 is a sample of observed motion in the lung from various publications which is adapted and shown in Table 19.2. Most of the studies quoted involved from 10 to 30

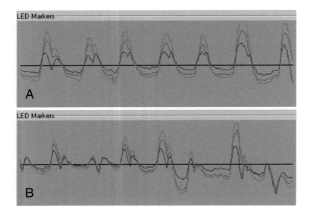

**Figure 19.1** Variation in respiratory cycle for a single patient taken during two different sessions. Each color represents one of the three external markers used.

TABLE 19.2 ▒ **Lung Tumor Motion Data from AAPM TG-76**

| Lobe | SI | AP | LR | TG-76 ref |
|---|---|---|---|---|
| Lower | 18.5 (9-32) | | | 85 |
| | (2-9) | | | 28 |
| | | 1 (0-4) | 10.5 (0-13) | 76 |
| | 9.5 (4.5-16.4) | 6.1 (2.5-9.8) | 6.0 (2.9-9.8) | 220 |
| Middle | | 0 | 9 (0-16) | 76 |
| | 7.2 (4.3-10.2) | 4.3 (1.9-7.5) | 4.3 (1.5-7.1) | 220 |
| Middle/upper | 7.5 (2-11) | | | 85 |
| | (2-6) | | | 28 |
| Upper | | 1 (0-5) | 1 (0-3) | 76 |
| | 4.3 (2.6-7.1) | 2.8 (1.2-5.1) | 3.4 (1.3-5.3) | 220 |
| Not specified | (0-50) | | | 84 |
| | 3.9 (0-12) | 2.4 (0-5) | 2.4 (0-5) | 26 |
| | 12.5 (6-34) | 9.4 (5-22) | 7.3 (3-12) | 101 |
| | (2-30) | (0-10) | (0-6) | 91 |
| | 12 (1-20) | 5 (0-13) | 1 (0-1) | 77 |
| | 7 (2-15) | | | 87 |
| | 5.8 (0-25) | 2.5 (0-8) | 1.5 (0-3) | 67 |
| | | 6.4 (2-24) | | 52 |
| | (0-13) | (0-5) | (0-4) | 92 |
| | 4.5 (0-22) | | | 66 |
| Maximum all (including not specified) | 50 | 24 | 16 | |
| Maximum lower | 32 | 9.8 | 13 | |
| Maximum middle | 10.2 | 7.5 | 16 | |
| Maximum upper | 7.1 | 5.1 | 5.3 | |

Mean range of motion and the (minimum-maximum) ranges in mm for the three dimensions. SI: superior-inferior; AP: anterior-posterior; LR: left-right.

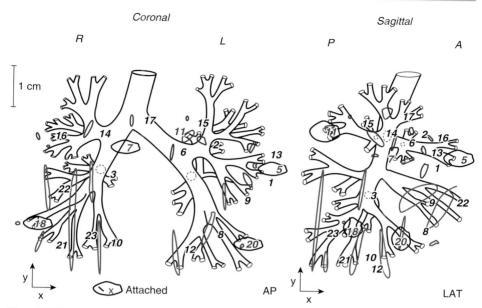

**Figure 19.2** Variation of tumor trajectory during inhale and exhale, hysteresis. Each number indicates different patient studied. (Reproduced from: Seppenwoolde Y, Shirato H, Kitamura K, et al., Precise and real-time measurement of 3D tumor motion in lung due to breathing and heartbeat, measured during radiotherapy. Int J Radiat Oncol Biol Phys 2002;53:822-834, with permission from Elsevier.)

patients. Though the data are representative and were not intended to be exhaustive, several trends are observed. First, the range of motion can be quite large (up to 50 mm in some patients). Second, the maximum range depends on the lobe in the lung, with the lower lobe showing the largest range and the upper lobe the smallest. This intuitively makes sense because the lower lobe is bounded by the diaphragm inferiorly. Third, the SI direction shows the greatest range, followed by the anterior-posterior (AP) direction and then the left-right (LR) direction.

Many studies demonstrated hysteresis in the tumor trajectories. This means that the trajectory during inhalation is different from the trajectory during exhalation and that the maximum range of motion may not be demonstrated at full inhalation. Figure 19.2 shows an example of this. This will have an impact on the motion management strategies discussed in subsequent sections of this chapter.

AAPM TG-76 states that in general abdominal organ motion is in the SI direction with no more than 2 mm range in the AP and LR directions, though this was based on early 4D CT data and is probably not correct (see reference 1). They do qualify that in some individuals the kidneys may display more complex motions.

## 19.3 Tracking the Respiratory Cycle Through Anatomic Surrogates

With most current technology, it is not possible to directly visualize tumor motion or respiratory motion during the course of treatment (or even during a simulation scan). For this reason it has been important to establish anatomic surrogates to serve as a means of tracking the respiratory cycle. These include the chest wall and abdominal displacement as observed by the change in the patient's external contour. This is achieved by placing a marker on the patient surface and tracking with a camera (infrared or visible light), a pressure-sensitive belt placed around the

TABLE 19.3 ▪ **Respiratory Cycle Tracking Solutions**

| Method | Product, Vendor |
|---|---|
| Infrared marker tracking; marker placed on abdomen just below xiphoid process | RPM, Varian |
| Pressure belt | Anzai belt, Philips |
| 3D surface mapping with stereo cameras | Gate-RT, Vision RT |
| 3D surface mapping with swept laser | Sentinel, C-Rad |
| Spirometry | SDX, Dyn'R |
| Diaphragm detection on planar images | 4D CBCT "Symmetry," Elekta Inc. |

patient's abdomen, or direct capture and tracking of the patient surface (stereo cameras or lasers). In addition, spirometry and detection of the diaphragm have been used. Table 19.3 shows some of the available technology used to track the respiratory cycle.

With any of these methods it cannot be assumed that there is a direct coupling of the motion of the surrogate anatomy with the tumor itself or that they are in phase with each other. AAPM TG-76 describes many studies in which the phase offset was in the range of 0.5 to 1 second. Furthermore, the phase offset between the surrogate and the tumor itself has been shown to change over the course of treatment.[3] Therefore the use of any surrogate will introduce uncertainty.

## 19.4 Motion Encompassing

As shown in Table 19.1, there are several ways to visualize the extent of motion and thereby delineate a volume that encompasses the extent of the motion. Each of these will be discussed in the following sections.

### SLOW CT

This method involves running the CT scanner at a slow revolution rate or acquiring multiple scans and averaging them. Either way should allow for the collection of data for several respiratory cycles (around 5 seconds), throughout the imaging volume. The result is in essence a time-averaged blurring of the data. Therefore the entire range of motion is encompassed in the scan. Slow CT has the advantage that it represents an average state for the patient and is therefore well suited for accurate dose calculation. Slow CT has the disadvantage of blurry images that are often difficult to visualize for delineation. An average intensity projection scan can also be created by combining different respiratory phases of a 4D CT scan (below).

### 4D CT/RESPIRATORY-CORRELATED CT

4D CT (or respiration-correlated CT) is a key tool in the measurement and management of respiratory motion. It provides a phase-resolved visualization of tissue motion in 3D, essentially a 3D "movie." The first paper describing the technique was published in 2003,[4] and vendor adoption was rapid. The technology is now widely available.

To acquire 4D image data sets, knowledge of the point in the respiratory cycle for each projection is required. For this purpose a respiratory trace is acquired (either via a belt or an infrared (IR) marker place on the thorax) during the time when the CT data are acquired. Respiratory sorting is then done retrospectively (correlating each projection with a point in the respiratory cycle) or prospectively (acquiring projections at a defined point in the respiratory cycle). When

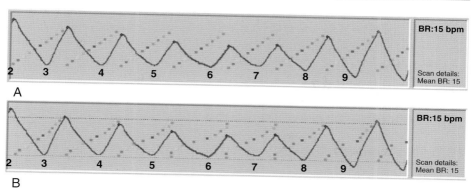

**Figure 19.3** Amplitude- vs. phase-based respiratory cycle binning. *(From Li et al., Clinical evaluations of a novel amplitude-based binning algorithm for 4DCT reconstruction in radiation therapy. Med Phys 2012;39(2):922-932.)*

acquiring a retrospective 4D data set, the respiratory cycle is split into bins, usually 10 bins per breathing cycle, and the slices are sorted by bin. Each bin is then reconstructed into a 3D data set. The 4D motion can then be observed by looping through the 3D images for each bin. In this way the entire range of motion can be visualized. Since there are approximately ten 3D data sets, the labor required to contour would increase by a factor of 10. Vendors have developed algorithms to propagate contours drawn on one set to the rest of the sets to alleviate this situation. Once the automated contours are created they should be reviewed to determine their accuracy. One advantage of 4D CT over slow CT, mentioned above, is that the image in each respiratory bin is quite sharp. There is, however, typically more noise in 4D CT images versus a standard helical scan because vendor protocols typically reduce the mA in 4D CT scans in order to limit the dose.

There is ongoing debate as to how to determine the respiratory bins. This can be done by the phase or by the amplitude. In phase-based binning the bins are determined by their temporal relationship to the cycle, whereas in amplitude-based binning the bins are determined by the fraction of maximum amplitude. Figure 19.3 demonstrates the difference between the two methods. Each method has advantages, although some studies suggest that amplitude-based binning produces fewer or a comparable amount of image artifacts compared to phase-based binning. The algorithm is based on observing if there are irregularities in the amplitude and/or the pattern of the respiratory cycle and then determining the best method based on the combination of the irregularities.[5,6]

4D images can also be acquired with cone beam CT (CBCT), positron emission tomography (PET), and magnetic resonance (MR) imaging techniques using similar methods. In current technologies, 4D CBCT is acquired by automatically detecting the position of the diaphragm in the planar images acquired during CBCT acquisition.

## 19.5 Limiting Respiratory Motion

Forced shallow breathing techniques are designed to limit the diaphragm motion by applying a reproducible pressure on the abdomen. Originally this was accomplished using the body frame system that incorporated an abdominal compression plate.[7] Another system is the Body Fix system, which employs a body length vacuum cushion and the pressure plate with a vacuum-sealed thin plastic sheet.[8] The vacuum-sealed sheet is designed to hold the patient in place while applying uniform pressure over the abdomen and thorax. This may limit respiratory motion.

Other methods involve the use of Velcro belts that are wrapped to a consistent length around the patient's abdomen.[9] Pressure is then applied using an air-filled bladder as used in a blood pressure cuff. The pressure in the bladder is monitored during treatment to ensure that there is not a leak in the system. With any of these methods, a trial and error process is employed as the pressure is increased until the motion is reduced to desirable ranges, typically 5 to 10 mm. Maintaining patient comfort is important. If the pressure is increased too much the motion may actually increase due to patient discomfort. One issue to consider is whether the treatment beams will pass through the devices used to limit respiration.

## 19.6 Respiratory Gating

Respiratory gating involves the image acquisition for planning and "gating" the beam (i.e., turning it on and off) during delivery only at a specified segment of the respiratory cycle. For both imaging and treatment the patient breathes normally, which is a major advantage of this approach (nearly all patients are suitable candidates). The images are acquired using the prospective method described in Section 19.4. The position and width of the segment of the respiratory cycle to be used, called the gate, are determined by observing the amount of motion and restricting it to below a specified limit during the gate, typically 5 mm. This can be done using fluoroscopy or a full 4D CT scan. The percentage of time that the respiratory signal is within the gate is called the duty cycle and is usually about 30% when gating on the end-expiration portion of the breathing cycle. This means that gated treatment beam delivery times are typically at least 3 times longer than conventional treatments. The advantage of this method is that it allows for smaller treatment volumes since the treatment is only delivered over a limited range of the tumor motion.

It must be noted that respiratory gating uses a surrogate anatomic marker to track the respiratory cycle (e.g., a marker block on the abdomen). For gating to be accurate, the relative phase between the position of this surrogate and the tumor must remain constant over time. Recent studies, however, have shown that this is not the case, which probably explains some of the variability observed in early experiences with respiratory gating (e.g., large interfraction variability in the position of the diaphragm even when the same gating window was used). These and other considerations have led some centers to discontinue the use of gating.

## 19.7 Breath-Hold Techniques

Breath-hold techniques allow one to essentially "freeze" the motion of a tumor during the time a beam is on. In the case of the lung, they also provide a dosimetric advantage if full inspiration is used because more normal lung is expanded away from the high dose region. However, performing breath holds is a complex process that many patients find difficult to comply with, either for social or language issues or for medical reasons, especially in the case of patients with lung cancer. It is ideal to evaluate patients for possible breath-hold techniques well prior to simulation. The exact equipment and technique used at simulation must also be used during treatment. Audiovisual (AV) feedback has become quite common. Older techniques use video goggles. When the VisionRT is available, a popular method is to use a Kindle or iPad in the room so the patient can see where his or her ideal breath-hold position is. Some centers have also begun to explore the use of a combination breath-hold/gating approach where the patient executes breath holds that conform to a gating window. There are, however, many challenges with this approach that are not yet fully explored.

### DEEP INSPIRATION BREATH HOLD

This technique is used to change the internal anatomy so that optimal organ at risk (OAR) sparing can be achieved, most commonly for left-sided breast cancers. The deep inspiration causes less lung and heart tissue to be irradiated. The lung volume and positioning are reproducible because the patient is driven to a nearly maximal lung tidal volume with each breath hold. It requires a compliant patient who can actively participate in the process. It is helpful to provide AV feedback in these cases so that the patient can more reproducibly achieve the proper level of inspiration. Several studies have found 3D surface mapping solutions such as Align RT (Vision RT) to be superior methods for monitoring the level of inspiration.[10,11]

## ASSISTED BREATH HOLD

This method was developed at William Beaumont Hospital and is now marketed as Active Breathing Control (ABC) by Elekta. The device consists of a digital spirometer that is used to measure the respiratory volume. A balloon valve is also present in the airway. The valve can be closed to suspend the breathing at a particular point in the respiratory cycle, effectively forcing a breath hold. There must be a proper seal on the mouthpiece and a nasal clip to prevent air leakage during the breath hold. There are mixed data as to how this system performs relative to voluntary breath-hold techniques. One randomized study showed insignificant differences but included only a limited number of patients (23).[12]

## SELF-HELD BREATH HOLD

As the name implies, self-held breath hold involves voluntary breath hold by the patient. This technique faces many challenges in terms of reproducibility and other factors, but it is mentioned in AAPM TG-76 and so is included here.

According to AAPM TG-76, the self-held breath-hold technique can be used with or without respiratory monitoring. If done without monitoring, the patient is asked to hold the breath at a consistent point in the respiratory cycle. At that point the patient depresses a switch that deactivates an interlock, allowing the therapist to turn on the beam. Just before releasing the breath the patient releases the switch, activating the interlock and turning off the beam. This method requires a very compliant patient who can actively participate in the treatment delivery. This is extremely important. The patient dependency makes this a less than optimal solution. Varian currently offers an interface to C-series and above linacs to implement this technique. Elekta also offers a gating interface called "Response," which can accomplish some of these goals. Alternatively, the breathing can be monitored automatically using external marker systems or 3D surface mapping systems. These can be interfaced directly to the linacs, automating the beam on/off process. For either method deep inspiration is usually chosen to utilize dosimetric advantages like those described in Section 19.6. The use of a high dose rate on the linac makes these methods easier to deliver. A typical patient can hold his or her breath for 10 to 15 seconds. At 600 monitor units (MU)/min, 100 MU can be delivered in 10 seconds. At 400 MU/min it would take 15 seconds to deliver the same 100 MU. A full delivery of the treatment can be done in 1 to 2 breaths for fixed gantry angle beams, making this method reasonably efficient.

# 19.8 Respiratory Motion and Treatment Planning

## TARGET VOLUMES

When using motion encompassing techniques, a 4D CT dataset is used to generate an internal target volume (ITV). For SBRT the ITV is usually defined as the maximum range of motion volume plus 5 mm.[13]

Several derived data sets can be obtained from the 4D data. One is called the maximum intensity projection (MIP). This involves reporting the maximum intensity across all bins for each voxel to create a single 3D data set. In theory this should then delineate the full range of motion as the higher density tumor intensity values are painted throughout the respiratory cycle. Bradley et al. have shown this to be a superior method in determining the extent of motion.[14] Another, nominally equivalent method is to register all phases of the 4D data set in the planning system and use these to contour the maximal extent of excursion.

The average intensity projection (AIP) is simply an average intensity for each voxel across each bin. A slow CT closely approximates the AIP. Both of these are closer to reality in terms of treatment delivery and are the preferred data sets to be used for dose calculation.[15,16] They are also more representative of the (slow) CBCT that will be acquired during IGRT on a linac. This may aid in alignment accuracy. The MIP should not be used for dose calculation because it distorts the inhomogeneity in the body.

The minimum intensity projection (MinIP) is the inverse of the MIP. It may be useful in determining the extent of motion for targets outside the lung such as liver.[17]

## IMRT

There have been many studies evaluating the possible interplay of IMRT deliveries and respiratory motion.[18-24] The dynamic motion of the multi-leaf collimator (MLC) leaves creates gradients inside the target volume. The interplay of the motion of the leaves with the motion of the tumor may create hot or cold spots. Despite this concern, many studies have shown that the dose errors introduced by the MLC/target motion interplay will average out over a course of delivery.[18,21,25] AAPM TG-76 cautions against using IMRT for targets subject to respiratory motion, particularly in few fraction treatments such as SBRT.

# 19.9 Imaging and Tracking During Treatment

The ideal method to deliver treatments to targets that move during the respiratory cycle would be to track the motion in real time. This allows for greater treatment volume reduction as in gating but without the efficiency loss required by the duty cycle. The CyberKnife system was the first to accomplish this goal.[26] The system uses cross-firing fluoroscopic imagers to detect the tumor position in near real time (approximately one image per second). The linac is mounted to a robotic arm that can move in synchronization with the tumor. A key component of the system is the ability to predict future motion by some small amount of time because of the relatively coarse time sampling of the images and because there is a delay time from the detection of the tumor position to the moment when the beam turns on. Initially the tumor position was detected using an implanted fiducial, but recently a method to detect the tumor position without fiducials has been introduced.[27] A vest with markers is used to establish a real-time surrogate for model tracking.

The use of conventional linacs to track tumor motion by adjusting the MLC shape has also been investigated.[28] Systems such as Calypso can be used for real-time tracking but require an implanted fiducial. Calypso tracks the position of an electromagnetic beacon in 3D. While Calypso is most widely used for the prostate, studies are under way to implement this technique in the lung.[29] Recently the Vero system has been introduced with real-time tracking capability.[30] Finally, the emerging MR-enabled treatment units (e.g., ViewRay Inc.) provide real-time MRI imaging during treatment. This provides visualization without the need for implanted fiducials.

# 19.10 Quality Assurance

## 4D IMAGING

A phantom capable of reproducing realistic breathing motion is needed. An object of known size and shape is imaged without motion as a baseline. 4D images are then acquired for a range of breathing patterns. The congruence of the reconstructed object to the baseline images can then be checked. The agreement should be within a few millimeters and should be consistent with departmental margins.

## GATING

Specialized phantoms are needed to test the accuracy of gated treatments. AAPM TG-76 lists the desired characteristics of a phantom.

1. The phantom should be able to reproduce cyclical and random motions found in human respiration.
2. The gating feedback mechanism must be able to detect the phantom motion.
3. The phantom should be constructed of low density materials for CT and x-ray compatibility.
4. The device should be large enough to accommodate detectors such as ion chambers and diodes.
5. The phantom should be reliable and cost effective.

Phantoms are available from CIRS, Modus Medical, and Sun Nuclear, among others.

## BREATH-HOLD METHODS

Patient selection is one key to achieving reproducible results with breath-hold techniques. The patient must be compliant and able to actively participate in the process. Test runs, AV feedback, and training can improve patient consistency. There can be changes in the respiratory pattern over the course of treatment, including changes in patient condition and increased familiarity with the system. The consistency of the respiratory cycle should be monitored throughout the course of treatment.

## RESPIRATORY SYNCHRONIZATION METHODS

These methods are largely still under development, and the QA is not well described. AAPM TG-264, Safe Clinical Implementation of MLC Tracking in Radiotherapy, is in progress. End-to-end testing with specialized phantoms as described in the section on gating would be a useful approach. The addition of film dosimetry capability to confirm dose coverage should be considered.

## EQUIPMENT-RELATED QA

Beam on/off techniques should be tested for operation and for the impact of dose delivery. For example, is the same dose delivered for 100 MU uninterrupted versus 10 MU with several on/off cycles?

Spirometers should be tested for accurate air volume measurements by using syringes of known volume to inject air through the spirometer and to draw air out.

Any machine interlocks and interfaces should be tested for proper operation.

## FOR THE PHYSICIAN

With advances in radiation treatment technology, it is now possible to assess and manage respiratory motion as part of the treatment process. With proper use of this technology, one can potentially reduce treatment margins, minimize toxicity, and potentially escalate target dose. Multiple methods exist to assess respiratory motion, as well as manage motion if needed, such as slow CT, 4D CT, abdominal compression, gating, and breath hold (self or assisted). Each method has strengths and weaknesses, many of which are outlined in the AAPM TG-76 document. Regardless of the method employed, some key concepts include patient tolerance of management method, reproducibility of motion between simulation and each treatment session, treatment delivery times, motion of both tumor and normal tissues, complexity of use, and need for ongoing QA to ensure system function.

Because it is often not feasible to directly visualize motion during treatment, anatomic surrogates are used to track the respiratory cycle, such as infrared markers on the abdomen, pressure belts, or spirometry. However, it is important to note that there may not be perfect concordance between motion of the surrogate and tumor motion, and there can be phase offsets, which can also change over time. Some systems such as CyberKnife and Calypso have the ability to track tumor motion in real time/near real time, and other systems are under development. The various advantages and disadvantages of each system are detailed in this chapter.

Various strategies are available for generating the target volume, including using a MIP scan versus contouring on each phase of the respiratory cycle. However, for treatment planning, AIP is the recommended image set over the MIP because it more accurately represents reality during treatment delivery. There have been concerns over dose errors with the use of IMRT with dynamic MLC leaves on tumors with respiratory motion, but most studies have shown that this will be averaged out over a treatment course and is not clinically significant.

Given the complexity of respiratory motion management and assessment technology, proper QA is needed to ensure treatment safety. A phantom capable of reproducing realistic breathing motion is needed to assess the imaging technology and method of reconstruction. If performing gated treatments, further specialized phantoms capable of accommodating detectors and testing with the gating feedback mechanism are needed.

## References

1. Goldstein SD, Ford EC, Duhon M, et al. Use of respiratory-correlated four-dimensional computed tomography to determine acceptable treatment margins for locally advanced pancreatic adenocarcinoma. Int J Radiat Oncol Biol Phys 2010;76(2):597–602.
2. Keall PJ, Mageras GS, Balter JM, et al. The management of respiratory motion in Radiation Oncology report of AAPM Task Group 76. Med Phys 2006;33(10):3874–900.
3. Redmond KF, Song DY, Fox JL, et al. Respiratory motion changes of lung tumors over the course of radiation therapy based on respiration-correlated four-dimensional computed tomography scans. Int J Radiat Oncol Biol Phys 2009;75(5):1605–12.
4. Ford EC, Mageras GS, Yorke E, et al. Respiration-correlated spiral CT: A method of measuring respiratory-induced anatomic motion for radiation treatment planning. Med Phys 2003;30(1):88–97.
5. Olsen JR, Lu W, Hubenschmidt JP, et al. Effect of novel amplitude/phase binning algorithm on commercial four-dimensional computed tomography quality. Int J Radiat Oncol Biol Phys 2008;70(1): 243–52.
6. Li H, Noel C, Garcia-Ramirez J, et al. Clinical evaluations of an amplitude-based binning algorithm for 4DCT reconstruction in radiation therapy. Med Phys 2012;39(2):922–32.
7. Negoro Y, Nagata Y, Aoki T, et al. The effectiveness of an immobilization device in conformal radiotherapy for lung tumor: Reduction of respiratory tumor movement and evaluation of the daily setup accuracy. Int J Radiat Oncol Biol Phys 2001;50(4):889–98.
8. Han K, Cheung P, Basran PS, et al. A comparison of two immobilization systems for stereotactic body radiation therapy of lung tumors. Radiother Oncol 2010;95(1):103–8.

9. Lovelock DM, Zatcky J, Goodman K, et al. The effectiveness of a pneumatic compression belt in reducing respiratory motion of abdominal tumors in patients undergoing stereotactic body radiotherapy. Technol Cancer Res Treat 2014;13(3):259–67.

10. Tang X, Zagar TM, Bair E, et al. Clinical experience with 3-dimensional surface matching-based deep inspiration breath hold for left-sided breast cancer radiation therapy. Prac Radiat Oncol 2014;4(3): e151–8.

11. Rong Y, Walston S, Welliver MX, et al. Improving intra-fractional target position accuracy using a 3D surface surrogate for left breast irradiation using respiratory-gated deep-inspiration breath-hold technique. PLoS ONE 2014;9(5):e97933.

12. Bartlett F, Colgan R, McNair H, et al. The UK HeartSpare Study: Randomised evaluation of voluntary deep-inspiratory breath-hold in women undergoing breast radiotherapy. Radiother Oncol 2013;108(2): 242–7.

13. deKoste JR, Lagerwaard FJ, de Boer HC, et al. Are multiple CT scans required for planning curative radiotherapy in lung tumors of the lower lobe? Int J Radiat Oncol Biol Phys 2002;53(5):1211–15.

14. Bradley JD, Nofal AN, El Naqa IM, et al. Comparison of helical, maximum intensity projection (MIP), and averaged intensity (AI) 4D CT imaging for stereotactic body radiation therapy (SBRT) planning in lung cancer. Radiother Oncol 2006;81(3):264–8. [Epub 2006 Nov 20].

15. Tian Y, Wang Z, Ge H, et al. Dosimetric comparison of treatment plans based on free breathing, maximum, and average intensity projection CTs for lung cancer SBRT. Med Phys 2012;39(5): 2754–60.

16. Glide-Hurst CK, Hugo GD, Liang J, et al. A simplified method of four-dimensional dose accumulation using the mean intensity projection. Med Phys 2008;35(12):5269–77.

17. Liu J, Wang J-Z, Zhao J-D, et al. Use of combined maximum and minimum intensity projections to determine internal target volume in 4-dimensional CT scans for hepatic malignancies. Radiat Oncol 2012;7:11.

18. Yu CX, Jaffray DA, Wong JW. The effects of intra-fraction organ motion on the delivery of dynamic intensity modulation. Phys Med Biol 1998;43(1):91–104.

19. Kissick MW, Boswell SA, Jeraj R, et al. Confirmation, refinement, and extension of a study in intrafraction motion interplay with sliding jaw motion. Med Phys 2005;32(7):2346–50.

20. Pemler P, Besserer J, Lombriser N, et al. Influence of respiration-induced organ motion on dose distributions in treatments using enhanced dynamic wedges. Med Phys 2001;28(11):2234–40.

21. Bortfeld T, Jokivarsi K, Goitein M, et al. Effects of intra-fraction motion on IMRT dose delivery: Statistical analysis and simulation. Phys Med Biol 2002;47(13):2203–20.

22. Kubo HD, Wang L. Compatibility of Varian 2100C gated operations with enhanced dynamic wedge and IMRT dose delivery. Med Phys 2000;27(8):1732–8.

23. Keall PJ, Kini VI, Vedam SS, et al. Motion adaptive x-ray therapy: A feasibility study. Phys Med Biol 2001;46(1):1–10.

24. Van Dyk J, Barnett RB, Cygler JE, et al. Commissioning and quality assurance of treatment planning computers. Int J Radiat Oncol Biol Phys 1993;26(2):261–73.

25. George R, Keall PJ, Kini VR, et al. Quantifying the effect of intrafraction motion during breast IMRT planning and dose delivery. Med Phys 2003;30(4):552–62.

26. Brown WT, Wu X, Amendola B, et al. Treatment of early non-small cell lung cancer, stage IA, by image-guided robotic stereotactic radioablation—CyberKnife. Cancer J 2007;13(2):87–94.

27. Bibault JE, Prevost B, Dansin E, et al. Image-guided robotic stereotactic radiation therapy with fiducial-free tumor tracking for lung cancer. Radiat Oncol 2012;24(7):102.

28. Ge Y, O'Brien RT, Shieh CC, et al. Toward the development of intrafraction tumor deformation tracking using a dynamic multi-leaf collimator. Med Phys 2014;41(6):061703.

29. Wu J, Ruan D, Cho B, et al. Electromagnetic detection and real-time DMLC adaptation to target rotation during radiotherapy. Int J Radiat Oncol Biol Phys 2012;82(3):e545–53.

30. Depuydt T, Poeis K, Verellen D, et al. Treating patients with real-time tumor tracking using the Vero gimbaled linac system: Implementation and first review. Radiother Oncol 2014;112(3):343–51.

# CHAPTER 20

# Intracavitary Brachytherapy

## 20.1 Introduction

Intracavitary brachytherapy can be performed using low dose rate (LDR), pulsed dose rate (PDR), or high dose rate (HDR) sources. LDR implants expose the patient care team to more radiation than HDR and require longer hospitalization of the patient and more resources dedicated to source storage and radiation safety measures. There is also an increased risk of error, for example, by selecting the incorrect source strength when retrieving source capsules from storage or implanting sources in the incorrect order. For these reasons, intracavitary brachytherapy has largely moved to HDR delivery using remote afterloaders.

The main issue in converting from LDR to HDR was in establishing equivalent dose fractionation regimens. LDR had a long clinical history with well-established dose fractionation, survival rates, and complication rates. Theoretically, HDR has a lower therapeutic ratio than LDR because of the short duration of the treatments. HDR with computerized treatment planning has the ability to optimize the dose to targets and critical structures, which can overcome this deficit. In fact, studies have shown the equivalence of LDR and HDR.[1]

In evaluating HDR treatments it is sometimes useful to convert to radiobiologically equivalent doses (most commonly the $EQD_2$, or equivalent dose in 2 Gy fractions), though it is important to remember the caveats and assumptions that come with such model-based conversions. Numerous biologically equivalent dose (BED) calculators are available online and as apps; the American Brachytherapy Society (ABS) provides Excel worksheets to convert HDR doses to 2 Gy equivalent doses (http://www.americanbrachytherapy.org/guidelines/index.cfm). These worksheets should be used with caution and can support, but not supplant, careful clinical assessment.

## 20.2 Intracavitary Treatment Sites

Intracavitary brachytherapy takes advantage of anatomic pathways to place radioactive sources directly adjacent to tumor sites. This is less invasive than interstitial implants and can in many cases be done without general anesthesia.

Standard gynecological (gyn) applicators are made from surgical steel with plastics used for the build-up caps and vaginal cylinder segments. Magnetic resonance imaging (MRI)-compatible applicators replace surgical steel with either titanium or carbon fiber; neither of these materials has the same mechanical strength as surgical steel, and therefore they require extra care in handling during sterilization and the procedure.

### GYNECOLOGICAL SITES

#### Endometrial

One common application of intracavitary brachytherapy is the treatment of endometrial cancers. Figure 20.1 shows the anatomy for reference. The ABS consensus guidelines for adjuvant vaginal

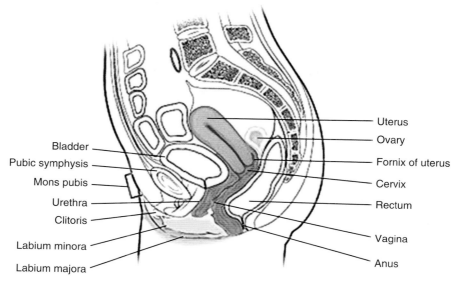

Bladder

Pubic symphysis

Mons pubis

Urethra

Clitoris

Labium minora

Labium majora

Uterus

Ovary

Fornix of uterus

Cervix

Rectum

Vagina

Anus

Human female reproductive system: lateral view

A

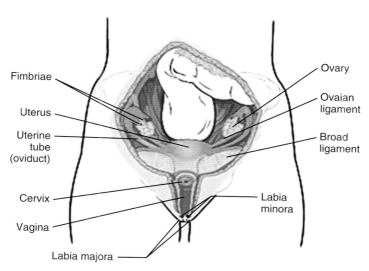

Fimbriae

Uterus

Uterine
tube
(oviduct)

Cervix

Vagina

Ovary

Ovaian
ligament

Broad
ligament

Labia
minora

Labia majora

Human female reproductive system: anterior view

B

**Figure 20.1** Anatomy of the vagina, cervix, and uterus. *(http://en.wikipedia.org/wiki/Uterus).*

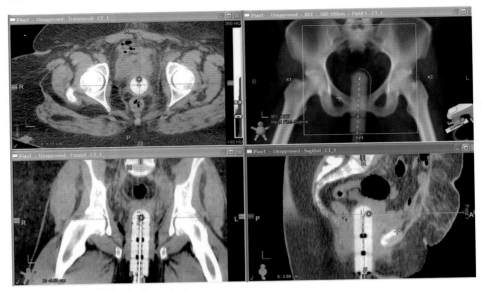

**Figure 20.2** Typical HDR cylinder implant.

cuff brachytherapy after hysterectomy[2] contains the most recent society recommendations on this procedure. According to National Comprehensive Cancer Network (NCCN) guidelines, for Stage I patients with no adverse risk factors brachytherapy can be the sole adjuvant therapy after surgery. For Stage I patients with adverse risk factors and Stage II patients, pelvic external beam therapy of 4500 to 5000 cGy is given in addition to brachytherapy. After surgical removal of the uterus, the standard applicator is a segmented cylinder with one central catheter. A standard cylinder set consists of cylinders of different diameters (2 cm to 4 cm) with several segments each and one or two types of cylinder end caps. The physician chooses the appropriate cylinder based on the patient anatomy; the goal is to use the cylinder shape that minimizes any air gaps between cylinder and tissue. In practice the largest diameter cylinder that is comfortable for the patient is used. This has the added benefit of reducing the rate of dose fall-off due to the inverse square law. Figure 20.2 shows a typical cylinder implant. A variation of the standard cylinder is the shielded cylinder, in which tungsten shielding segments of 90°, 180°, and 270° can be inserted. Shielded cylinders have the disadvantage that the CT simulation image for treatment planning cannot be taken with the shields in place because of the large artifacts the shielding would cause. Some shielded applicators have removable shields so that they can be placed after imaging. A solution to the imaging challenges that come with shielded cylinders, the Miami applicator was designed to allow for noncylindrical dose distribution without the use of metal shielding. Its design is similar to a cylinder, but in addition to the central channel, six peripheral channels allow for customization of the dose distribution. Most cylinder and Miami applicator designs allow for the central channel to be replaced with a tandem to treat patients who were medically inoperable and in whom the uterus was not removed. Figure 20.3 shows typical cylinder applicators. A tandem and ovoid applicator can also be used for these patients as described in Section 2.1. More recently, 3D printing technology has been used to custom-print cylinder applicators,[3] and an inflatable vaginal cylinder has been introduced.[4]

## Cervix

The ABS consensus guidelines for locally advanced carcinoma of the cervix, Part I General[5] and Part II HDR,[1] cover pretreatment evaluation, treatment, and dosimetric issues for locally advanced

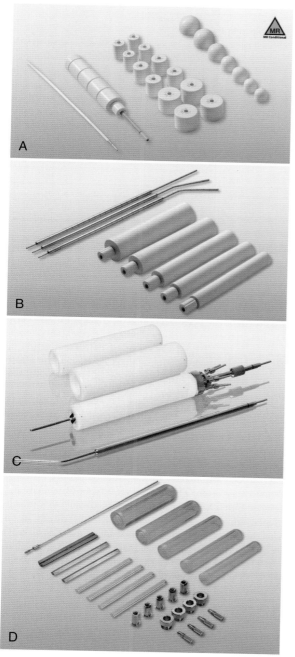

**Figure 20.3 A,** Segmented cylinder applicator set (Varian Medical Systems). **B,** Cervix applicator set (Varian Medical Systems). **C,** Miami-style applicator set (Varian Medical Systems). **D,** Shielded applicator set (Varian Medical Systems).

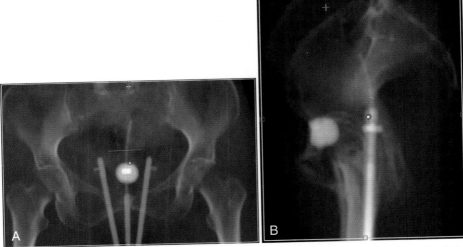

**Figure 20.4** **A,** AP image of a tandem and ovoid implant. **B,** Lateral image of a tandem and ovoid implant.

cervical cancer. The guidelines also recommend adoption of the Groupe Europeen Curietherapie-European Society of Therapeutic Radiation Oncology (GEC-ESTRO) guidelines for contouring, image-based treatment planning, and dose reporting (see Section 20.3). Except for very early stage endometrial cancer (FIGO IA-IB1), brachytherapy is delivered either directly after external beam radiotherapy (EBRT) or in conjunction with EBRT (4 fractions of EBRT/1 fraction of brachytherapy per week). The external beam dose is usually around 4500 cGy, whereas the HDR dose is typically 550 cGy to 600 cGy for five fractions. The total treatment duration should not exceed 8 weeks, including brachytherapy.

For the treatment of cervical cancer, the classic intracavitary applicator is the tandem and ovoid (T&O). The tandem is inserted through the cervical os into the uterus. The two ovoids (or colpostats) are placed laterally in the vaginal fornices. Figure 20.4 shows a typical T&O implant. T&O applicator sets come with an assortment of tandems of varying length and bend angles of 30°, 45°, and 60°. Ovoid caps, whose purpose is to remove cervical tissue from the very high dose area, come in different diameters to be customizable to the patient anatomy. Shielded ovoid caps are also available but are not used very often. There are several types of tandem and ovoid applicators. The Fletcher and Fletcher-Suit-Delclos ovoids orient the dwells in a mostly anterior/posterior direction. The Henschke and Manchester ovoids orient the dwells in an inferior/superior direction. A variation of the T&O applicator is the tandem and ring (T&R) applicator, in which the ovoids are replaced by a ring. Figure 20.5 shows typical applicators. The ring is also capped, similar to the ovoids. The advantage of the ring is that it is easier to place, especially for patients with a shallow cervical os. For unilaterally bulky tumors, it is more challenging to get a good ring placement, and a (slightly asymmetric) T&O might be the better choice. For bulky disease, T&O/T&R applicators are sometimes complemented by adding two to three interstitial needles using free-hand (no template) needle placements. Combination T&O/T&R applicators with a limited number of interstitial needles built into the applicator are also available. T&O/T&R applicators also have a rectal retractor, which is used to increase the distance between the implant and the rectum. The space between the rectal retractor and the applicator is packed with wet gauze. Packing is also placed anteriorly to help reduce bladder doses.

Good packing and obtaining good geometry are key to achieving a high quality implant. To do this, the ovoids or ring needs to be as close to the cervical os in the superior direction but as

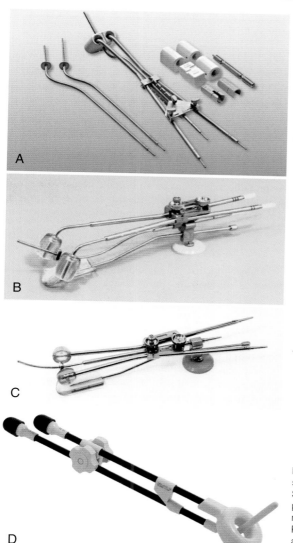

**Figure 20.5 A,** Fletcher-style applicator set-defined geometry (Varian Medical Systems). **B,** Fletcher-Suit-Delclos applicator (Mick Radio-Nuclear Instruments). **C,** Henschke applicator (Mick Radio-Nuclear Instruments). **D,** Ring and tandem applicator (Image courtesy of Elekta AB).

far laterally as possible. The reason to do this is so that the distance from the ovoid or ring dwells to the prescription point or volume is less than the distance from the dwell points to the rectum. If the ovoid dwells are positioned too close to the midline, they are more likely to deliver a higher dose closer to the rectum. If this is the case then the contribution in dose from the dwell position to the rectum will always be higher than the contribution to the prescription point, making it very difficult to achieve a good dose distribution. As mentioned previously, the rectal retractor and packing can help push the rectum away from the ovoids and ring, but obtaining good geometry is also advisable. For women with a narrow fornix this can be quite challenging. In these cases sometimes a cylinder with protruding tandem is used.

The ABS consensus guidelines for locally advanced carcinoma of the cervix, Part I General,[5] define the criteria for an adequate implant to be the following:

- The tandem should be centered between the ovoids on an anterior-posterior (AP) image and bisect them on a lateral image.
- On a lateral image, the ovoids should not be displaced inferiorly from the flange (cervical stop) and should be as symmetrical as possible (should overlap one another).
- The tandem should be approximately one half to one third the distance between the symphysis and the sacral promontory, approximately equidistant between a contrast-filled bladder and rectum.
- The superior tip of the tandem should be located below the sacral promontory within the pelvis.
- Radio-opaque packing will be visible on radiographic images and should be placed anterior and posterior to the ovoids, with no packing visible superior to the ovoids. Superior packing represents an unwanted inferior displacement of the applicator and indicates the need to repack properly before source loading.

## Vaginal Cancers

The treatment for vaginal cancers is similar to that of endometrial cancers in that a vaginal cylinder is also used. If the disease is confined to a limited area a shielded cylinder may be used.

## Uterine Cavity

For treatment of the uterine cavity in Stage I inoperable patients, a tandem alone would not be able to provide good dose coverage. One solution was the use of Heyman capsules, which consisted of a number of low dose rate $^{137}$Cs capsules packed into the uterus. Originally the dose was estimated based on the number of capsules and the treatment time, but no accurate dose calculation was available. With the advent of computerized treatment planning, dose calculations were performed. The Heyman capsules were also available in an afterloading format for use with $^{192}$Ir. Heyman capsules have been replaced by Y applicators, which consist of two tandems mounted on an applicator with the tandem tips tilted away from each other in the shape of a Y. Like tandems, the double tandems for the Y applicators come in a selection of lengths and angles. In addition, sometimes a straight central tandem is used. Figure 20.6 shows a typical applicator. Currently 3D CT or MR-based planning is done to accurately identify the target volume and critical structures.

## ENDOBRONCHIAL, ESOPHAGEAL, AND NASOPHARYNX TREATMENTS

Tumors in the bronchial tree, esophagus, and nasopharynx can also be treated with intracavitary brachytherapy. A single catheter is inserted under fluoroscopic guidance to just beyond the location of the tumor. The length of the catheter is measured and must be carefully verified before each esophageal or nasopharynx treatment. For endobronchial treatments the catheter is placed as far down the airway as possible to anchor it in place. If this is not done the catheter can become dislodged if the patient coughs. The dose distribution is usually cylindrically symmetric, and due to only one channel being used there is limited flexibility in dose shaping. Endobronchial lesions near the carina may require two channels, with one going down each main stem bronchus. The prescription point for endobronchial treatments can vary. Usually it is 5 mm from the center of the catheter. The main airways can be significantly larger than 5 mm radius, so sometimes 10 mm is used. The difficulty in using larger prescription distances is that the catheter does not stay centered in the airway but rather rests against a portion of the airway wall. Pushing the dose out to 10 mm can cause portions of the wall to receive excessive dose. Catheters have been designed

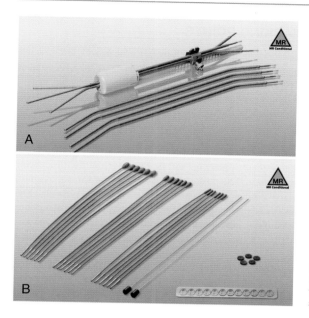

**Figure 20.6 A,** Universal endometrial applicator set (Varian Medical Systems). **B,** Heyman packing applicator set (Varian Medical Systems).

with retractable centering mechanisms to counter this effect. This points out one of the major flaws of endobronchial treatments. The catheter is confined to the airway, and therefore only small lesions can be treated because pushing the dose out to treat larger lesions would cause excessive dose to the airway wall. For this reason, intracavitary brachytherapy in these regions has been largely replaced by intensity-modulated radiation therapy (IMRT) approaches or, sometimes, photodynamic therapy. The ABS consensus guidelines for brachytherapy of esophageal cancer[6] provide details on patient selection, dose fractionation regimens for definitive, adjuvant, and palliative brachytherapy, and applicator selection.

## RECTUM

The most recent development in intracavitary applicators is the development of rectal applicators. New developments in materials, single-use applicators, and 3D imaging for treatment planning were the preconditions needed to facilitate clinical implementation. Because of the proximity of critical structures and the radiation sensitivity itself, efforts are under way to develop rectal applicators that allow selective shielding of areas that do not need to be treated.

# 20.3 Treatment Planning

## IMAGING

The ABS consensus guidelines for locally advanced carcinoma of the cervix, Part I General,[5] recommend the use of cross-sectional imaging (CT or MRI). While the superior soft tissue contrast available in MRI provides better information on tumor extent and parametrial involvement, CT imaging is more widely available. PET imaging is used to study nodal involvement. All imaging equipment must undergo periodic QA to ensure spatial accuracy and correct transfer of images to the TPS (see Chapter 7). Based on surveys performed in 2010,[7] approximately 55% of brachytherapy practitioners use CT for simulation imaging.

## CONTOURING AND DOSE TRACKING POINTS

Treatment planning must take into consideration dose delivered by both the EBRT and brachytherapy components of the radiation therapy. Dose prescriptions must follow the rules for written directives set out in 10 CFR 35 in the Code of Federal Regulations of the United States and contain information on the isotope and source configuration, target, target dose and fractionation, and applicator type. Dose constraints to organs at risk (OARs) should also be listed.

### ICRU-38

The ICRU-38, Dose and Volume Specification for Reporting Intracavitary Therapy in Gynecology, published in 1985, used a dose prescription method that was even at the time rarely used.[8] It is only described here for completeness. The dose prescription uses the three maximum dimensions of the 60 Gy isodose surface (minus any dose delivered by external beam). The maximum length is measured based on the plane containing the tandem, while the maximum width is measured perpendicular to the height measurement, usually at the height of the ovoids.

The *bladder point* is defined at the trigone of the bladder as visualized by a Foley balloon filled with 7 cm$^3$ of diluted contrast. This point does not in general correlate with the maximum dose to the bladder. The ICRU *rectal point* is defined as on a vertical line directly posterior to the center of the ovoids/ring and 0.5 cm posterior to the posterior vaginal wall. The most accurate method of visualizing this point on radiographs is with the use of barium contrast; lead rectal markers are not as reliable and will systematically lower the reported dose. Again, this rectal point does not always coincide with the maximum dose to the rectum.

The *pelvic wall points* are determined by the intersection of the following two lines on the AP radiograph: (1) the line connecting the superior aspects of the acetabula and (2) the tangents to the medial aspects of the acetabula intersecting at right angles with (1). On the lateral radiograph, the position would be approximated by the midpoint of (1).

### Manchester System

The Manchester system was originally developed in the mid-20th century based on the older source loading techniques of the Paris system and the fractionation schemes of the Stockholm system. It defines the prescription and OAR dose tracking points that are still being used today to characterize T&O/T&R and tandem and cylinder (T&C) implants. The major new development of the Manchester system was the realization that the dose-limiting anatomic structure was the area in which the uterine vessels cross the ureter. Since these anatomic landmarks could not be visualized on imaging technology of the time, a method was developed to approximate the position of these landmarks relative to the radio-opaque applicator as seen on orthogonal x-rays for a wide patient population. The treatment plan was then designed to deliver the prescribed dose rate to these points, $A_{left}$ and $A_{right}$.

*Point A (left and right)* are localized as defined by the 2011 ABS recommendation:[5] "On the TPS, connect a line through the center of each ovoid or the lateral-most dwell position in a ring. From the point on the tandem where this line intersects, extend superiorly the radius of the ovoids or for the rings move superiorly to the top of the ring and then move 2 cm along the tandem. Define point A on each side as 2 cm laterally on a perpendicular line from this point on the tandem. For tandem and cylinders, begin at the flange or seeds marking the os and move 2 cm superiorly along the tandem and 2 cm laterally on a perpendicular line." Note that the line connecting points A is always perpendicular to the tandem. For implants in which the ovoids/ring are forced by the anatomy to be slightly asymmetric relative to the tandem, the points A will have different distances to the sources in the ovoids/ring. In clinical practice, the dose prescription is then often set to the average of the points A.

To define the lateral dose falloff, the Manchester system uses *point B (left and right)* defined as follows. On the TPS, connect a line through the center of each ovoid or the lateral-most dwell position in a ring. From the point on the tandem where this line intersects, extend superiorly the radius of the ovoids or for the rings move superiorly to the top of the ring and then move 2 cm along the midline of the patient. Define point B on each side as 5 cm laterally on a perpendicular line from this point on the patient midline. Note that the line connecting points B is always perpendicular to the patient midline.

Within the Manchester system, different loading (LDR) or dwell time (HDR) patterns can be used to shape the dose distribution. Therefore, the practitioner should be aware that the same dose prescription to points A does not constrain the variation in the roughly pear-shaped isodose distribution.

## American Brachytherapy Society and GEC-ESTRO Contouring Guidelines

The GEC-ESTRO group has published a set of contouring guidelines for cervical cancer using both CT and MRI imaging.[9-12] These guidelines have been widely adopted internationally, with 32% of physicians internationally using them, based on data from a practice pattern survey performed in 2010.[7] For definitive treatment using a combination of EBRT and brachytherapy, the changing topography requires an adaptive imaging and contouring approach to brachytherapy treatment planning. The GEC-ESTRO group spent significant effort studying the different treatment approaches across four major European brachytherapy centers and after several intensive workshops provided the following recommendations for volume definitions:[6]

- The GTV contains the visible gross tumor volume as defined by ICRU-50, -62, and -83.[13-15]
- The high risk CTV (HR-CTV) contains the cervix and any visible macroscopic disease (GTV).
- The intermediate risk CTV (IR-CTV) contains areas of initial macroscopic disease at the start of treatment but at the time of contouring has at most microscopic disease extension.
- The low risk CTV (LR-CTV) encompasses areas of potential microscopic disease.

These volumes are further subdivided by disease extension at time of diagnosis (subscript D) and at each subsequent brachytherapy fraction (subscripts B1, B2, ...).

All critical organs should be contoured. For gyn and genitourinary (GU) brachytherapy, this includes the rectum, sigmoid colon, and bladder. The ABS recommends tracking $D_{2cc}$, $D_{0.1cc}$, and $D_{max}$ for each critical organ. The ABS does not make a specific recommendation for tracking dose to the lymph nodes, but concedes that points B (pelvic wall points) as defined by ICRU-38 might be used.

## TREATMENT PLANNING AND TREATMENT PLANNING SYSTEM (TPS) ALGORITHMS

In treatment planning, two types of planning strategies can be used: (1) standard plans or (2) custom plans.

*Standard plans* are at this time only recommended for use in cylinder-based intracavitary brachytherapy, because the prescription reference line is fixed relative to the applicator geometry at either the applicator surface or 5 mm away from the applicator surface. To create a standard plan, a CT of a cylinder is created and imported in the treatment planning system. Cylinder plans are characterized by:

- Dose per fraction
- Cylinder diameter, type of cap, and number of segments. The type of cap will determine the superior coverage. For more extensive disease it may be desirable to push the dose more superiorly, and using a cap with a more distal dwell position can facilitate this.

TABLE 20.1 ▦ **Sample Criteria in the Most Common Clinical Settings for HDR Brachytherapy**

| Type of Implant | Typical Brachy Prescription | Organs at Risk (OAR) | Constraints | Other Considerations |
|---|---|---|---|---|
| Vaginal cylinder | 700 cGy × 3 to 5 mm depth if HDR alone; 550 cGy × 2 to 5 mm depth if EBRT 4500 cGy | Rectum | None typically. If Rx to 5 mm then rectal dose will usually be ≥Rx | Larger vaginal cylinders will help decrease normal tissue dose. Can use shielded cylinder or multichannel cylinder to minimize rectal dose if disease is confined to the anterior areas. |
| Tandem & ovoid/ tandem & ring | 600 cGy × 5 with EBRT 4500 cGy for point A EQD$_2$ 8000-9000 cGy | Rectum Bladder Bowel | If 3D planning, D$_{2cc}$ rectum and sigmoid bowel <75 Gy equivalent quadratic dose (EQD)$_2$; bladder <90 Gy EQD$_2$. If 2D planning, typically rectal and bladder point doses <75% | Good positioning of applicator and packing is essential to cover tumor and minimize normal tissue dose. If tandem tip is close to bowel, do not use most distal 1-2 dwells to minimize bowel dose. |

- Length of treatment
- Location of prescription line (cylinder surface and/or 5 mm away from surface)
- Dwell position and dwell times

*Custom plans* can be used for cylinders and should be used for all other intracavitary treatment plans. If a treatment is delivered in a fractionated pattern the applicator location should be verified through imaging before each fraction. The repeat placement of the tandem is facilitated by placing a uterine stent and suturing it in place at the time of the first fraction. This makes it possible to place the applicator for future fractions without the use of anesthesia. The available dose optimization algorithms for HDR TPS allow for a considerably larger flexibility of dose shaping compared to LDR brachytherapy with its limited number of sources and source strength.

The ABS recommends that treatment plans for cervical treatments (T&O, T&R, T&C) should contain and report the following parameters:

- Dose per fraction and total dose
- Type of applicator
- Radionuclide, including source strength
- Dwell position and dwell times
- Dose to points A and/or D$_{90}$, D$_{100}$, and V$_{100}$ for the HR-CTV
- ICRU rectal and bladder points and/or D$_{2cc}$, D$_{0.1cc}$, and D$_{max}$ for each critical organ (D$_{5cc}$ for organ wall if used)
- Isodose distributions in the sagittal, oblique frontal coronal through points A and axial through the vaginal sources

The dose to critical organs is handled differently based on the area being treated and the type of applicator. Table 20.1 shows some sample criteria in the most common clinical settings.

The majority of TPS use the AAPM TG-43 formalism for dose calculations. Model-based dose calculation algorithms are becoming available. AAPM TG-186 on model-based dose calculation algorithms[16] recommends reporting doses and dose prescriptions in the AAPM TG-43 formalism with model-based dose calculation results reported in addition to the AAPM TG-43 calculations. This approach is analogous to the Radiation Therapy Oncology Group (RTOG) approach to implementing new inhomogeneity correction algorithms in lung treatments: report both methods in parallel to ensure a systematic transition in dose prescription, and allow time for thorough experimental and clinical validation of the new dose calculation algorithms.

There are several techniques used for HDR brachytherapy planning. In forward planning, the dwell times and dwell positions can be set to emulate the loading patterns of an LDR implant. It should be noted that although the isodose lines will look identical to an LDR implant, the biologically equivalent dose (BED) at different points of the implant will be different. The more common forward planning method is to start with dwell positions and dwell times emulating an LDR implant, and then manually adjust the dwell positions until the desired dose distribution shape is reached. This dose distribution is then normalized either to points A (cervix) or to the reference line for cylinder treatments. For intracavitary implants using volumetric contours based on GEC-ESTRO, inverse planning can be used to optimize dose coverage of the HR-CTV. In addition to reporting dose to volume, dose to the points A as well as dose to the ICRU rectal and bladder points should be reported to provide continuity with traditional dose prescription systems.

## FOR THE PHYSICIAN

Intracavitary brachytherapy is increasingly moving from LDR to HDR due to a variety of reasons, including less radiation exposure to staff with remote afterloaders and less inpatient time for patients. When comparing studies of LDR versus HDR, it is important to be mindful of equivalent dose conversions and apply standards such as $EQD_2$. For the common sites utilizing intracavitary brachytherapy, good guidelines exist from ABS and other societies.

Intracavitary brachytherapy is often used to treat gynecologic cancers. In vaginal cylinder brachytherapy, it is important to use the largest cylinder diameter that the patient can tolerate to decrease surface dose and risk of air gaps. Various cylinder systems exist, some with shielding for normal tissue protection. Similarly for cervical cancer treatment, various systems can be used for T&O treatment, and T&R systems are becoming more popular. Key to effective treatment in this setting is good placement of the T&O/T&R and packing to help stabilize the equipment and move normal tissues such as the rectum away from the high dose region. Other less common applications of brachytherapy include inoperable uterine cancers, endobronchial tumors, esophageal tumors, and nasopharynx tumors.

CT- or MR-based treatment planning is more routinely used to help delineate target volume and normal tissues. Traditionally, brachytherapy records point doses (such as point A, bladder point, rectal point). The Manchester system has been used to define many of the points of interest in traditional planning and is still being used. With 3D planning, it is clear that these points do not always coincide with the max dose to the organ. Isodose plans provide additional information to point doses when evaluating treatment plans, although exact guidelines for isodose plan evaluation are still evolving. ABS has guidelines for treatment parameters to record. For simple treatments such as a vaginal cylinder, a standard plan can be used because the applicator geometry and patient anatomy are fixed. Otherwise, custom plans should be generated to reflect applicator location relative to local anatomy. For fractionated treatments, application position should be verified prior to each fraction.

Dose calculations are improving for brachytherapy, with model-based algorithms becoming available. These still need more validation but should improve dose accuracy in the future.

## References

1. Viswanathan AN, Beriwal S, De Los Santos JF, et al. American Brachytherapy Society consensus guidelines for locally advanced carcinoma of the cervix. Part II: High-dose-rate brachytherapy. Brachyther 2012;11(1):47–52.
2. Small W Jr, Beriwal S, Demanes DJ, et al. American Brachytherapy Society consensus guidelines for adjuvant vaginal cuff brachytherapy after hysterectomy. Brachyther 2012;11(1):58–67.

3. Cunha JA, Mellis K, Sethi R, et al. Evaluation of PC-ISO for Customized, 3D Printed, Gynecologic $^{192}$Ir HDR Brachytherapy Applicators. J Appl Clin Med Phys 2015;16(1).
4. Gloi A. First clinical implementation of the Capri applicator. J Appl Clin Med Phys 2014;15(1).
5. Viswanathan AN, Thomadsen B. American Brachytherapy Society consensus guidelines for locally advanced carcinoma of the cervix. Part I: General principles. Brachyther 2012;11(1):33–46.
6. Gaspar LE, Nag S, Herskovic A, et al. American Brachytherapy Society (ABS) consensus guidelines for brachytherapy of esophageal cancer. Int J Radiat Oncol Biol Phys 1997;38(1):127–32.
7. Viswanathan AN, Creutzberg CL, Craighead P, et al. International brachytherapy practice patterns: A survey of the Gynecologic Cancer Intergroup (GCIG). Int J Radiat Oncol Biol Phys 2012;82(1): 250–5.
8. ICRU. Report No. 38. Dose and volume specification for reporting intracavitary therapy in gynecology. Bethesda, MD: ICRU; 1985.
9. Haie-Meder C, Pötter R, Van Limbergen E, et al. Recommendations from Gynaecological (GYN) GEC-ESTRO Working Group* (I): Concepts and terms in 3D image based 3D treatment planning in cervix cancer brachytherapy with emphasis on MRI assessment of GTV and CTV. Radiother Oncol 2005;74(3):235–45.
10. Pötter R, Haie-Meder C, Van Limbergen E, et al. Recommendations from gynaecological (GYN) GEC ESTRO working group (II): Concepts and terms in 3D image-based treatment planning in cervix cancer brachytherapy—3D dose volume parameters and aspects of 3D image-based anatomy, radiation physics, radiobiology. Radiother Oncol 2006;78(1):67–77.
11. Hellebust TP, Kirisits C, Berger D, et al. Recommendations from Gynaecological (GYN) GEC-ESTRO Working Group: Considerations and pitfalls in commissioning and applicator reconstruction in 3D image-based treatment planning of cervix cancer brachytherapy. Radiother Oncol 2010;96(2):153–60.
12. Dimopoulos JC, Petrow P, Tanderup K, et al. Recommendations from Gynaecological (GYN) GEC-ESTRO Working Group (IV): Basic principles and parameters for MR imaging within the frame of image based adaptive cervix cancer brachytherapy. Radiother Oncol 2012;103(1):113–22.
13. Jones D. ICRU Report 50: Prescribing, recording and reporting photon beam therapy. Med Phys 1994;21:833–4.
14. ICRU. Report 62: Prescribing, recording and reporting photon beam therapy (supplement to ICRU Report 50). Bethesda, MD: International Commission on Radiation Units and Measurements; 1999.
15. ICRU. Report 83: Prescribing, recording, and reporting photon-beam intensity-modulated radiation therapy (IMRT). J ICRU 2010;(10):27–40.
16. Beaulieu L, Tedgren ÅC, Carrier JF, et al. Report of the Task Group 186 on model-based dose calculation methods in brachytherapy beyond the AAPM TG-43 formalism: Current status and recommendations for clinical implementation. Med Phys 2012;39(10):6208–36.

# CHAPTER 21

# Interstitial Brachytherapy

## 21.1 Introduction

Interstitial brachytherapy has a long tradition, starting with radium needles being implanted in superficial tumors in the 1930s. The implant systems developed at the time, Manchester and Quimby, still guide the needle placement patterns used in implants today.

Though radium needles where initially used for interstitial implants, other radioactive nuclei were developed over time. Table 8.1 in Chapter 8 contains a list of the most commonly used brachytherapy sources. Low dose rate (LDR) ribbons of $^{192}$Ir or $^{137}$Cs were the most popular devices for interstitial brachytherapy until remote high dose rate (HDR) afterloaders were developed. Compared to LDR brachytherapy, HDR afterloaders reduce the exposure to physicians and staff treating the patient, reduce the time a patient has to spend immobile as an inpatient, and allow more flexibility in customizing treatment plans. In addition, the number of sources that need to be kept, calibrated, and stored securely is significantly reduced in HDR compared to LDR.

The transition from LDR to HDR raised some concerns about the change in cell kill based on the difference in radiobiology between the two methods. Therefore, some centers developed a transitional pulsed dose rate (PDR) delivery method, in which HDR afterloaders were used to deliver fractions of the total dose at preset time intervals, typically 1 hour. As outcome and toxicity data from interstitial HDR have matured, PDR and LDR treatments are being phased out of clinical use.

Interstitial brachytherapy can be used either as monotherapy or as an adjuvant boost to external beam radiotherapy. Its strength lies in delivering highly conformal doses with steep dose gradients to tumors that are not surgically resectable because of the close proximity to critical organs. Interstitial brachytherapy can also be used in patients who are not surgical candidates. These advantages have to be carefully weighed against the risks of the procedure, including risk from local anesthesia, infection, and patient immobilization over the duration of treatment.

## 21.2 Clinical Targets

### GYNECOLOGICAL TARGETS

This section focuses on diseases treated with interstitial brachytherapy. Earlier stage disease is sometimes treated with intracavitary implants (e.g., tandem and ovoid); more information can be found in Chapter 20.

Interstitial brachytherapy for the treatment of cervical cancer is used as a last resort if external beam treatment does not reduce the tumor size sufficiently to get satisfactory coverage with an intracavitary implant. There are several options for designing the interstitial implant, including those that are a blend of intracavitary with interstitial components:

- Tandem & ring (T&R)/tandem & ovoid (T&O) with two to three free-hand interstitial needles

- T&O applicators with combined interstitial channels
- Perineal implant with central vaginal cylinder, tandem and concentrically arranged catheter template. A common applicator is the Syed-Neblett template consisting of 12 interstitial catheters around a central cylinder, though other applicators are available.

Though it is more invasive, planning studies suggest a better coverage with the latter applicator.[1] A variety of dose and fractionation schedules are used in interstitial brachytherapy for gynecologic cancers, ranging from 1 to 8 fractions, either daily or twice daily (BID), typically to biologically weighted dose of 75 to 85 Gy.

For vaginal cancer, the American Brachytherapy Society (ABS) consensus guidelines for interstitial brachytherapy for vaginal cancer[2] recommend that patients with bulky disease (≥0.5 cm) be considered for interstitial implants. Because of the rarity of the disease, the consensus guidelines are based on the results of single-institution studies since no randomized prospective trial data are currently available. A cylindrically symmetric perineal implant template with a vaginal cylinder is recommended for this type of implant. The typical needle spacing is not more than 1 cm between needles. Table I of the consensus documents summarizes the dose fractionation schemes used by experts or reported in small single-institution studies. Dose fractionation schemes include 2 Gy × 18 fractions of external beam radiation therapy (EBRT) followed by 6 Gy × 5 fractions of brachytherapy or 1.8 Gy × 28 fractions of EBRT followed by 7 Gy × 3 fractions of brachytherapy.

## BREAST

The purpose of interstitial breast brachytherapy is to deliver accelerated partial breast irradiation (APBI) to the lumpectomy cavity following surgery. Interstitial breast treatments fall into two categories: interstitial HDR using two planes of implanted needles and partial breast HDR brachytherapy using applicators implanted in the surgical cavity. Intra-operative radiation therapy (IORT) is also used (see Chapter 23).

A variety of applicators have been developed for placement in the lumpectomy cavity. The MammoSite device (shown in Figure 21.1) has several sizes of a pressurized applicator (e.g., spheres of 4 to 5 cm and 5 to 6 cm in diameter, an ellipsoid of 4 cm × 6 cm), which is filled with saline solution. A silicone catheter is located in the center of the balloon. The purpose of the balloon is to mold the lumpectomy cavity tissue into a spherical shape, which can then be irradiated. The implant of the balloon applicator can either be performed at the time of surgery or shortly after. Ideally, there should be a few days' wait between implant and imaging for treatment

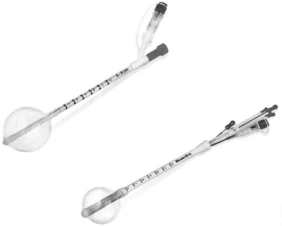

**Figure 21.1** MammoSite applicator (*Image courtesy of Hologic, Inc.*).

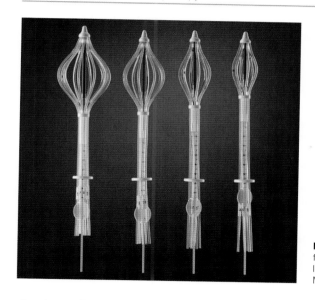

**Figure 21.2** SAVI applicators in four different sizes to match different size lumpectomy cavities. (Courtesy Cianna Medical.)

planning to allow for air pockets to resolve and seroma to drain. A limiting factor for the original MammoSite applicator treatments is the proximity of the lumpectomy cavity to the skin of the patient. At least 7 mm of spacing is required to avoid potential late-term toxicity with an unsatisfactory cosmesis outcome. To overcome the skin sparing issue, several multilumen catheters have been developed to enable asymmetric dose shaping to improve skin sparing. These include multilumen balloon catheters, as well as multilumen catheters without the use of a balloon (e.g., the SAVI applicator; see Figure 21.2).

Interstitial breast implants using catheters are utilized if the lumpectomy cavity is too small for the implant of other applicators or the cavity has closed before the applicator was implanted. Typically 10 to 20 catheters are placed in a planar arrangement through the tumor region. The treatment regimen is similar to lumpectomy cavity treatments (i.e., a week of 10 fractions delivered BID). To minimize unnecessary radiation exposure to the patient, especially the contralateral breast, it is important to place the catheters such that the catheter tips are located toward the patient midline.

In addition to these techniques, IORT can be used to deliver a boost to the lumpectomy site during surgery. This is supported by the recently reported 5-year results of the TARGIT-A trial.[3] More information can be found in Chapter 23 on IORT. The main systems in use are the Zeiss Intrabeam device, a low kV target and applicator on a mobile arm, and the Xoft/Axxent system, a low kV x-ray tube in a catheter that is used in combination with a balloon applicator. Because of the similarity in beam energy of these devices to traditional brachytherapy sources, they are often classified as "electronic brachytherapy." American Association of Physicists in Medicine Task Group (AAPM TG)-182 is developing recommendations for electronic brachytherapy quality management.

Published dose fractionation schemes for most interstitial targets rely on the experience of relatively small, single-institution studies. The notable exception is interstitial treatments for the breast, which follow a very well-defined APBI protocol.[4] The dose constraints are listed in Table 21.1.

## PROSTATE

The interstitial implant of LDR prostate seeds is a well-established procedure which is covered in Chapter 22. Interstitial HDR treatments are also used for prostate treatments, initially as boost

TABLE 21.1 ▦ **Dose Constraints for APBI**

| | |
|---|---|
| Planning target volume (PTV) | 1 cm margin from device minus chest wall, ribs, and skin<br>$V_{90}$ >90%<br>$V_{200}$ <10 cm³ (balloon) or $V_{200}$ <20 cm³ (interstitial)<br>$V_{150}$ <50 cm³ (balloon) or $V_{150}$ <70 cm³ (interstitial) |
| Dose | 3.4 Gy × 10, delivered BID at least 6 hours apart |
| Conformance | Volume of cavities not occupied by breast tissue or applicator ≤10% |
| Skin dose | <100% of prescribed dose (interstitial) or <145% (balloon) |
| Lung dose | <75% of prescribed dose |

TABLE 21.2 ▦ **Current Dose Fractionation Schemes for HDR Prostate Brachytherapy from the ABS Consensus Guideline[4]**

| Institution | Monotherapy | Boost | Salvage |
|---|---|---|---|
| MSKCC | 9.5 Gy × 4 | 7 Gy × 3 | 8 Gy × 4 |
| UCSF | 10.5 Gy × 3 | 15 Gy × 1 | 8 Gy × 4 |
| William Beaumont | 9.5 Gy × 4 (historical)<br>12-13.5 Gy × 2 (current) | 10.5 Gy × 2 | 7 Gy × 4 combined<br>with hyperthermia |
| Texas Cancer Center | N/A | 6 Gy × 2, two sessions | N/A |
| GammaWest<br>Brachytherapy | 6.5 Gy × 3, two sessions | 6.5 Gy × 3 | N/A |
| Toronto | N/A | 15 Gy × 1 | N/A |
| UCLA | 7.25 Gy × 6 | 6 Gy × 4 | N/A |

for adjuvant external beam radiotherapy, but increasingly also as monotherapy. A body of literature has been published, which is summarized in the ABS consensus guideline for HDR prostate brachytherapy.[5]

The rationale for HDR brachytherapy for prostate is to provide local control, which has shown to be a major factor in disease outcome for low, intermediate, and high risk prostate cancer. Assuming the linear-quadratic model of biologically effective dose (BED) is valid in hypofractionated regimens, an argument can be made that high doses delivered in fewer fractions will be advantageous in achieving better local control while at the same time improving normal tissue sparing. Therefore, dose escalation combined with hypofractionation has been the major goal in the development of new treatment regimens for prostate cancer. HDR brachytherapy provides very high localized dose delivery and steep dose gradients toward critical organs.

Currently, the literature on prostate HDR is limited to single-institution or pooled data with a wide variety of dose fractionation schemes, an extensive list of which can be found in Table I of the ABS consensus guidelines. Currently used dose fractionation schemes are listed in Table 3 of the same document. The prescription doses of this table are summarized in Table 21.2. The Radiation Therapy Oncology Group (RTOG)-0321 trial was the first multi-institutional prospective trial studying Grade 3 toxicity for HDR prostate boost following external beam radiotherapy. Preliminary follow-up results showing acceptable levels of adverse events were published.[6] Catheter placements for prostate HDR follow established practice patterns from prostate LDR (Chapter 22). Catheters are placed under trans-rectal ultrasound (TRUS) guidance; square implant templates with needle spacing of 0.5 cm between rows and columns are used to guide needle placement. Depending on the dose fractionation scheme used, the patient may either be treated in a single day or admitted for an overnight stay using epidural anesthesia with the catheters left in place.

## OTHER SITES

Interstitial brachytherapy has also been used for base of tongue and head and neck cancers, sarcomas, and lung cancers. The implementation of intensity-modulated radiation therapy (IMRT) for head-and-neck (H&N) cancers, and both IORT and IMRT for sarcoma treatments, has reduced the use of the more time- and personnel-intensive brachytherapy techniques. In addition, the newer techniques are less invasive, thereby reducing the risk of adverse events such as infections secondary to interstitial implants or adverse reactions to antibiotics.

The ABS recommendations for HDR brachytherapy for H&N carcinoma[7] contain a summary of interstitial implant techniques for H&N brachytherapy. Catheters are placed as parallel and equidistant in the implant plane as possible, given the geometric limitations of clear access to base of tongue or other interstitial H&N sites. Since the publication of the ABS guidelines, IMRT has been widely implemented into clinical practice and has largely replaced H&N brachytherapy.

Brachytherapy for sarcomas is a technique closely related to IORT. At the time of surgery, interstitial catheters are sutured to the surgical bed in areas where clear margins cannot be achieved for technical reasons. The catheter geometry is usually single plane or, occasionally, two parallel planes. The ABS recommendations for brachytherapy of soft tissue sarcomas[8] recommend catheter placements of 1 to 2 cm beyond the clinical target volume (CTV) laterally and 2 to 5 cm beyond the CTV in the longitudinal direction. Catheter entry points should be at a distance to the surgical incision, with catheters either in parallel or transverse to the direction of the incision. Radio-opaque markers such as surgical clips are used to demarcate the CTV as well as organs at risk (OARs) in the vicinity of the tumor. Dose and fractionation regimens vary among institutions. The technique has been largely replaced by IORT or postoperative IMRT.

Interstitial brachytherapy can also be delivered by implantation of radioactive sources in the lung during wedge resections for early stage lung cancer. Stranded low dose rate $^{125}$I seeds fixed to a vicryl mesh are implanted next to the surgical staples with the intent to sterilize possible positive margins or surgical contamination.[9] The spacing of the strands can vary based on the seed activity, or alternatively, a range of acceptable activity can be established for 1 cm spacing. AAPM TG-222, Operative Interstitial Lung Radiotherapy (in progress), is charged with providing the following information:

1. Review the steps in the procedure (educational)
2. Describe the treatment planning and dosimetric aspects of the procedures (educational)
3. Recommend dosimeteric parameters useful for evaluating and specifying the treatments (recommendations)
4. Make recommendations for quality management unique to the procedures (recommendations)
5. Recommend a definition for medical events involving these procedures (recommendations)

# 21.3 Day of Implant Procedure

## TRANSPORT OF PATIENT THROUGHOUT THE PROCEDURE

In many facilities, the location of implant, imaging, and treatment delivery may not be in the same room or allow the use of the same treatment couch. In those cases, the patient needs to be moved without shifting the position of the implant. Several commercial systems have been developed to assist in patient movement. These range from sliding couch tops to hover technologies. Independent of which technology is used, the implant should be checked before and after each move to ensure its integrity. Especially for genitourinary (GU) and GYN implants, the patient's bed should be kept flat to avoid any pressure from the mattress acting on the catheters, potentially shifting position or bending. A cover is often placed over the implant catheters if they protrude from the patient, with an extended length to minimize the potential for something to catch on a catheter. This is of most concern for interstitial implants because of the number of catheters involved.

## IMAGING FOR NEEDLE PLACEMENT AND TREATMENT PLANNING

Needles for interstitial implants are made of surgical steel, titanium, or flexible plastic. Titanium needles are MR compatible up to 3 T, whereas plastic needles are fully MR compatible. Steel needles, though having the best mechanical strength, also create the most artifacts in CT imaging. In some devices a central metal stylus is used to provide rigidity. The central stylus can be removed for CT scanning, which reduces artifacts.

Interstitial implants, especially in the GU/GYN areas, are often performed in close proximity to critical organs. Therefore, implants are performed under image guidance. Ultrasound, fluoroscopy, CT, and MR imaging can all be used for this purpose depending on access and availability.

CT imaging is most often used for treatment planning because of its availability in most Radiation Oncology departments. Magnetic resonance imaging (MRI), if available, will provide better soft tissue contrast for imaging but can make identification of interstitial needles more challenging than it is in computed tomography (CT). CT/MR fusion can be used to combine the advantages of easy catheter identification on CT with the soft tissue contrast available through MRI. Because the MRI is often performed without the implant in place, the image fusion needs to be able to perform a nonrigid transformation. The localization errors for nonrigid transformations are on the order of several millimeters. The upcoming AAPM TG-132 report, Use of Image Registration and Data Fusion Algorithms and Techniques in Radiotherapy Treatment Planning, will give further guidance on this matter. Alternatively, orthogonal x-ray images can be used to plan the treatment. This is rarely done with the advent of CT and MR imaging and is difficult to evaluate for implants with many catheters or needles. In addition, it offers limited information regarding OARs.

## CATHETER RECONSTRUCTION

Accurate catheter reconstruction in the treatment planning imaging set forms the basis for accurate treatment planning. At simulation, documentation should be created to show needle implant location in the template and the desired needle numbering scheme for templates that do not provide premarked grid positioning. For implants without a template, a photo of the implant site with the desired catheter numbering added is a good visual aid to match HDR channels to the treatment plan. The planning imaging set should extend inferiorly to include the needle template (if one was used), so the treatment planner can follow the individual needles from the template to the tip.

Uncertainties in needle matching are introduced by artifacts from metal implants or gold marker seeds and crossing needles. Artifacts are highest for stainless steel needles and lowest for the plastic catheters. Imaging should be done with the obturators removed. Flexible, low electron density dummy wires such as aluminum wires can be used in either all or some of the needle catheters to provide a visual aid.

Uncertainties due to crossing needle paths depend on the elasticity of the needles and are therefore larger for titanium needles compared to stainless steel and can be quite prominent for plastic needles. Catheters—especially those passing close to the pubic arch—are sometimes deflected by bone or cartilage. Several practical strategies exist to minimize uncertainties. If crossing needles can be identified during simulation, a dummy marker can be inserted in one of the crossing needles to clearly distinguish needle paths. If needle tips are obscured by metal artifacts, the length of the needle beyond the template can be measured, and from that the length of the needle section implanted into the patient can be extrapolated. On the treatment planning image, it is usually helpful to mark all needles with clearly visible needle paths first before working on the obscured needle path. The 3D image view available in many commercial treatment planning systems (TPS) is an excellent visual aid to check the catheter reconstruction.

## QUALITY ASSURANCE OF TREATMENT PLANS

In treatment planning, either forward or inverse planning techniques can be used. Brachytherapy has higher dose heterogeneity than external beam techniques, but the $V_{200}$ (volume receiving 150% of the dose) should be limited to areas immediately adjacent to the needles and ideally not connect between needles. Dose fractionation schemes for most interstitial targets vary considerably among institutions and among patients depending on the specific clinical situation. Carefully verifying the prescribed dose against the written directive is therefore essential to avoid possible misadministrations.

As in external beam, a secondary independent plan check should be performed for interstitial brachytherapy. The verification of the catheter reconstruction should be independently verified before the start of treatment planning to reduce the risk of needing to replan the patient due to errors made at this stage.

After the plan is completed and approved by the physician, a complete independent second check of the plan should be performed. This second check should include:

- Written directive
- Catheter reconstruction, including length of catheter and distance of first source to needle tip
- Dose prescription matches target coverage and dose inhomogeneity
- OAR dose
- Correct location of dose tracking points (if used)
- Secondary dose checks, using either commercial or self-developed software. In addition to verifying the ability of the planning system to calculate dose correctly, it can also catch any changes made to the treatment plan between documentation and secondary dose check.

## QUALITY ASSURANCE CHECKS PRIOR TO TREATMENT

The ACR-ASTRO practice guideline for the performance of HDR brachytherapy[10] recommends that before the start of the treatment, the physician or physicist should independently verify the correct order of transfer tube connections from the remote afterloader unit to the catheters. The length of each channel should also be confirmed. In addition, the physicist should verify the correct transfer of treatment parameters from the TPS to the afterloader console, including dwell times, dwell position, and source strength. The physician should verify that the implant position has not moved compared to the position at simulation. One practical method to do so is to note the distance of catheter extension beyond the implant template on the simulation spreadsheet marking the catheter positions. Alternatively, the catheter could be marked where it exits the skin. Before the treatment start with the active source, a dummy source should be run through all channels to verify the channel length and detect any potential channel obstructions. Figure 21.3 shows a sample checklist containing recommended pretreatment checks according to the ACR-ASTRO practice guideline, NRC regulatory requirements, and institutional safety policies. AAPM TG-59 on HDR brachytherapy treatment delivery[11] published in 1998 also provides an extensive quality assurance checklist. Although sections of that report refer to older technology, the general recommendations are in agreement and are somewhat more detailed with respect to the physics section and emergency procedures than the ACR-ASTRO practice guideline.

## GammaMed HDR Treatment Check Sheet

**Treatment date:**
**Plan name:**

**\*\*\*Initial all lines\*\*\***

| Therapist | Pretreatment General Checks |
|---|---|
| | Intercom and CCTV functional |
| | Pretreatment survey:_____mR/hr    Tolerance <1 mR/hr<br>Survey meter #:_____  Cal due date:_____<br>\*\*\*If radiation level is >1 mR/hr, give explanation:_____ |
| | Confirm Radiation Oncologist and Physicist are authorized for HDR |

| Therapist | Physicist | Treatment Plan Checks | |
|---|---|---|---|
| | | Patient name correct | |
| | | Date and time correct | |
| | | Source strength correct | on Planned Treatment |
| | | Total scaled Curie-seconds are correct | Report |
| | | Dwell position and times correct | |
| | | Signatures of RadOnc. Physicist and RTT | |
| | | RadOnc approved prescription | in MOSAIQ |
| | | RadOnc and physicist approved plan pdf | |

| Therapist | Physicist | Patient Checks | |
|---|---|---|---|
| | | Patient identified by two methods | |
| | | Guide tube integrity | |
| | | Guide tube/applicator length | |
| | | Connection to indexer channel correct | |
| | | SAVI pretreatment check sheet complete | For SAVI only |
| | | SAVI expansion tool in place | |
| | | Flexible probe extension _____cm<br>Tolerance 6.3 ± 0.1 cm | Cylinder only |
| | | Procedural pause at time: | |

| Therapist | Post-Treatment Checks |
|---|---|
| | Treatment delivered as planed |
| | Post-treatment survey:_____ mR/Hr<br>\*\*\* If post-Tx reading > pre-Tx reading, confirm reading then implement emergency procedures \*\*\* |
| | SAVI expansion tool removed |
| | Treatment delivery report printed |
| | Treatment recorded in MOSAIQ |

**In case of error or treatment emergency, document error(s) and total treatment interruption time:**

**Figure 21.3** Sample pretreatment QA checklist.

# 21.4 Staff Training and Supervision Requirements

The ACR-ASTRO practice guideline for the performance of HDR brachytherapy Section III[10] contains detailed recommendations on qualifications of personnel to perform HDR brachytherapy in general. Because interstitial brachytherapy is more complex than most intracavitary brachytherapy, it is important for the delivery of a safe and high quality procedure to have an experienced patient care team in place. The regulatory requirements for brachytherapy as summarized in Chapter 8 apply to interstitial brachytherapy.

---

**FOR THE PHYSICIAN**

HDR has been gaining in popularity in recent years due to a variety of factors, including reduced dose to staff with afterloading and less inpatient time for patients. Common clinical applications of interstitial brachytherapy are listed below:

- Gynecologic cancers: Such as with the Syed-Neblett template. There are a range of dose and fractionation schemes in use, and HDR doses must be adjusted for comparison against LDR or external beam doses.
- Breast cancers: Several options exist, including lumpectomy cavity irradiation with a balloon (e.g., MammoSite), interstitial catheters, or intraoperative radiation. Skin dose needs to be considered in this setting for cosmetic outcome.
- Prostate cancers: Although LDR is still more common, use of HDR is rising. This can be used as monotherapy, as a boost to external beam, or for salvage treatment of recurrent cancers. Multiple dose regimens have been published in single-institution series, although RTOG-0321 prelim results are encouraging with 19 Gy in 2 fractions as a boost after external beam.
- Other cancers: Less commonly used
  - H&N cancers
  - Sarcomas
  - Lung cancers

For HDR treatment delivery, volumetric imaging is typically performed to ensure target coverage while minimizing normal tissue dose. Because it is often necessary to transport patients during the treatment day (i.e., from OR to simulation to treatment room), patients are often kept flat and relatively immobile to keep catheters in place. Catheter positions must be reconstructed for treatment planning. With the high dose per fraction delivered and potential for harm with misadministration, independent plan checks should be done, and catheter reconstruction must be independently verified. ACR-ASTRO has published guidelines for pretreatment QA, including checking the connections from afterloader to the catheters and treatment parameters such as dwell times, positions, and source strength. A dummy source is used to verify channels and detect potential obstructions.

## References

1. Hsu I, Chow J, Speight J, et al. A comparison between tandem and ovoids and interstitial gynecologic template brachytherapy dosimetry using a hypothetical computer model. Int J Radiat Oncol Biol Phys 2002;52:538–43.
2. Beriwal S, Demanes DJ, Erickson B, et al. American Brachytherapy Society consensus guidelines for interstitial brachytherapy for vaginal cancer. Brachyther 2012;11:68–75.
3. Vaidya JS, Wenz F, Bulsara M, et al. Risk-adapted targeted intraoperative radiotherapy versus whole-breast radiotherapy for breast cancer: 5-year results for local control and overall survival from the TARGIT-A randomised trial. Lancet 2014;383:603–13.
4. Shah C, Vicini F, Wazer DE, et al. The American Brachytherapy Society consensus statement for accelerated partial breast irradiation. Brachytherapy 2013;12:267–77.

5. Yamada Y, Rogers L, Demanes DJ, et al. American Brachytherapy Society consensus guidelines for high-dose-rate prostate brachytherapy. Brachytherapy 2012;11:20–32.
6. Hsu I, Bae K, Shinohara K, et al. Phase II trial of combined high-dose-rate brachytherapy and external beam radiotherapy for adenocarcinoma of the prostate: Preliminary results of RTOG 0321. Int J Radiat Oncol Biol Phys 2010;78:751–8.
7. Nag S, Cano ER, Demanes DJ, et al. The American Brachytherapy Society recommendations for high-dose-rate brachytherapy for head-and-neck carcinoma. Int J Radiat Oncol Biol Phys 2001;50:1190–8.
8. Nag S, Shasha D, Janjan N, et al. The American Brachytherapy Society recommendations for brachytherapy of soft tissue sarcomas. Int J Radiat Oncol Biol Phys 2001;49:1033–43.
9. Odell DD, Kent MS, Fernando HC. Sublobar resection with brachytherapy mesh for stage I non-small cell lung cancer. Semin Thorac Cardiovasc Surg 2010;32–7.
10. Erickson BA, Demanes DJ, Ibbott GS, et al. American Society for Radiation Oncology (ASTRO) and American College of Radiology (ACR) practice guideline for the performance of high-dose-rate brachytherapy. Int J Radiat Oncol Biol Phys 2011;79:641–9.
11. Kubo HD, Glasgow GP, Pethel TD, et al. High dose-rate brachytherapy treatment delivery: Report of the AAPM Radiation Therapy Committee Task Group No. 59. Med Phys 1998;25:375–403.

# CHAPTER 22

# Prostate Seed Implant

## 22.1 Introduction

Prostate brachytherapy is one of several treatment techniques available for patients with localized disease. Prostate brachytherapy is currently practiced using two different techniques: (1) prostate seed implant (PSI) using low dose rate (LDR) sources and (2) high dose rate (HDR) brachytherapy. Because prostate HDR is one variation of interstitial implants, it is grouped with other interstitial implants in Chapter 20.

Like other technologies in Radiation Oncology, PSI has undergone major changes both in implementation of technology and in clinical recommendations based on knowledge from clinical trials. Initially, $^{103}$Pd loose seeds were the only available radiation source for implant. In 1999, the National Institute of Standards and Technology (NIST) changed its calibration standard, leading to a 9% adjustment in dose calibration.[1] $^{125}$I, $^{131}$Cs, and $^{198}$Au expanded the practitioner's choice of sources. Better ultrasound technology and computing technology allowed the move to 3D-based preplanning or live planning in the operating room (OR). Vendors developed preloaded needles, stranded seed configurations, and stranding technology that could be used to assemble strands in the OR itself. Third-party vendors are now offering independent assays of seeds, which led AAPM to change the recommendation for clinical seed assays.[2]

Patient selection criteria and treatment regimens for PSI are constantly evolving as more clinical data become available. The "classic" PSI monotherapy patient has low grade, early stage disease. PSI is also a choice for intermediate risk patients, either as monotherapy or in combination with other therapies. The American College of Radiology (ACR)-American Society for Radiation Oncology (ASTRO) practice guideline for the transperineal permanent brachytherapy of prostate cancer[3] suggests "that each facility establish and follow its own practice guidelines. Ongoing clinical trials will help to better define indications." The American Brachytherapy Society's (ABS) recommendations for transperineal permanent brachytherapy of prostate cancer[4] published in 1999 discusses in more detail patient selection criteria based on clinical rationales drawn from literature review and the authors' extensive clinical experience. This guideline was updated in 2012.[5] In general, patients with lower risk disease, good life expectancy, acceptable urinary function, and favorable anatomy are good candidates for prostate brachytherapy as monotherapy. Select patients with intermediate or high risk disease might also be candidates for brachytherapy, especially as boost therapy in conjunction with external beam radiotherapy.

Medical physicists must abide by the legal requirements of using radioactive by-product material for medical purposes in their region of practice. In the United States, agreement states adopt the Nuclear Regulatory Commission (NRC) Regulations Title 10 Part 35 Use of Byproduct Material within the Code of Federal Regulations (10 CFR 35). Non-agreement states (http://nrc-stp.ornl.gov/rulemaking.html) adopt their own regulations, which are usually based on the NRC regulations.

Several societies have developed recommendations on many aspects of PSI. The ACR and ASTRO have collaborated to publish practice guidelines aimed at the whole treatment team and high level technical guidelines for physicists.[3,6] The ABS has a series of recommendations addressed to both physicians and physicists.[5,7] American Association of Physicists in Medicine (AAPM) Task Group (TG)-64 on PSI brachytherapy and AAPM TG-128, Quality Assurance Tests for Prostate Brachytherapy Ultrasound Systems[8,9] and white papers[2] offer recommendations on dosimetry and quality assurance (QA) for the physicist.

## 22.2 Sources

### LDR SOURCES, CHARACTERISTICS, ADVANTAGES, AND DISADVANTAGES

Cesium is the most recent isotope developed for PSI (see Table 22.1). Because of its very short half-life, there may be a biological advantage in faster dose delivery with possibly lower long-term complication rates. This rationale is similar to arguments driving clinical trials for prostate stereotactic body radiation therapy (SBRT) and HDR.

While some studies have shown an advantage of one isotope over another in very select clinical presentations, other studies have contradicted these findings. Clinical studies have not shown any statistically significant difference between the isotopes based on outcome or toxicity. The time to urethral and rectal toxicity development is shorter for shorter half-life isotopes. Lower energy isotopes cause the delivered dose to be more sensitive to the seed spacing.

AAPM TG-43 on brachytherapy,[10] Dosimetry of Interstitial Brachytherapy Sources, specifies the calculation of dose to tissue for the various source isotopes and source models (see Chapter 8). In 1999, NIST discovered a significant error of about 9% in determining the air kerma strength for $^{103}$Pd. The new 1999 NIST air kerma strength standard, $S_{K,N99}$, was subsequently implemented and $^{103}$Pd dose calculations adjusted accordingly. The reader should be aware of this when referencing publications on the dosimetry and clinical use of $^{103}$Pd published before the corrected standard.

### LOOSE AND STRANDED SEEDS

In the early years of PSI, sources were only available as loose seeds, either unsterilized or sterilized. Seed designs vary between vendors, which causes differences in dose distribution that are large enough that they need to be accurately modeled in treatment planning, but not so large that they would impact the decision about which seed to buy. AAPM TG-43-U1, A Revised AAPM Protocol for Brachytherapy Dose Calculations,[11] contains detailed drawings for several seed models. The general seed schema is shown in Figure 22.1. The radioactive material is packaged inside a titanium capsule with welded end caps; the cap shape and outside surface texture may vary. The isotope is mounted on a carrier substrate and packaged into pellets, rods, or cylinders. Most capsules also contain a high electron density material such as lead, silver, gold, or tungsten as markers to improve seed visibility on x-ray images.

Loose seeds provide ultimate flexibility in designing an implant. Specialized devices (e.g., the Mick applicator, Figure 22.2B) are available to automate the process of loading loose seeds into

TABLE 22.1   List of Sources and Source Characteristics

| Source | $^{103}$Pd | $^{125}$I | $^{131}$Cs | $^{198}$Au |
|---|---|---|---|---|
| Half-life (days) | 17 | 59.4 | 9.7 | 2.7 |
| Energy (keV) | 21 | 28 | 30 | 412 |
| Initial dose rate (monotherapy) (cGy/h) | 18-20 | 7 | 1.9 | N/A |
| Relative biological effectiveness (RBE) | 1.9 | 1.4 | Not known | Not known |

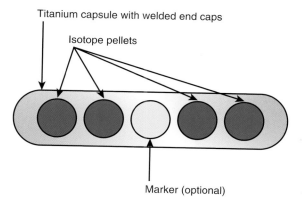

Titanium capsule with welded end caps

Isotope pellets

Marker (optional)

**Figure 22.1** Schematic of a generic prostate seed.

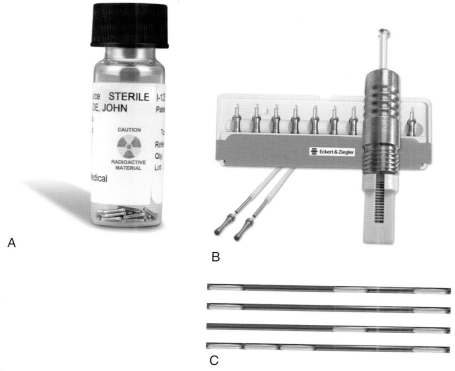

A

B

C

**Figure 22.2 A,** Loose, sterile seeds in vial for seed assay; **B,** loose seeds in Mick cartridge; **C,** stranded seeds including different spacers. *(Images courtesy of Eckert & Ziegler.)*

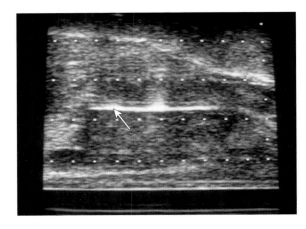

**Figure 22.3** Sagittal ultrasound image of an echogenic seed strand. *(Image courtesy of Eckert & Ziegler.)*

the applicator needle and to reduce staff exposure. However, loose seeds do migrate more easily along the needle track[12] and potentially could be lost into the bladder or, more rarely, embolize into the lung or even the brain. Different surface textures and shapes were developed to prevent seed migration. Over time, stranded seeds became available in different configurations: strands/braids of 10, chains of up to 70 seeds, preloaded needles, and devices to custom-strand seeds in the OR. The material used for strands or braids is bioabsorbable suture material. More recently, echogenic strands have been developed to increase the visibility of seed strand placement during implant (Figure 22.3). These strands consist of braided strings of bioabsorbable material, thereby increasing the complexity of the surface, which increases the visibility on ultrasound (US) (U.S. Patent US7874976 B1).

Figure 22.2 shows loose seeds (A), loose seeds in Mick cartridges (B), and stranded seeds (C). Each system has advantages and disadvantages depending on the technology and implant technique used. For example, preloaded needles require a preplan; this results in source order efficiency because the exact numbers of sources with a small additional margin of seeds needed for a patient are ordered versus creation of a source estimate using a nomogram.[13-15] It should be noted that these nomograms are seed model and potentially institution specific. On the other hand, with preordered strands there is inflexibility in adjusting the plan while in the OR. Such adjustments might be necessary in the following situations:

- Previously undetected pubic arch interference with the placement of anterior lateral needles
- Change in gland size between initial planning study and actual implant date
- Positioning change (e.g., between magnetic resonance imaging (MRI) preplan and transrectal ultrasound (TRUS) imaging during implant) causes the urethra and rectal avoidance geometry to change

Table 22.2 summarizes the uses, advantages, and disadvantages of currently available seed systems.

## SEED ASSAY

AAPM TG-40,[16] AAPM TG-56, Code of Practice for Brachytherapy Physics,[17] and AAPM TG-64[8] all contain recommendations on prostate seed source calibrations and physicist responsibilities. These task groups were published before third-party independent source assays became available. At the time, preassembled sterile sources were not in use; third-party independent assay services were not available yet. To update and clarify recommendations, the AAPM Low Energy

**TABLE 22.2 ■ Uses, Advantages, and Disadvantages of Different Seed Systems**

| Seed Type | Loose | | Stranded | | |
|---|---|---|---|---|---|
| | Unsterilized | Sterilized | Stranded in OR | Strands of 10 | Chain of up to 70 Seeds | Preloaded Needles |
| Use | Preplanned or live plan Nomogram for live plan | Preplanned or live plan Nomogram for live plan | Preplanned or live plan Nomogram for live plan | Preplanned or live plan Nomogram for live plan | Preplanned or live plan Nomogram for live plan | # of needles, seeds/ needle, and spacing determined by preplan |
| Advantage | Flexibility of implant planning in OR Direct assay of seeds used Adapt in OR based on actual location | Planning flexibility Adapt in OR based on actual location | Planning flexibility Efficient seed order Limits seed migration | Planning flexibility Limits seed migration | Planning flexibility Compact storage Efficient for # of seeds ordered Limits seed migration | Efficient implant time Limits seed migration |
| Disadvantage | Sterilization required Potential seed migration | Batch assay Potential seed migration | Batch assay Time required for stranding Possible stranding errors | Batch assay Preset spacers Less efficient for # of seeds ordered | Batch assay Preset spacers | No flexibility to adapt plan in OR |

TABLE 22.3 ■ Overview of Assay Recommendations from AAPM TG-40, AAPM TG-56, and AAPM TG-64, with LEBSC WG Superseding Earlier Recommendations

| | AAPM TG-40 (1994)/AAPM TG-56 (1997) | AAPM TG-64 (1999) | LEBSC WG (2008) |
|---|---|---|---|
| Loose, unsterilized | 10% | Random sample of at least 10% of seeds | ≥10% of total or 10 seeds, whichever is larger |
| Cartridge, unsterilized | N/A | N/A | ≥10% of total, either whole cartridge assay or individual sources |
| Stranded/ cartridge, unsterilized | 10% or 2 strands, whichever is larger | N/A | 10% or 2 strands, whichever is larger; or 5% or 5 loose seeds from same batch, whichever is larger |
| Stranded, sterilized | 1 single source from each strength batch | N/A | 10% of total, whole cartridge assay in sterile environment; or 5% or 5 loose seeds from same batch, whichever is larger |

N/A denotes no specific recommendations given.

Brachytherapy Source Calibration Working Group (LEBSC WG) was formed. The white paper on third-party brachytherapy source calibrations and physicist responsibilities[2] published by this working group contains updated recommendations for currently available source configurations and supersedes recommendations made by earlier task groups (see Table 22.3).

After a vendor manufactures the seeds, third-party assay services have the technical capabilities to assay all seeds within an order and then assemble them into the customer order either as preloaded needles or strands. The user is provided with an assay report, which provides valuable information on the distribution of seed strength within the order. The International Standards Organization/International Electrotechnical Commission (ISO/IEC) standard 17032[5] covers requirements for testing and calibration laboratories; accreditation under this standard can serve as an indicator for the quality of the third-party assay vendor. As the authors of AAPM LEBSC WG points out, there is still a residual risk of errors made by the third-party assay vendor. An example is event No. 54 in the IAEA report on accidental exposures in radiotherapy,[18] where a mismatch in units specified in the order versus vendor delivery reached the patient because the vendor assay was not double-checked. Therefore, it is the responsibility of the clinical medical physicist to verify the assay. Seed assays are performed at least a day before the implant procedure to give enough time to respond to survey results that may be outside the recommended tolerance. Table 22.4 summarizes the tolerance levels given by the AAPM LEBSC WG.

## 22.3 Treatment Planning

### PREIMPLANT PLANNING

The preimplant planning can take place either several weeks or days before the implant or in the OR on the day of implant (also called "live planning"). The ABS recommends TRUS for preimplant planning.[4] Implants performed before about 1990 relied on the Quimby[19] system, which calculates exposure rates for regular implant array patterns of linear, uniform activity sources. The source spacing was either 1 cm or 2 cm. More modern dose calculation methods and treatment planning methods have led to a technique using peripheral loading of needles with limited internal needles. This modified peripheral technique reduces the dose to the urethra.

TABLE 22.4 ▪ **Recommended Actions Based on the Sample Size Assayed and the Relative Difference, $\Delta S_K$, Found Between the Manufacturer's Source Strength Certificate and the Physicist's Source Assay**[a]

| Sample Size for Assay of Sources by End-User Medical Physicist | $\Delta S_K$ | Action by End-User Medical Physicist |
|---|---|---|
| Individual source as part of an order of ≥10 sources[b] | $\Delta S_K \leq 6\%$ | Nothing further. |
| | $\Delta S_K > 6\%$ | Consult with the radiation oncologist regarding use of the outlier source: Dependent on the radionuclide, intended target, source packaging, and availability of extra sources. |
| ≥10% but <100% of order, or batch measurements of individual sterile strands, cartridges, or preloaded needles | $\Delta S_K \leq 3\%$ | Nothing further. |
| | $5\% \geq \Delta S_K > 3\%$ | Investigate source of discrepancy or increase the sample size. |
| | $\Delta S_K > 5\%$ | Consult with manufacturer to resolve differences or increase the sample size. For assays performed in the operating room, consult with the radiation oncologist regarding whether to use the measured source strength or to average with the manufacturer's value. |
| 100% of order, or batch measurements of each and every individual sterile strand, cartridge, or preloaded needle | $\Delta S_K \leq 3\%$ | Nothing further. |
| | $5\% \geq \Delta S_K > 3\%$ | Investigate source of discrepancy. |
| | $\Delta S_K > 5\%$ | Consult with manufacturer to resolve differences. For assays performed in the operating room, consult with the radiation oncologist regarding the consequences of proceeding with the implant using the measured source strength. |

[a]Assay results obtained at sites other than the end-user institution should not replace the source strength value on the manufacturer's certificate. The source strength value to be used in planning may be either that stated on the manufacturer's certificate or the value determined by institutional medical physicist when the difference is ≥5%.
[b]For orders consisting of <10 sources, the action threshold is $\Delta S_K > 5\%$ for individual sources.
Adapted from AAPM LEBSC WG.[2]

# IMAGING FOR TREATMENT

TRUS, MRI, or CT imaging can be used for treatment planning. CT imaging is being slowly phased out as MRI, with its improved soft tissue contrast, is becoming more available in clinical practice. Because the implant itself will in most cases be performed under TRUS guidance, the shape of the prostate at the time of implant will be somewhat deformed due to the presence of the TRUS probe. Therefore, the planning image set should be one most closely resembling the prostate shape and position during implant (i.e., TRUS in most cases). Other imaging studies such as MRI can be fused to the planning image set. MRIs of the prostate can be taken either using a body coil placed over the patient's pelvic area or using an endorectal coil. While the endorectal coil does deform the prostate, the resulting anatomy may be close to the implant anatomy under TRUS, depending on coil diameter and positioning. The physician and physicist should evaluate the uncertainty of deformable registration used for image fusion to choose appropriate margins for contours.

One important component of the preplan imaging study is to assess possible pubic arch interference. A narrow pubic arch combined with a relatively large gland can make it difficult to impossible to get good needle access to the anterio-lateral sectors of the prostate. Patients with this specific anatomy are not good candidates for PSI.

If a preplanning technique is used, the positioning of the patient and the TRUS probe must be reproduced during the implant because leg position and probe position will greatly affect the anatomy. Another issue is the identification of the urethra if a Foley catheter is not used. Some institutions inject an aerated lidocaine gel solution into the urethra to make it visible on TRUS. Care must be taken to avoid rectal gas, and rectal clearing is often performed prior to the imaging study and the implant. Good contact between the probe and the rectal wall is required to achieve good imaging. A gel is often injected into the probe cover to help achieve this contact. Other systems use a solid or saline-filled probe cover. The reader is cautioned to test each system to ensure that they do not introduce scaling or distance errors as some have shown.[21]

One of the difficult aspects of imaging is the identification of the boundaries of the prostate gland, particularly at the base (superior) and apex (inferior). If a Foley catheter is used, it can help identify the base of the gland through visualization of the Foley balloon. It is common to identify the base and apex and determine the number of axial slices that contain the prostate. The length is then confirmed on sagittal views.

Institutions that are using live planning only will use the preimplant prostate volume and dimensions to estimate the number and strength of seeds to be ordered for implant. A nomogram[13-15] is the most commonly used method to derive these data. A nomogram is defined by Merriam-Webster as "A graphic representation that consists of several lines marked off to scale and arranged in such a way that by using a straight edge to connect known values on two lines an unknown value can be read at the point of intersection with another line." For a prostate seed implant, the nomogram is a two-dimensional graph relating the prostate volume for a given seed strength and prescription dose to determine the estimated number of seeds required for the implant. Figure 22.4 shows an example of a nomogram developed for prostate seed implants to determine the total activity of $^{125}$I seeds needed to deliver 145 Gy to D90 as a function of prostate diameter d.

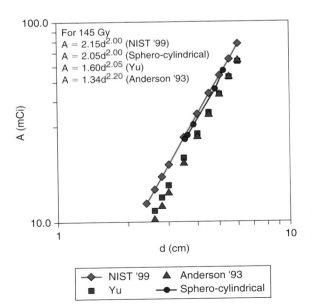

**Figure 22.4** Example of a nomogram developed for prostate seed implant. *(Adapted from Wu A, Lee C-C, Johnson M, et al. A new power law for determination of total $^{125}$I seed activity for ultrasound-guided prostate implants: clinical evaluations. Int J Radiat Oncol Biol Phys 2000;47(5):1397-1403.)*[20]

TABLE 22.5 ▪ **PSI DVH Constraints from Selected Literature**

| Organ | DVH Constraint (Rx to D90) | Isotope | Source |
|---|---|---|---|
| Prostate | 125 Gy (monotherapy)<br>100 Gy (boost) + 45 Gy (external) | [103]Pd | ABS recommendation on implementing NIST 1999[1] |
| | 144 Gy (monotherapy) | [125]I | Bice et al.[22] |
| | 140-160 Gy for D90 (monotherapy) | [125]I | Stock et al.[23] |
| | 140-200 Gy BED (low risk)<br>>200 Gy (BED) (intermediate/high risk) | [103]Pd, [125]I | Stone et al.[24] |
| | 115 Gy (monotherapy)<br>$V_{150}$ <45%<br>1.6-2.2 U source strength | [131]Cs | ABS recommendation on [131]Cs[25] |
| | 145 Gy (monotherapy) | [125]I | RTOG-9805 |
| | 108 Gy (boost) + 45 Gy (external) | [125]I | RTOG-0019 |
| | 145 Gy (monotherapy with [125]I)<br>125 Gy (monotherapy with [103]Pd)<br>110 Gy (boost with [125]I) + 45 Gy (external)<br>100 Gy (boost with [103]Pd) + 45 Gy (external) | [103]Pd, [125]I | RTOG-0232, ABS recommendation on prostate implant dose prescriptions[26] |
| Rectum* | $D_{max}$, $V_{100}$ (outer rectal wall defines volume) | [103]Pd, [125]I | RTOG-0232 |
| Urethra* | $D_{max}$ <200% of prescription dose | [103]Pd, [125]I | RTOG-0232 |

The rectum and urethra doses (*) are not planning dose constraints but parameters to be tracked in postimplant dosimetry. In clinical practice, they may be used as planning DVH constraints.

## PRESCRIPTION DOSES AND DOSE VOLUME HISTOGRAM CONSTRAINTS

Because of the differences in half-life, doses delivered by the isotopes used for PSI cannot be directly compared. Publications and protocols either recommend different doses for each isotope or calculate BEDs (biologically effective doses) using an $\alpha/\beta$ ratio of 2. Table 22.5 shows various dose volume histogram (DVH) constraints from selected publications, but typical doses for brachytherapy as monotherapy are 145 Gy with [125]I and 125 Gy with [103]Pd, and typical doses for brachytherapy boosts with external beam are 110 Gy with [125]I and 90 to 100 Gy with [103]Pd.

## WRITTEN DIRECTIVE

The NRC Regulations Title 10, Code of Federal Regulations Part 35[27] (10 CFR 35) regulates the use of by-product material. 10 CFR 35.40 covers the requirements and contents for the written directive used for the patient treatment. The written directive has two components: (1) before implant and (2) after the implant to allow for possible changes in implant strategy due to unforeseen medical circumstances arising during the implant procedure. Figure 22.5 shows a sample written directive fulfilling formal 10 CFR 35 Part 40 requirements for a permanent prostate seed implant using [125]I seeds.

The NRC has not given specific guidance on what constitutes the completion of a PSI procedure from the perspective of completing the written directive. It is therefore recommended that each institution clearly defines the end of the procedure in its Policies and Procedures (P&P) manual. Commonly used time points are (1) the patient leaving the OR or (2) the patient being released from recovery. What constitutes an accurate completion of the written directive is somewhat controversial. In the past, a dosimetric-based definition such as the dose received by 90% of the target (D90) >75% of the prescription dose was used. More recently an implanted

Doe, John
MR 11-22-33
DOB 01-01-1900

Preimplant:
Treatment Site:                           Prostate + margin (<5mm)
Intended Number of $^{125}$I Seeds: _____
Prescribed Activity (mCi):        _____
Treatment Time:                            Permanent
Date:                                          _____
AU Signature:                           _____
AU Name:                                     Dr. Who, MD

Postimplant:
Treatment Site:                           Prostate + margin (<5mm)
# of $^{125}$I Seeds Implanted:   _____
Implanted Activity (mCi):          _____
Treatment Time:                            Permanent
Date:                                          _____
AU Signature:                           _____
AU Name:                                     Dr. Who, MD

**Figure 22.5** Sample written directive.

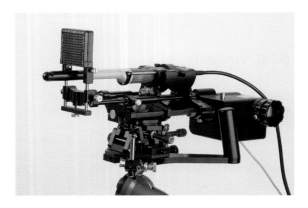

**Figure 22.6** Stepper/stabilizer with implant grid and US probe in place. *(Image courtesy of Analogic Corporation.)*

activity-based definition has been adopted.[28] As of this writing, the NRC has proposed but not finalized a new definition of what would constitute a deviation from the written directive, http://www.gpo.gov/fdsys/pkg/FR-2014-07-21/pdf/2014-16753.pdf.

## 22.4 OR Procedure

### NEEDLE INSERTION

The needle insertion takes place under image guidance to ensure the needles are implanted all the way to the prostate baseplane but not beyond, to avoid bladder perforation. The urethra and bladder bulb are often visualized using a Foley catheter filled with contrast.

A stepper/stabilizer unit attached to the OR table is used to hold the TRUS probe and the implant grid (Figure 22.6). The stepper allows the TRUS probe to be positioned in the three translational dimensions and pitch rotation to align with the patient. The implant grid used for needle guidance is mounted on the stepper at a fixed position and right angle relative to the

TRUS. At commissioning and during periodic QA, the grid position is calibrated relative to the TRUS probe and the electronic display of the implant grid on the TRUS image display. AAPM TG-128[9] Test 7 describes how to perform this test.

Computed tomography (CT)-guided needle insertion increases the imaging dose to the patient and staff compared to TRUS; lack of soft tissue contrast is another disadvantage. Magnetic resonance imaging (MRI)-guided needle implantation optimizes soft tissue contrast but is available at very few clinics and requires MR-compatible equipment. Thus the predominantly used technology for image guidance during the procedure is TRUS. The TRUS probe should have biplanar detector arrangements to provide a sagittal and transverse image. The prostate should be centered on the implant grid. The TRUS probe should be angled such that the posterior border of the prostate is parallel to the needle path. It is important to adjust the anterior-posterior position of the probe such that there is good ultrasound contact, but the pressure on the prostate should not be so high as to create a convex shape of the posterior prostate border. When using a preplan, great care must be taken to position the TRUS as closely as possible to the position of the preplan. This is achieved by matching the anatomy as closely as possible; the curvature of the urethra in the sagittal plane and calcifications in the gland are good landmarks.

The order of placing needles depends on physician preference: individual placement, placement by row, peripheral and central locations, or all at once. A portable C-arm is often used as an ancillary imaging device to the TRUS to help aid in needle visualization. The prostate does swell due to edema caused by needle positioning and can also shift position relative to the location of where the needle fixes one part of the anatomy, which can possibly cause localization uncertainties for some implant techniques.

One technique that can reliably fix prostate anatomy is the following:

- Placement of two central needles to the left and right of the urethra to fix the center of the gland.
- Implant rows from anterior to posterior rows; this has the advantage that eventual pubic arch interference is spotted early during implant, where adjustments to the plan or the implant are easiest.
- Within a row, alternate needle implant starting from midline moving out, alternating sides.

## SEED HANDLING AND SURVEY

On the day of the procedure, an authorized physicist will remove the sources from the source room and transport them in the appropriate shielding containers to the OR. The sources must be under personal supervision of an authorized user at all times. As part of the equipment, the authorized user should have a forceps, survey meter, and extra pig readily available to recover seeds that may be accidentally dropped during the procedure. Immediately after the procedure, a seed count must be performed to account for all radioactive seeds.

The following radiation surveys must be performed and documented during the procedure:

1. OR survey before the patient arrives to establish background levels
2. Survey patient before the procedure starts to establish patient background
3. OR survey of waste bins, cystoscopy bag, instrument tables, floor
4. Patient survey to determine if criteria for release of the patient are met

# 22.5 Postprocedure Follow-Up Imaging and Plan Analysis

The ACR-ASTRO practice guideline for the transperineal permanent brachytherapy of prostate cancer[3] states that postimplant dosimetry is a mandatory component of PSI for every patient, and surveys indicate that compliance with this is very high.[29] The purpose of postimplant follow-up is to verify seed count, location of seed placement, and dosimetry. The ABS recommendations for permanent prostate brachytherapy postimplant dosimetry analysis[30] are a resource for designing guidelines on postimplant dosimetry in clinical practice. Similar to external beam therapy, PSI has technical and dosimetric uncertainties that should be evaluated. In external beam, this is achieved using routine technical QA as well as studies of Type A and Type B errors (random and systematic errors) during patient treatment. Because PSI is a single-fraction treatment, the challenge lies in assessing total delivered dose during the lifetime of the implant. Seed migration (limited with the use of stranded seeds) and edema are the dominant factors introducing uncertainties. Postimplant dosimetry serves to evaluate the quality of the implant and dosimetric coverage, provides an ongoing quality control metric, and gives the clinician the opportunity to anticipate potential complications or implant additional seeds/supplement with external beam irradiation if areas of significant underdose are identified. This is particularly important since the postimplant D90 value has been shown to correlate with disease-free survival.[31,32] The importance of postimplant dosimetry was underscored by PSI misadministrations at the Philadelphia Veterans Administration hospital reported in 2009.[33] Over a period of 6 years, 92 patients received inadequate implants. Though the causal factors are complex in this case, one important finding was the weaknesses in the postimplant dosimetry program.

The timing of postimplant dosimetry varies between institutions, starting from a postimplant verification image on the same day to around day 30 after the procedure. At this time, there are no clinical data on the optimum time for follow-up. Edema and bleeding cause the gland to swell during the procedure; the average half-life of edema resolution is about 10 days, with fairly large variations between patients. Postimplant dosimetry immediately after the procedure (TRUS) or within 24 hours (CT) is often the most practical, as well as having the advantage of identifying possible underdosed areas immediately. The swelling of the gland will cause the total delivered treatment dose to be underestimated by about 10%. A follow-up study at day 30 after implant provides the most accurate dosimetric information for $^{125}$I; a 2 week follow-up study would be more appropriate for $^{103}$Pd, but the error introduced by performing a 30-day follow-up study is minor. In summary, while the exact timing of postimplant studies is still somewhat controversial, general guidelines are starting to emerge. A 2010 survey by the ABS indicates that the vast majority of practices (73%) perform postimplant dosimetry at day 30.[29] Each clinic should develop a consistent procedure for timing of postimplant imaging studies based on established practices.

Although orthogonal films can be used to visualize and confirm seed count after an implant procedure, the method is suboptimal for postimplant dosimetry because it does not allow for organ contour and DVH evaluation. TRUS is commonly used for postprocedure evaluation immediately after the implant in the OR. Modern TRUS systems, especially if used in conjunction with C-arm fluoroscopy, allow good enough visualization of implanted strands to create a good quality plan for in-OR assessment of implant quality. Access to the TRUS system outside the OR, reproducibility of TRUS positioning, and the invasive nature of the imaging modality make TRUS a rarely utilized technique for postimplant dosimetry outside the OR.

In the early days of prostate seed implants, postimplant x-rays were taken to check for possible seeds in the lung and/or brain. This procedure has been largely abandoned for several reasons:

- Seed migration into the lung or brain was a rare event for implants with loose seeds;
- Increased use of stranded seeds has lowered the probability of seed migration even further;
- Even if a seed was found to have migrated, the information was usually not acted upon because the risk of an invasive procedure to remove the stray seeds was far greater than the relatively small radiation dose from one errant seed;
- The x-ray generated unnecessary imaging dose to the lungs and brain.

TABLE 22.6 ▤ **Postimplant Reporting Recommendations**

| Source | Time (days) | Prostate | Urethra | Rectum |
|---|---|---|---|---|
| ABS recommendation on $^{131}Cs$[25] | 14 | $V_{150} < 45\%$<br>$D_{90} >$ Reference dose | 100%-140% of reference dose | $V_{100} < 0.5$ cm$^3$ |
| ABS recommendation on postimplant dosimetry[30] | Per policy | 200%, 150%, 100%, 90%, 80%, and 50% isodose lines<br>D100, D90, and D80<br>V200, V150, V100, V90, and V80<br>Prostate volume | Urethral dose length of urethra receiving >200% of the prescribed dose | Rectal dose |

$D_{90}$ has been shown to be correlated with outcome as defined by PSA levels.

CT and MRI are well suited for postimplant dosimetry, both being noninvasive and allowing for 3D image reconstruction for contour and dosimetric evaluation. Seeds are more difficult to localize on MR than on CT because they image as "no signal" areas similar to calcifications and no signal areas immediately outside the gland capsule. As a practical matter, no respondents to the 2010 ABS survey were using MRI.[29] The main challenge for CT-based postimplant dosimetry is the added contouring uncertainty at the base and apex due to the lack of soft tissue contrast compared with the other imaging modalities. Multimodality image fusion could provide additional uncertainty; however, changes in anatomy between imaging sessions will require deformable image registration, which also introduces uncertainty.

Table 22.6 summarizes recommendations on postimplant reporting parameters.

# 22.6 Safety, Policies, and Procedures

## ADMITTING PATIENTS VERSUS RELEASE

Per 10 CFR 35, the patients may be released (with written and oral instructions) if the dose to any other individual from exposure to the patient is not likely to exceed 5 mSv (0.5 rem). NUREG-1556, Vol. 9, Rev. 2, "Program-Specific Guidance About Medical Use Licenses"[34] states that a dose rate ≤1 mrem/hr at 1 meter for patients with $^{125}I$ implants meets the criteria. Instructions do not need to be provided if the dose rate at 1 m is ≤1 mrem/hr. See Chapter 10 for more information related to release criteria.

If the dose rate exceeds 1 mrem/hr, the patient needs to be admitted until the source activity has decayed below the release criteria. Policies and procedures should be in place to describe the legally required radiation signage as well as nursing and other staff education about radiation exposure to staff and visitors. A special situation can arise when the patient is fulfilling the dose rate criteria for release but develops medical issues in recovery that require admittance. The clinic should develop a process to ensure the attending physicians notify the clinical physicist.

## EQUIPMENT QA AND MAINTENANCE

AAPM TG-128[9] provides in-depth guidance on QA for PSI TRUS systems. The ACR technical standard for diagnostic medical physics performance monitoring of real-time ultrasound equipment[35] provides general guidance on ultrasound QA for diagnostic radiology. The treatment planning system QA should follow the general concepts outlined in AAPM TG-53, Quality Assurance for Clinical Radiotherapy Treatment Planning,[36] with dose calculations referring to the recommendations given by AAPM TG-43[8] and its updates[11] and supplement.[37]

TABLE 22.7 ■ Sample List of Procedures and Guidance Documents for PSI

| Staff | Policy |
|---|---|
| All | PSI procedure overview<br>Follow-up procedure |
| Physician | Written directive<br>Preimplant volume study<br>Patient wallet card<br>Patient selection criteria/DVH goals |
| Nursing | Nursing care for patients admitted after PSI |
| Physics | Emergency procedure<br>OR survey form<br>Day of implant procedure<br>Radioactive source handling, storage, and assay<br>TPS QA procedure<br>TRUS QA procedure<br>Nomogram description<br>Physics checklist |

PSI equipment has to undergo sterilization between procedures and is often stored away from the Radiation Oncology department near the OR (e.g., stepper, TRUS). It is essential to educate all staff involved on appropriate handling and the fragility of equipment. Parts that are mechanically calibrated (e.g., the washers defining the position of the grid above the TRUS) need to be checked periodically for integrity and accuracy. If possible, the correct mechanical position of calibrated parts should be marked.

## POLICIES AND PROCEDURES

PSI is a complex procedure involving two medical specialties (urology and Radiation Oncology), OR and departmental nurses, medical physicists, OR technicians, and radiation therapists. In the commissioning phase of a new prostate seed implant program, it is important to develop clear guidance on the roles and responsibilities of each staff member. Performing a dry run of the complete treatment process from initial US imaging to final postimplant planning is a useful tool to test procedures and find possible weak links or identify areas where further clarification is needed. Using commercial prostate seed implant phantoms and dummy seeds, test runs of the implant procedure are quite feasible to perform and provide useful training opportunities for the patient care team.

Table 22.7 shows a sample set of procedures and guidance documents that are helpful in defining procedural standards and ensuring regulatory requirements are followed. The procedures and guidance documents should be stored in a place where they are easily accessible to all staff members involved in the PSI program. If documents are stored digitally, they should be locked down to prevent any changes unless under formal review. Procedures and guidance documents should be formally reviewed annually; any changes should be communicated to all staff involved through a read-and-sign process.

## STAFF REQUIREMENTS AND TIME

Qualifications and responsibilities of personnel are outlined in the ACR-ASTRO practice guideline for the transperineal permanent brachytherapy of prostate cancer.[3] Specifically, the guideline states the radiation oncologist should have either formal training on PSI during an Accreditation Council for Graduate Medical Education (ACGME)-approved residency or fellowship or have

TABLE 22.8 ▪ **Sample Time Estimates for Each Prostate Seed Implant Procedure Step and Staff Involved for Real-Time Planning**

| Procedure | Step | Duration | Staff |
|---|---|---|---|
| >14 days before procedure | Treatment planning imaging | 1-2 hours | Urologist, radiation oncologist |
| 10 days before | Nomogram and seed order | 1-2 hours | Physicist |
| 3 days before | Source receipt | 1 hour | Radiation safety officer, medical physicist |
| 2 days before | Source assay | 1 hour | Physicist |
| Day of procedure | Seed transport to OR, equipment setup and survey | 1 hour | Physicist |
| | Patient preparation, anesthesia, preimplant imaging | 1 hour | Physicians, nurses, physicist |
| | Contouring | 15 minutes | Physician |
| | Treatment planning | 30 minutes | Physicist |
| | Needle placement and source implant | 1 hour | Physician/physicist |
| | Postimplant imaging and documentation | 10 minutes | Physician/physicist |
| | Postimplant survey, source transport to storage, documentation | 30 minutes | Physicist |
| | Postimplant physics documentation | 1 hour | Physicist |
| 30 days after | Postimplant imaging | 1 hour | Radiation therapist |
| | Contour | 30 minutes | Physician |
| | Postimplant plan and documentation | 2 hours | Physicist |

received appropriate training in TRUS, CT, and/or MR imaging as applicable and have been proctored for at least five cases to gain personalized supervised experience with the procedure. The medical physicist is strongly recommended to have board certification, should meet continuing medical education (CME) criteria specified in the ACR practice guideline for CME, and adhere to all local requirements for staff credentialing and licensing.

The time for each step in the process can vary based on the technique used and the relative skill of the team members. Table 22.8 shows sample time estimates for each step in a sample procedure using stranded seeds and intraoperative treatment planning, including the staff involved. It is helpful for each center to analyze the time and staffing required for each procedural step to allow for adequate allocation of resources.

### FOR THE PHYSICIAN

A prostate seed implant program is a highly specialized procedure requiring a well-trained team and specialized equipment. Like any surgical procedure, a minimum number of proctored cases are required for training, and enough procedures should be performed per year to maintain skill levels. This is underscored by surveys which indicate that the majority of physicians practicing brachytherapy have not received formal training in residency.[29] As resources, ACR, ASTRO, AAPM, and ABS all have recommendations and guidelines on various aspects of the brachytherapy process.

The implementation of a prostate seed implant program requires significant investment in equipment and administrative support:

- A stepper/stabilizer, US, and treatment planning unit
- Hot lab for the secure storage of sources, including source safe, survey meters, and well chambers for source assay

- Imaging equipment
- Facility radiation use permit
- Development of policies and procedures

A thorough, in-depth understanding of equipment functionality is the basis for safe use during the procedure by both physician and physicist. Commercial prostate phantoms are available for use in dry runs of the procedure. These dry runs can serve as end-to-end tests to verify that all procedures and equipment are in place, staff roles are clearly identified, and any remaining questions are resolved before the first patient implant.

For staffing, the medical physicist(s) should be certified by the ABR or equivalent organization in the appropriate subspecialty (i.e., therapeutic medical physics). In addition, the physicist should participate in Maintenance of Certification (MOC) and follow all licensing and/or credentialing requirements. Since a variety of options are available for seeds and applicators, the physicist must be aware that different seed assay requirements exist for seeds that are loose versus stranded versus preloaded into needles. There are also third-party vendors that provide assay services, although mistakes can still occur and the clinical medical physicist should still verify the assay.

In light of previously reported misadministrations during prostate seed implants discussed above, it cannot be emphasized enough that imaging during and after the implant procedure is an essential part of ensuring a high quality implant and optimal outcomes for the procedure. The low soft tissue contrast of many imaging modalities (i.e., TRUS, MRI, CT) used for prostate seed implants requires a trained eye to correctly and accurately identify the treatment target and critical structures during the contouring and implant process. If a preplanning technique is used, the positioning of the patient and the TRUS probe must be reproduced during the implant because leg position and probe position will greatly affect the anatomy.

Multiple surveys are required on the day of the implant procedure: OR survey before the patient arrives; patient survey before the procedure starts; OR survey after the procedure including waste bins, cystoscopy bag, instrument tables, and the floor; and patient survey to determine if criteria for release of the patient are met. Postimplant dosimetry should be performed to verify seed count, location of seed placement, and implant dosimetry.

There are also guidelines on QA for PSI TRUS systems. PSI equipment has to undergo sterilization between procedures. It is essential to educate all staff involved on appropriate handling of the equipment. Parts that are mechanically calibrated need to be checked periodically for integrity and accuracy.

## References

1. Beyer D, Nath R, Butler W, et al. American Brachytherapy Society recommendations for clinical implementation of NIST-1999 standards for [103]palladium brachytherapy. Int J Radiat Oncol Biol Phys 2000;47(2):273–5.
2. Butler WM, Bice WS Jr, DeWerd LA, et al. Third-party brachytherapy source calibrations and physicist responsibilities: Report of the AAPM Low Energy Brachytherapy Source Calibration Working Group. Med Phys 2008;35(9):3860–5.
3. Rosenthal SA, Bittner NH, Beyer DC, et al. American Society for Radiation Oncology (ASTRO) and American College of Radiology (ACR) practice guideline for the transperineal permanent brachytherapy of prostate cancer. Int J Radiat Oncol Biol Phys 2011;79(2):335–41.
4. Nag S, Beyer D, Friedland J, et al. American Brachytherapy Society (ABS) recommendations for transperineal permanent brachytherapy of prostate cancer. Int J Radiat Oncol Biol Phys 1999;44(4):789–99.
5. Davis BJ, Horwitz EM, Lee WR, et al. American Brachytherapy Society consensus guidelines for transrectal ultrasound-guided permanent prostate brachytherapy. Brachytherapy 2012;11:6–19. http://www.americanbrachytherapy.org/guidelines/Guidelines_Transrectal_Ultrasound.pdf.
6. ACR-ASTRO practice parameter for transperineal permanent brachytherapy of prostate cancer, 2014, http://www.acr.org/~/media/ACR/Documents/PGTS/guidelines/Brachy_Prostate_Cancer.pdf.

7. http://www.americanbrachytherapy.org/guidelines/prostate_low-doseratetaskgroup.pdf.
8. Yu Y, Anderson LL, Li Z, et al. Permanent prostate seed implant brachytherapy: Report of the American Association of Physicists in Medicine Task Group No. 64. Med Phys 1999;26(10):2054–76.
9. Pfeiffer D, Sutlief S, Feng W, et al. AAPM Task Group 128: Quality assurance tests for prostate brachytherapy ultrasound systems. Med Phys 2008;35(12):5471–89.
10. Meigooni AS. Dosimetry of interstitial brachytherapy sources: Recommendations. Med Phys 1995; 22(2):2.
11. Rivard MJ, Coursey BM, DeWerd LA, et al. Update of AAPM Task Group No. 43 Report: A revised AAPM protocol for brachytherapy dose calculations. Med Phys 2004;31(3):633–74.
12. Reed DR, Wallner KE, Merrick GS, et al. A prospective randomized comparison of stranded vs. loose [125]I seeds for prostate brachytherapy. Brachytherapy 2007;6(2):129–34.
13. Pujades MC, Camacho C, Perez-Calatayud J, et al. The use of nomograms in LDR-HDR prostate brachytherapy. J Contemp Brachytherapy 2011;3(3):121.
14. Cohen GN, Amols HI, Zelefsky MJ, et al. The Anderson nomograms for permanent interstitial prostate implants: A briefing for practitioners. Int J Radiat Oncol Biol Phys 2002;53(2):504–11.
15. Li T, Fountain BL, Duffy EW. Physical derivation of nomograms in permanent prostate brachytherapy. Brachytherapy 2010;9(1):50–4.
16. Kutcher GJ, Coia L, Gillin M, et al. Comprehensive QA for Radiation Oncology: Report of AAPM Radiation Therapy Committee Task Group 40. Med Phys 1994;21(4):581–618.
17. Nath R, Anderson LL, Meli JA, et al. Code of practice for brachytherapy physics: Report of the AAPM Radiation Therapy Committee Task Group No. 56. Med Phys 1997;24(10):1557–98.
18. Ortiz P. Lessons learned from accidental exposures in radiotherapy. IAEA Safety Reports Series. Vienna: International Atomic Energy Agency; 2000.
19. Quimby EH. The grouping of radium tubes in packs and plaques to produce the desired distribution of radiation. Am J Roentgenol 1932;27:18–36.
20. Wu A, Lee C-C, Johnson M, et al. A new power law for determination of total [125]I seed activity for ultrasound-guided prostate implants: Clinical evaluations. Int J Radiat Oncol Biol Phys 2000;47(5): 1397–403.
21. Diamantopoulos S, Milickovic N, Butt S, et al. Effect of using different U/S probe standoff materials in image geometry for interventional procedures: the example of prostate. J Contemp Brachytherapy 2011;3(4):209–19.
22. Bice WS Jr, Prestidge BR, Prete JJ, et al. Clinical impact of implementing the recommendations of AAPM Task Group 43 on permanent prostate brachytherapy using [125]I. American Association of Physicists in Medicine. Int J Radiat Oncol Biol Phys 1998;40(5):1237–41.
23. Stock RG, Stone NN, Tabert A, et al. A dose–response study for [125]I prostate implants. Int J Radiat Oncol Biol Phys 1998;41(1):101–8.
24. Stone NN, Potters L, Davis BJ, et al. Customized dose prescription for permanent prostate brachytherapy: Insights from a multicenter analysis of dosimetry outcomes. Int J Radiat Oncol Biol Phys 2007;69(5):1472–7.
25. Bice WS, Prestidge BR, Kurtzman SM, et al. Recommendations for permanent prostate brachytherapy with [131]Cs: A consensus report from the Cesium Advisory Group. Brachytherapy 2008;7(4):290–6.
26. Rivard MJ, Butler WM, Devlin PM, et al. American Brachytherapy Society recommends no change for prostate permanent implant dose prescriptions using iodine-125 or palladium-103. Brachytherapy 2007;6(1):34–7.
27. Commission NR. Medical use of byproduct material. 10 CFR Part 35. Washington, DC, 2007.
28. Nag S, Demanes DJ, Hagan M, et al. Definition of medical event is to be based on the total source strength for evaluation of permanent prostate brachytherapy: A report from the American Society for Radiation Oncology. Pract Radiat Oncol 2011;1(4):218–23.
29. Buyyounouski MK, Davis BJ, Prestidge BR, et al. A survey of current clinical practice in permanent and temporary prostate brachytherapy: 2010 update. Brachytherapy 2012;11(4):299–305.
30. Nag S, Bice W, DeWyngaert K, et al. The American Brachytherapy Society recommendations for permanent prostate brachytherapy postimplant dosimetric analysis. Int J Radiat Oncol Biol Phys 2000;46(1): 221–30.
31. Potters L, et al. A comprehensive review of CT-based dosimetry parameters and biochemical control in patients treated with permanent prostate brachytherapy. Int J Radiat Oncol Biol Phys 2001;50(3): 605–14.

32. Zelefsky MJ, Kuban DA, Levy LB, et al. Multi-institutional analysis of long-term outcome for stages T1-T2 prostate cancer treated with permanent seed implantation. Int J Radiat Oncol Biol Phys 2007;67(2):327–33.
33. Bogdanich W. At V.A. Hospital, a Rogue Cancer Unit. New York Times; June 20, 2009.
34. http://www.nrc.gov/reading-rm/doc-collections/nuregs/staff/sr1556/v9/nureg-1556-9.pdf.
35. ACR technical standard for diagnostic medical physics performance monitoring of real time ultrasound equipment. American College of Radiology (ACR), 2011.
36. Fraass B, Doppke K, Hunt M, et al. American Association of Physicists in Medicine Radiation Therapy Committee Task Group 53: Quality assurance for clinical radiotherapy treatment planning. Med Phys 1998;25(10):1773–829.
37. Rivard MJ, Butler WM, DeWerd LA, et al. Supplement to the 2004 update of the AAPM Task Group No. 43 Report. Med Phys 2007;34(6):2187–205.

# CHAPTER 23

# Intraoperative Radiotherapy (IORT)

## 23.1 Introduction

The goal of intraoperative radiotherapy (IORT) is to deliver a single high dose of radiation at the time of surgery to enhance tumor control. IORT is typically useful in cases where a complete surgical resection will be difficult. For example, a locally invasive tumor might surround a nerve or blood vessel that cannot be resected, or a tumor may invade into a bone that cannot be fully cut away. In such cases, irradiation of the tumor site during surgery may play a role in controlling disease. IORT also has a role in cases in which previous external beam radiotherapy (EBRT) has been delivered and critical structures have already reached tolerance doses. There are advantages to irradiating in the intraoperative setting, among them the ability to directly visualize the tumor bed and the ability to directly shield or move sensitive structures out of the treatment field. Further clinical background can be found in the textbook *Intraoperative Irradiation.*[1]

Support for the use of IORT comes mainly from single-institution studies; large randomized trials have been difficult to conduct. In the 1990s, for example, the Radiation Therapy Oncology Group (RTOG) began a phase III trial of IORT for pancreas and colorectal cancer but could not complete enrollment, and the IORT committee was subsequently disbanded. Nevertheless, there are numerous institutional studies and also pooled retrospective studies from Europe that support IORT. Some applications include colorectal cancer (locally advanced or unresectable for curative intent), pancreas and gastric cancer (where there is residual disease after resection), sarcomas of the abdomen or pelvis, breast cancers, and gynecological cancers that are locally recurrent.

An important disease site for IORT is breast cancer. IORT is one way of providing accelerated partial breast irradiation (APBI). The rationale for this treatment is to provide local control following breast conserving surgery since the site of recurrence is often the lumpectomy cavity. Recently, 5-year outcomes data were reported from the TARGIT-A trial,[2] a large international randomized control trial that compares adjuvant whole breast EBRT to IORT. The 5-year local recurrence rates in the IORT-only arm were not statistically different from the EBRT arm, and there were fewer non-cancer deaths (e.g., related to cardiovascular disease). The authors conclude that IORT has a role in select breast cancer patients. IORT has also been used in breast cancer as a replacement for the boost portion of the course of treatment.[3] One theory used to explain the positive results is that the sterilization of the wound fluid during surgery with radiation helps to prevent residual tumor cell growth.[4]

In many situations outside of breast cancer IORT is used in combination with EBRT, with EBRT often being delivered prior to surgery. In this setting, typical IORT doses are:[1]

- 7.5 to 10 Gy for negative or close margins
- 10 to 12.5 Gy for positive margins
- 15 to 20 Gy for gross residual disease or tumor that is unresectable

The margin status can be determined intraoperatively via frozen tissue pathology. In patients with recurrent disease who have received previous irradiation, it may not be safe to deliver high doses of EBRT, and so higher doses of IORT (15 to 20 Gy) may be delivered in order to compensate. The dose limiting structures depend on the site. In the pelvis, for example, the dose of IORT that can be safely delivered is limited by peripheral neuropathy and urethral stenosis. Surgical anastomoses are another at-risk structure. In many cases (roughly a half to a third of cases at some institutions), surgeries that begin as possible IORT candidates end up not being candidates for IORT because of the operative results.

## 23.2 Technologies and Techniques for IORT

A variety of technologies are available for delivering IORT, as summarized in Table 23.1. Each has clinical and practical advantages and disadvantages.

### INTRAOPERATIVE ELECTRON RADIOTHERAPY WITH LINEAR ACCELERATORS

Intraoperative electron radiotherapy (IOERT) uses electron beams (up to 12 MeV) produced from a linear accelerator (linac). Up until the 1990s, and in some instances later, some centers had a dedicated linac vault that could serve as an OR for this purpose. The development of mobile linacs has enabled more widespread use of IOERT. IOERT is the subject of two American

TABLE 23.1 ▦ **Technologies for Delivering IORT and Associated Advantages and Disadvantages**

| Technology | System Description | Advantages | Disadvantages |
|---|---|---|---|
| HDR brachytherapy | $^{192}$Ir remote afterloader + surface applicator or interstitial needles | • Conformal planning is possible & structure avoidance<br>• Accessibility of tumor bed (e.g., abdominal wall or base of skull)<br>• Can treat large tumor | • Restricted to treating a 0.5 cm thick tumor bed (surface applicator)<br>• Shielded OR room is needed<br>• Long treatment times (>1 hr in some cases).<br>• Source replacement each 90 days |
| Low kV | Intrabeam. Electron beam on a gold target inside a spherical applicator | • Shielded OR not required<br>• Well suited to spherical targets<br>• Surface and shallow depth applicators available<br>• Has independent dose monitoring system | • Limited to small volumes<br>• Moderately long treatments (15-30 minutes) |
| Low kV | Electronic brachytherapy, Xoft/Axxent, 50 kVp miniature x-ray tube inside a catheter | • Shielded OR not required<br>• Well suited to spherical targets | • Limited to small volumes<br>• Spherical applicators mainly (others under development)<br>• Moderately long treatments (15-30 minutes)<br>• No independent dose monitoring system |
| Intraoperative electron radiotherapy (IOERT) | Mobile linear accelerator, Mobetron, Novac-7, or LIAC | • Treats deep tumors<br>• Short treatment times (2-5 minutes)<br>• Minimal OR shielding requirements | • Cone and linac can limit access to tumor bed<br>• Placing cone can be a challenge<br>• Field size typically limited to 10 cm × 10 cm, though patching is possible |

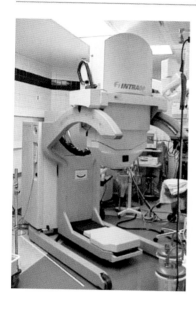

**Figure 23.1** Mobile IOERT linac Mobetron (IntraOp Inc.) generating electrons from 6 to 12 MeV. The linac couples with a metal applicator cone in the patient using a "soft-docking" mechanism. The beam stop (bottom) shields for photon contaminants making it possible to deploy in unshielded ORs. *(From Beddar AS, Biggs PJ, Chang S, et al. Intraoperative radiation therapy using mobile electron linear accelerators: Report of AAPM Radiation Therapy Committee Task Group No. 72. Med Phys 2006;33(5):1476-1489.)*

Association of Physicists in Medicine (AAPM) Task Groups (TG): up until the 1990s, and in some instances later, (1) AAPM TG-48 from 1995[5] and (2) AAPM TG-72 on IORT with mobile linacs published in 2006,[6] which largely supplants AAPM TG-48.

Three mobile IOERT units are commercially available: Mobetron (Intraoperative Medical Systems, Inc., Santa Clara, CA), Novac-7 (Hitesys SRL, Aprilia, Italy), and LIAC (Italy). The Mobetron (Figure 23.1) was first used at University of California San Francisco in 1997 and is the most widely used system in the United States. It is described in detail in AAPM TG-72, though the system has been modified somewhat since that report was published. It uses a compact linac operating in the X-band 10 GHz frequency (most other linacs are S-band accelerators at 3 GHz, making them approximately 3 times larger). As currently marketed, it provides electron beams at energies of 6 MeV, 9 MeV, and 12 MeV at high dose rates (approximately 10 Gy/min), which facilitates procedures in the operating room (OR). The effective source-to-surface distance (SSD) is 50 cm. The linac is mounted on a C-arm that allows it to be positioned with a ±45° gantry tilt (in the left-right axis for a patient whose head is pointed toward the gantry) and head tilt of +10 to −30° (superior-inferior axis). This enables easier positioning during the procedure, although positioning is often still a challenge. Metal applicators are used to collimate the electron beam. Applicator sizes range from 3 cm to 10 cm circles, available in 0.5 cm increments. The end of the applicator is either flat or beveled at 15° or 30°. The bevel provides better access to some locations such as the pelvic sidewall. Typically a 1 cm margin is used around the involved tumor area. During the procedure, the appropriate (sterile) applicator is selected and affixed to the OR table with a Buckwalter clamp. After the applicator is in place in the patient, the linac is then aligned to the upper face of the applicator. The Mobetron employs a laser-based "soft-docking" mechanism for this purpose, while the Novac-7 and LIAC systems use hard-docking to attach the applicator to the linac. Soft-docking means that the accelerator is physically decoupled from the applicator in the patient, thereby reducing the chance of direct interaction with the patient. Respiratory motion can be a challenge when creating a docking; the dock must be set at mid-inhale to stay within tolerance.

Shields are sometimes used to reduce the dose to critical structures in IOERT. A common shield is lead covered in saline-soaked gauze, the goal of which is to reduce transmitted dose by 90%. Some IOERT texts claim to use a 1 to 2 mm thick lead sheet,[1] though this is likely not enough given the Rp/10 (Rp is the practical range of the electron beam) rule of thumb for lead shields. Gauze packing can also be used to effectively move structures out of (or occasionally into) the irradiation field. In IOERT prescriptions are typically set to the 90% isodose line. Bolus (0.5 cm, 1.0 cm thick) can be used to increase surface dose and/or reduce the depth of penetration. It is important to include the shield and bolus items in the OR instrumentation count.

Acceptance testing and commissioning of IOERT equipment are described in AAPM TG-72 with institutional experience reported in Mills et al.[7] The following measurement tasks are required: percent depth dose (PDD), profiles, applicator factors (relative to a standard 10 cm applicator, typically specified at $d_{max}$ and often measured with an electron diode), and air gap factors (since applicators cannot always be placed in direct contact with the tissue). Given the number of applicators, the measurement tasks involved can be extensive. Additionally, leakage outside the applicator should be measured; this can be as high as 25% of the prescribed dose. Finally, the output should be calibrated with AAPM TG-51, Protocol for Clinical Reference Dosimetry of High-Energy Photon and Electron Beams,[8] or equivalent. AAPM TG-72 notes the special case of the Novac-7, which has a large dose per pulse (>10 mGy/pulse). In such cases ion recombination effects can become extremely large and result in dose errors of up to 20%. AAPM TG-72 recommends against using ion chamber calibration protocols in this regime. Fricke dosimeters have been used.

Quality assurance tests and frequencies are outlined in Table VI.1 in AAPM TG-72. These largely adhere to AAPM TG-142, Quality Assurance of Medical Accelerators, recommendations for linear accelerators with some differences (e.g., daily check of beam energy).[9] The docking mechanism should be checked on a daily basis. It is considered acceptable to do the daily tests the night before to accommodate OR accessibility. The docking alignment should be measured monthly. Beam flatness should be measured monthly, as well as at least annually with the soft-docking system in place. AAPM TG-72 also specifically recommends that prior to the first patient treatment, an outside audit of dose calibration be employed. QA tests are often complicated by access to the OR and workload limits.

Shielding requirements for mobile linacs are minimal due to their low energy (12 MeV electrons). Mobile linacs do, however, produce some photon leakage and scatter, which must be considered in situating them in an OR, which typically does not have shielding. The Mobetron has a beam stop behind the patient to intercept photon contaminants, but extrafocal components are still present. Krechtov et al.[10] present a shielding study for the Mobetron unit and conclude that loads of 5 to 6 patients per week can fit within the workload limits of a typical OR, though this must be verified for each facility with shielding calculations and surveys. In considering workload it is important to include the daily warm-up and QA since this can be as large as or larger than the actual beam on-time used for treatments. Investigations have shown that below 12 MeV there is very little neutron contamination,[11] so this component can be safely ignored. If shielding is not sufficient it may be possible to use more than one OR room or to deploy mobile barriers. These considerations often result in the need to place the device in a shielded vault during commissioning because the number of monitor units is very large. There are other considerations for use of an IOERT linac in an OR, including availability of appropriate power and the structural load-bearing capacity of the floors.

## LOW kV IORT AND ELECTRONIC BRACHYTHERAPY

There are two low kV x-ray devices currently on the market. The ASTRO emerging technology committee published a report in 2010 that reviews these technologies.[12] Complete task group–level reports are lacking for these systems, but information on calibration and QA for these units can be found in AAPM Report 152 and in the 2007 AAPM response to the Conference of Radiation Control Program Directors, Inc. (CRCPD) request for recommendations for the CRCPD's model regulations for electronic brachytherapy. AAPM TG-182 on electronic

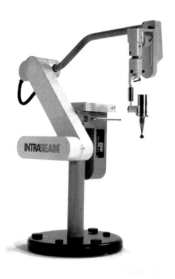

**Figure 23.2**  The Intrabeam device (Carl Zeiss Surgical, Oberkochen, Germany). A 50 kV electron beam is accelerated onto a gold target in the applicator to produce an x-ray dose distribution that is approximately spherically uniform. *(From Park CC, Yom SS, Podgorsak MB, et al. American Society for Therapeutic Radiology and Oncology (Astro) Emerging Technology Committee Report on electronic brachytherapy. Int J Radiat Oncol Biol Phys 2010;76: 963-972.)*

brachytherapy QA is in progress. Further information on the commissioning and QA of these systems can be found in Chapter 4. In the remainder of this section, the two currently available systems will be described separately. Though the systems share some similarities in the way x-rays are produced (a low kV electron source accelerated to a metal target), they are very different in their physical dimensions and methods of application.

The first device, the Intrabeam (Carl Zeiss Surgical, Oberkochen, Germany), was originally developed for the brain but is now commonly used for the breast. It is well suited for irradiating quasi-spherical cavities. The device, shown in Figure 23.2, accelerates an electron beam to the end of a 10 cm tube where it hits a 3.2 mm diameter gold target to produce x-rays that emerge in an approximately spherically uniform distribution. On the tip of the source pole one attaches a spherical polyetherimide plastic applicator available in sizes from 1.5 cm to 5 cm in steps of 0.5 cm (3 to 5 cm applicators are often used). The unit is mounted on a floor stand that accommodates 6-degrees-of-freedom positioning. A suture is used to close the cavity around the applicator, and the skin is retracted. Conformity of the tissue to the applicator is important and can be checked with ultrasound. Skin dose can be measured with radiochromic film or OSLD placed in sterile packaging. Care must be taken to suction out the seroma fluid in the lumpectomy cavity because this can have a strong impact on dose.

Dose is typically prescribed to 5 Gy at 1 cm depth, which results in approximately 20 Gy to the surface, depending on the applicator size. Treatment times are 15 minutes to 30 minutes. Internal shielding is typically not needed unless the applicator is within 1 cm of a rib or chest wall, which may happen in thin patients and/or medial lesions. Because it operates at low kV, the device does not require a shielded OR. Exposures have been measured at 12 to 15 mR/h at 2 m from the applicator.[12] No society-level reports have appeared on the dosimetry or QA of the Intrabeam device, but several single-institution studies are available.[13,14] In brain applications the treatment is delivered using the bare x-ray probe. Surface applicators are available for pelvic/abdominal treatments as well as skin treatments.

The Xoft Axxent electronic brachytherapy source (Xoft Inc., Fremont, CA) was FDA approved in 2006 and is being used for IORT, particularly for the breast. The system uses a miniature x-ray tube (2.2 mm diameter × 10 mm long) in a water-cooled catheter. As such it is classified as electronic brachytherapy. The sources have a 2.5 hr lifetime and are designed to be disposable. The tube operates up to 50 kV and is heavily filtered, providing a radial dose function similar to a low energy brachytherapy source. The relevant report on dosimetry of such beams is AAPM TG-61, Protocol for 40-300 kV X-Ray Beam Dosimetry in Radiotherapy and Radiobiology.[15]

For breast treatments the Xoft system is used with a balloon applicator (sizes 3 to 6 cm) for treatment of tissue 1 to 2 cm deep. This can be used either for a single dose IORT treatment, or if the balloon applicator is left in the cavity, it can be used to deliver fractionated treatments (typically 10 fractions of 3.4 Gy/fraction delivered BID). Further review of balloon applicators for fractionated breast treatment can be found in Chapters 20 and 21 and Strauss and Dickler.[16] These include the $^{192}$Ir-based MammoSite, Contura, and Savi applicators. The Xoft system has other applicators that may extend its use beyond breast IORT. These include flap applicators (like the HAM applicator discussed in the next section), surface cones, and expandable planar applicators for laparoscopic surgeries. The Xoft system does not require a shielded OR.

## HIGH DOSE RATE BRACHYTHERAPY

Finally, IORT can be delivered using high dose rate (HDR) brachytherapy. Surface applicators are placed in the patient and have guide tubes through which the HDR source travels. An example is the HAM applicator (Harrison-Anderson-Mick; Mick Radio-Nuclear Instruments Inc., NY),[17] an 8 mm thick silicone sheet with guide tubes at separations of 10 mm. The Freiburg Flap applicator is another example, which employs a mesh-like array of connected spheres. The applicator sheets can be cut to the necessary size in the OR. HDR-based IORT offers the advantage of being able to treat large tumor beds and to reach relatively inaccessible regions such as the pelvic sidewall and "go where no cone has gone before."

During an HDR IORT procedure a treatment plan is typically chosen from an atlas of plans of various square and rectangular sizes that are predefined to optimize the dose uniformity at the treatment depth. The prescription dose is typically set to a depth of 0.5 cm at the center of the applicator. As such, HDR-based IORT is most often used to treat superficial tissue, although some centers have used interstitial brachytherapy to treat tumor beds deeper than 0.5 cm. Lead disks (approximately 3 mm thick) may be placed to protect critical structures. The advantages of HDR IORT in terms of flexibility must be weighed against the need for a shielded OR and relatively long treatment time. Treatment time can be in excess of an hour in some cases, which has implications for anesthesia procedures and the arrangement of monitoring equipment.

Further information about HDR brachytherapy and applications can be found in Chapters 8, 20, and 21. A key reference is AAPM TG-59, High Dose-Rate Brachytherapy Treatment Delivery,[18] though this is not specific to IORT. As described there, rigorous quality assurance tests of the equipment and procedures are required. Staff should also undergo annual safety and emergency procedures training, which includes what to do with a stuck source failure.

# 23.3 Safety, Staffing, and OR Considerations

Because IORT takes place in the OR, special considerations are warranted. First are the requirements of the sterile environment, which is especially important given that postoperative infections are a leading cause of morbidity and mortality in the United States and elsewhere. Equipment must be sterile. IOERT applicators can be heat/flash sterilized if they are metal or gas EtOH sterilized if they are constructed of aluminum or PMMA. The latter can result in cracks after repeat sterilization. HDR applicators must also be sterile, which requires a sterilization procedure if they are opened for inspection and testing prior to the procedure. More generally, all staff must understand the protocols for sterile fields and maintaining a sterile environment in the OR. The Association of periOperative Registered Nurses (AORN) has developed a set of guidelines, a key component of which is communication and a team approach, which includes the Radiation Oncology delivery team.

Finally, good communications and training are important beyond just maintaining a sterile environment. Radiation oncologists and surgeons must work together closely to identify the area to be treated and any at-risk structures. The whole delivery team must work together in getting the applicators into place and, in the case of IOERT, docking the patients. This may require moving the patient in some cases. Cross-training of staff on the principles of radiation delivery and aspects of safety promotes the effectiveness of the team.

## FOR THE PHYSICIAN

Intraoperative radiotherapy (IORT) can be used to deliver large single doses of radiation up to 20 Gy to improve local control and potentially survival. Large randomized trials have been difficult to conduct, but encouraging results are emerging from the TARGIT-A trial on IORT for localized breast cancer, which has recently reported 5-year outcomes data. IORT is useful in other sites as well where a complete resection would be difficult. These can include locally advanced colorectal cancer, pancreatic cancer, gastric cancer, sarcomas of the abdomen or pelvis, and gynecologic cancers. Typical doses range from 7.5 to 20 Gy depending on the situation (e.g., negative margins versus gross residual disease). Techniques are available to control the dose to critical structures such as nerves, urethra, or surgical anastomoses. Surgical packing can be used to move structures out of the field. Lead shields (≈3 mm thick) can be placed to shield critical structures, such as the chest wall in a thin woman with breast cancer.

Three main technologies are available for delivering IORT:

1. A compact mobile linac delivering electrons of energy 6 to 12 MeV. This technique, commonly referred to as IOERT (intraoperative electron radiotherapy), employs an applicator cone placed into the patient that docks up to the mobile linac in the OR. Three units are commercially available: the Mobetron (widest use in the United States) and the Novak-7 and LIAC from Italy. IOERT is the subject of the AAPM TG-72 report.
2. High dose radiation (HDR) IORT using an HDR brachytherapy source coupled with a surface applicator (e.g., the HAM applicator with guide tubes). This is particularly useful where the access to the tumor bed is limited and there is no need to treat deep-seated tissue (dose prescription is typically to 0.5 cm depth).
3. IORT can also be accomplished with low kV x-rays. Two devices are currently on the market: the Xoft/Axxent system (Xoft Inc.), which is a miniature 50 kVp x-ray tube inside a catheter; and the IntraBeam system (Carl Zeiss Inc.), which uses an electron beam accelerated onto a gold target to produce x-rays that emerge in an approximately spherically uniform distribution from an applicator at the tip of a movable arm. Both low kV systems are most widely used for breast IORT with spherical applicators, though other IORT approaches are under development.

The various delivery systems mentioned above have advantages and disadvantages in the following endpoints: the depth of tissue that can be treated (deep for IOERT versus superficial for brachytherapy), accessibility to hard-to-reach regions such as the pelvic sidewall (a relative advantage for HDR), treatment times (short for IOERT versus longer for HDR), and the need for a shielded OR (HDR).

## References

1. Gunderson LL, Willett CG, Calvo FA, et al., editors. Intraoperative irradiation: Techniques and results (Current Clinical Oncology). 2nd ed. New York: Humana Press; 2011. p. 529.
2. Vaidya JS, Joseph DJ, Tobias JS, et al. Risk-adapted targeted intraoperative radiotherapy versus whole-breast radiotherapy for breast cancer: 5-year results for local control and overall survival from the TARGIT—A randomised trial. Lancet 2014;383(9917):603–13.

3. Vaidya JS, Baum M, Tobias JS, et al. Targeted intra-operative radiotherapy (Targit): An innovative method of treatment for early breast cancer. Ann Oncol 2001;12(8):1075–80.
4. Belletti B, Vaidya JS, D'Andrea S, et al. Targeted intraoperative radiotherapy impairs the stimulation of breast cancer cell proliferation and invasion caused by surgical wounding. Clin Cancer Res 2008;14(5): 1325–32.
5. Palta JR, Biggs PJ, Hazle JD, et al. Intraoperative electron beam radiation therapy: Technique, dosimetry, and dose specification: Report of task force 48 of the Radiation Therapy Committee, American Association of Physicists in Medicine. Int J Radiat Oncol Biol Phys 1995;33(3):725–46.
6. Beddar AS, Biggs PJ, Chang S, et al. Intraoperative radiation therapy using mobile electron linear accelerators: Report of AAPM Radiation Therapy Committee Task Group No. 72. Med Phys 2006;33(5): 1476–89.
7. Mills MD, Fajardo LC, Wilson DL, et al. Commissioning of a mobile electron accelerator for intraoperative radiotherapy. J Appl Clin Med Phys 2001;2(3):121–30.
8. Almond PR, et al. AAPM's TG-51 protocol for clinical reference dosimetry of high-energy photon and electron beams. MEDICAL PHYSICS-LANCASTER PA 1999;26:1847–70.
9. Klein EE, et al. Task Group 142 report: Quality assurance of medical accelerators. Med Phys 2009;36(9):4197–212.
10. Krechetov AS, Goer D, Dikeman K, et al. Shielding assessment of a mobile electron accelerator for intra-operative radiotherapy. J Appl Clin Med Phys 2010;11(4):3151.
11. Loi G, Dominietto M, Cannillo B, et al. Neutron production from a mobile linear accelerator operating in electron mode for intraoperative radiation therapy. Phys Med Biol 2006;51(3):695–702.
12. Park CC, Yom SS, Podgorsak MB, et al. American Society for Therapeutic Radiology and Oncology (Astro) Emerging Technology Committee Report on electronic brachytherapy. Int J Radiat Oncol Biol Phys 2010;76(4):963–72.
13. Avanzo M, Rink A, Dassie A, et al. In vivo dosimetry with radiochromic films in low-voltage intraoperative radiotherapy of the breast. Med Phys 2012;39(5):2359–68.
14. Eaton DJ. Quality assurance and independent dosimetry for an intraoperative x-ray device. Med Phys 2012;39(11):6908–20.
15. Ma CM, Coffey CW, DeWerd LA, et al. AAPM protocol for 40-300 kV x-ray beam dosimetry in radiotherapy and radiobiology. Med Phys 2001;28(6):868–93.
16. Strauss JB, Dickler A. Accelerated partial breast irradiation utilizing balloon brachytherapy techniques. Radiother Oncol 2009;91(2):157–65.
17. Harrison LB, Enker WE, Anderson LL. High-dose-rate intraoperative radiation therapy for colorectal cancer. Oncol (Williston Park) 1995;9(8):737–41, discussion 742–8 passim.
18. Kubo HD, Glasgow GP, Pethel TD, et al. High dose-rate brachytherapy treatment delivery: Report of the AAPM Radiation Therapy Committee Task Group No. 59. Med Phys 1998;25(4):375–403.

# CHAPTER 24

# Special Procedures

## 24.1 Introduction

Special procedures are defined by the following characteristics:

- Unique beam configuration, accessories, or radiation delivery device settings compared to other treatments such as 3D conformal radiation therapy (3D CRT) or intensity-modulated radiation therapy (IMRT)
- Relative number of patients treated is small
- Not widely offered in all clinics because of the relative effort to implement a special procedure compared to the number of patients seen

Some special procedures such as total body irradiation (TBI) and total skin electron treatments (TSET) have been staple tools of clinical treatment for many years, while others such as radioactive microspheres for liver metastases are relatively new. New device or drug developments can quickly change the number of patients treated with a special procedure; for example, the development of medicated stents eliminated the use of intravenous brachytherapy within a short time. Some special procedures are still in the process of settling with a medical specialty; for example, radioactive microsphere treatments are performed by radiation oncologists, nuclear medicine physicians, and interventional radiologists.

Also considered in this chapter is the issue of pregnant patients. This is a "special procedure" in the sense of assessing pregnancy status and designing specialized treatment if it is decided to proceed with treatment while the patient is pregnant.

## 24.2 Total Body Irradiation

The purpose of TBI is to prepare a patient for bone marrow (hematopoeitic stem cell) transplant, either allogeneic or from a donor. This transplant is employed in the treatment of leukemia, lymphoma, or occasionally for nonmalignant disease such as common variable immunodeficiency and aplastic anemia. High doses of TBI can eliminate residual cancer cells. The irradiation in combination with chemotherapeutic agents acts to one of two purposes: to ablate the patient's hematopoietic stem cells in the bone marrow (myeloablative TBI) or to suppress the immune system of the patient prior to transplant (nonablative). With improvements in chemotherapeutic agents, the number of TBI patients has been decreasing over recent years, although it remains a key component of some transplant protocols.

Nonablative TBI regimens typically use a dose of 200 cGy × 1 fraction, whereas the myeloablative TBI regimens typically use 1200 to 1550 cGy delivered over 3 to 5 days, typically BID. Various boosts (such as testicular boosts) may also be employed in addition to TBI. The common characteristic through most protocols is the use of a low dose rate (typically 5 to 15 cGy/min at midplane) to minimize toxicity such as pneumonitis. The extended treatment source-to-surface distance (SSD) usually is sufficient to bring the dose rate into the range of preset linear accelerator (linac) dose rates. For some pediatric setups, a shorter SSD may require special tuning of the linac to achieve the required dose rate. TBI treatments rely not only on accurate execution of the treatment plan, but also on precise timing of the treatment delivery. A second linac on which TBI treatments can be delivered should be available as backup in case of equipment failure. It is often not an option to delay the TBI treatment of a patient, because this irradiation is carefully timed in advance with the conditioning regimen and the transplant.

Because TBI patients are treated on a wide range of protocols in combination with other therapies, the dose fractionation scheme is often set by the choice of treatment protocol in oncology and carefully coordinated with the stem cell transplant (autologous or allogeneic). Incorrect dose delivery can lead to severe or even fatal toxicity. Good communication between oncology and Radiation Oncology is therefore essential to ensure the correct protocol is selected for treatment planning and treatment. Best practice is to request a copy of the treatment protocol for a dosimetry and physics check to verify the correct dose fractionation scheme was planned. Expected early side effects of treatment include the typical symptoms of whole body irradiation: nausea, fatigue, and/or headache.

The American College of Radiology/American Society of Therapeutic Radiation Oncology (ACR/ASTRO) practice guideline for the performance of total body irradiation[1] contains detailed descriptions of the qualifications of the patient care team (physicians, medical physicists, radiation therapists, nurses, and dosimetrists). This practice guideline emphasizes the importance of a well-qualified team of physician subspecialties and caregivers specifically trained for the administration of this high risk procedure. Incorrectly administered or medically supported TBI carries severe toxicity risks including death of the patient. In addition to being trained in their respective skills, all caregivers need to work as a team and verify that every caregiver has a thorough understanding of the procedure and his or her role in it. End-to-end dry runs of all protocols used in clinical practice are a highly effective training tool and can also be used to verify that policy and procedure guidelines are complete and accurate.

American Association of Physicists in Medicine Task Group (AAPM TG)-29, The Physical Aspects of Total and Half Body Irradiation,[2] was published in 1986 at a time when the results of large clinical trials incorporating TBI were not yet available. Nevertheless, much of the discussion on dose accuracy, clinical reasoning, and the basic principles of irradiation design are unchanged. The one exception is the use of hemi-body irradiation for widespread metastatic disease; better chemotherapy agents, earlier cancer detection, and new approaches to oligometastatic disease treatments have rendered this technique extinct except for limited applications in veterinary Radiation Oncology.

## PATIENT SETUP FOR TBI

The most commonly used setup for adults is in a standing position on a small pedestal. This position provides many advantages: easy positioning of beam spoiler and lung blocks, less variation in separation compared with the seated position, and good spacing away from walls and the floor to reduce backscatter. The major disadvantage is that it requires the patient to stand still for an extended time period of 20 min to 30 min or longer, which is very challenging for many TBI patients. TBI stands are often custom-built, and different clinics have developed adaptations to provide patient support:

- A custom-mounted bike saddle of adjustable height can support some of the patient's weight without interfering with the beam excessively.
- Railings or bars for the hands can assist the patient with keeping balance.
- To minimize the fall risk, the patient could wear a full-body climbing harness secured by a belay anchor in the ceiling. Other solutions include Velcro straps or lateral support bars.

The beam arrangement for a standing setup is at an extended SSD of approximately 400 cm. With an open 40 cm × 40 cm field and a collimator rotation of 45°, this results in a maximum field dimension of 225 cm. For patients who cannot stand for the duration of the treatment, an alternative is to be placed in a sitting or supine position on a gurney. Instead of anterior-posterior (AP/PA), the fields are treated from the lateral direction. Because there is a significant change in separation from the shoulders to the head/neck area, tissue compensators are almost always used. Lung blocks are not possible with this setup, although the arms provide some natural blocking. Some centers also use a decubitus lying-down setup for patients who cannot stand. This arrangement allows AP/PA treatment and can accommodate lung blocks, though positioning may be less stable.

Small children up to about 3 years of age can be placed in a frog-leg position on a special bed or vac-lock bag on the floor. The main consideration is whether they will fit into the field size projected onto the floor. The beam spoiler is mounted above the patient, and the lung blocks can be placed directly on the beam spoiler. Taller children can be on the floor and treated with two fields (gap on the thigh with feathering) or treated on a gurney. For older children, the choice between gurney and a standing position has to be made based on the maturity and cooperation of the child. Anesthesia is an option for immobilization, but a tablet computer with a game or movie in the child's hands can be a surprisingly effective immobilization device with considerably less associated morbidity than with anesthesia.

Some clinics have developed technologies to treat the patient on a moving couch or on a fixed couch with a radiation source sweeping over the patient. These techniques are exceedingly rare and will therefore not be discussed here.

## BEAM SPOILERS, TISSUE COMPENSATORS, AND LUNG BLOCKS

A beam spoiler is always used in TBI treatments for the purpose of increasing lower energy components in the beam to avoid skin sparing, which is **not** desirable in TBI protocols. The spoiler is typically made of clear plastic such as acrylic or Plexiglas. The spoiler is placed about 20 to 30 cm away from the patient.

In myeloablative TBI regimens, it is typically necessary to block the lungs to reduce the incidence of pneumonitis; this is the case for most treatments with the exception of single-fraction regimens. Lung blocks can be mounted either on the beam spoiler itself or on a special accessory tray between beam spoiler and patient. The purpose of the lung blocks, contrary to their name, is not to block dose to the lung completely (lungs may receive ≈70% of the prescription dose). They serve instead as tissue compensators to avoid overdose in an area of the body where low density lung tissue decreases the effective thickness significantly compared to the separation at the umbilicus. The position of the lung blocks is verified using a megavoltage (MV) radiograph and film during simulation and treatment. The position of the lung block shadows on the patient should be marked as reference points.

Depending on the protocol, tissue compensators may be required to increase homogeneity of delivered dose across the patient. A typical protocol goal is ±10% dose homogeneity to all tissues. A common method for compensator construction is the use of lead strips of about 2 mm thickness layered onto an accessory tray that is then mounted on the linac accessory tray.

## COMMISSIONING MEASUREMENTS AND IN-VIVO DOSIMETRY

AAPM TG-29[2] Section 3 describes in detail the measurements required to commission a TBI procedure using the reference dosimetry methods described in AAPM TG-21, A Protocol for the Determination of Absorbed Dose from High-Energy Photon and Electron Beams; these should be replaced by the reference dosimetry methods of AAPM TG-51, Protocol for Clinical

Reference Dosimetry of High-Energy Photon and Electron Beams.[3] Although the use of solid water phantoms for reference dosimetry is acceptable, it is best practice to use a large water phantom for annual calibrations to perform these measurements. Commissioning data (PDDs, output factors, beam profiles) should be gathered for the clinical setup used (i.e., at extended distance with the beam spoiler and compensator tray in place).

During commissioning of the TBI technique, the in-vivo dosimetry system should be placed on an anthropomorphic phantom in treatment setup to verify the dose calculation and dose inhomogeneity across the treatment field. Radiochromic film should be placed between axial slices in the phantom at the same levels as the in-vivo dosimeters to assess dose inhomogeneity as a function of separation. AAPM TG-29 Figure 2[2] shows the ratio of $Dose_{max}/Dose_{midline}$ as a function of patient thickness and beam energy. As the patient thickness increases, the ratio of peak to midline dose diverges with the lower energy beam ratio rising more quickly. For most patients, the choice of beam energy of 6 MV or 10 MV is appropriate; obese patients may require higher beam energies of 10 MV or 15 MV to achieve the ±10% dose homogeneity to all tissues. Therefore, all photon energies in this range should be commissioned for TBI.

## TREATMENT PLANNING

Current treatment planning systems do not include the accelerator settings and beam data used for dose calculation in TBI. Since the patient is often treated while standing, a CT scan of the patient in treatment position is often also not available unless the patient is to be treated on the couch either supine with lateral beams or in decubitus position. Treatment planning for TBI is therefore performed by hand calculation, usually in the form of spreadsheets or use of second monitor unit (MU) check programs. The input parameters are patient height, separation at the umbilicus (usually the widest area of the body), dose, and dose rate. The prescription point is usually chosen at midline at the level of the umbilicus in adults and the head in children because these are the thickest parts. When using a spreadsheet, the measured beam data on which the calculation is based must be password protected to avoid accidental changes to the data. Dose inhomogeneities across the treated field should be kept to ±10% of prescription dose. If a tissue compensator is used, the thicknesses of compensating lead can also be calculated in a spreadsheet. The tissue compensator must be part of the second check procedure to verify correct thickness and assembly. If a patient setup is used that allows CT simulation, the dose can be planned using a conventional treatment planning system. In this case, the multi-leaf collimator (MLC) can be used to modulate the beams to achieve dose homogeneity across the body.[4]

The MU and other settings per field are manually entered into the record & verify (R&V) system. Because the high number of MUs needed at extended SSD for TBI treatments usually exceeds the per-field MU safety limits set in the R&V software, a special TBI mode is often made available within the R&V software. The alternative would be to treat with multiple (up to 5 or 6) split fields, adding extra time to the already extended treatment time.

Treatments using multiple overlapping fields should be avoided for two reasons: (1) The overlapping fields create a larger dose inhomogeneity in the match area, and (2) cells circulating in the bloodstream may not receive the full dose per treatment fraction.

## TREATMENT QA AND IN-VIVO DOSIMETRY

The positioning of the lung blocks is confirmed before the first treatment. Film can be used, but it has the disadvantage of requiring time to develop. Computed radiography (CR) film cassettes use photo-stimulated phosphor plates to obtain x-ray images. Even though the CR cassettes require an up-front capital investment, the long-term cost savings of not having to maintain a film processor makes CR cassettes an economical choice. If the TBI stand is movable, an alternative option is to move the TBI stand to the accelerator with the couch moved out of the way and use the electronic portal imaging device (EPID) for kV image acquisition. This allows the lung blocks to be adjusted appropriately.

Typically diodes, metal oxide semiconductor field-effect transistors (MOSFETs), thermoluminescent dosimeters (TLDs), or optically stimulated luminescence dosimeters (OSLDs) are used for in-vivo dosimetry for the first TBI fraction to verify (1) the accurate mounting and thickness of the tissue compensators for treatment and (2) dose at several points across the body (see Chapter 3 for details on in-vivo dosimetry). The dosimeter is typically left on for the whole treatment (AP and PA beams) and readout at the end. Diodes that give instantaneous readout of dose have a large advantage in that the expected dose rate can be verified after the first minute of treatment, and the treatment can be halted if any significant deviations are noted. For a single-fraction TBI this may be particularly important. MOSFETs cannot provide dose rate information, but can provide instantaneous readout at completion of the first fraction. This information is helpful to confirm lung compensator thickness and accurate placement of tissue compensators. Typical locations for dosimeters are:

- On forehead (prescription point for children)
- Neck (thinnest point)
- Chest: entrance and exit dose to check lung block thickness
- Umbilicus (prescription point in adults, since it is typically the thickest part of the body)
- Optional: extremities, especially upper and lower legs if compensators are used
- Selected protocols require testes boosts for pediatric male patients

## 24.3 Total Skin Electron Treatments

Mycosis fungoides ("mushroom-like fungal disease") is a type of non-Hodgkin's lymphoma, more precisely a cutaneous B-cell lymphoma. Depending on the stage and extent of disease, superficial radiation is one of several available treatment options. The disease is generally rare to start with, and improvements in access to care and earlier diagnosis have further increased the number of patients who are treated with local superficial radiation and decreased the number of patients requiring total skin electron treatments. Therefore, the number of clinics commissioning a total skin electron treatment (TSET) procedure will likely remain small.

AAPM TG-30, Total Skin Electron Therapy: Technique and Dosimetry,[5] provides a detailed description of TSET techniques, commissioning of a TSET program, and in-vivo dosimetry. The goal of TSET is to superficially irradiate the whole skin with as much dose homogeneity as possible. Given the complex shape of the human body, there are limits on the achievable dose homogeneity of about 10% to 15%. Two main setup strategies have evolved: (1) rotational two-field techniques in which the patient is placed on a platform rotating at equal speed and (2) the Stanford 6-field technique. In the Stanford 6-field technique, the patient assumes six treatment positions; because of the length of the treatment, the treatment alternates between three of the six positions for each fraction. Rotational treatment is somewhat better in achieving a homogeneous skin dose but requires careful coordination of rotational speed and treatment delivery time. The Stanford technique can be performed on the same patient setup platform as that used in TBI and therefore requires less up-front investment in special equipment.

A variety of beam energies were used when the technique was first developed; in current use 6 MeV electrons have become the standard. Two matched fields that are pointed up and down from the horizontal axis by about 20° provide a 10% dose inhomogeneity over the surface of an anthropomorphic phantom. Pointing the beams upward and downward also reduces the photon contamination, which is greatest in the forward-scattered direction along the electron beam central axis. Similar to TBI, a beam spoiler is placed near the patient upstream from the incident beam, increasing wide-angle scatter to improve dose uniformity. Some accelerators offer a special high dose rate electron mode designed for TSET treatments at extended distances.

In-vivo dosimetry is used to verify the dose and dose homogeneity across the patient body during treatment. The scalp, chin, perineum, and soles of feet are areas that do not receive full dose with the standard setup techniques. If clinically necessary, these areas are boosted using a clinical electron setup technique. The scalp and perineum can be treated using vertex fields. The chin is more challenging to treat on a conventional linear accelerator because of the patient/beam geometry; a possible alternative is to use a superficial treatment modality such as superficial brachytherapy. Other areas of concern for underdosing are the skin folds of the buttock, inframammary folds, and abdominal skin folds in obese patients. The first approach to preventing underdosing of skin fold areas is careful taping to eliminate or reduce folds. If the folds are too deep, boost fields may be required. The determination should be made based on in-vivo dosimetry measurements in the affected areas.

The penetration depth of 6 MeV electron beams and the corresponding x-ray bremsstrahlung component will lead to some dose penetrating beyond the desired depth. For this reason, internal eye shields are used for the AP and AP oblique fields to lower the dose to the lenses. Very thin areas of the body may require shielding in the course of treatment to avoid overdosing. The primary areas of concern are the fingertips and toenails; overdosing could lead to skin toxicity up to temporary loss of nails. Lead shields can be manufactured to protect the sensitive areas.

In summary, developing a TSET program requires a significant commitment of staff time and resources. The treatment techniques are complex compared to TBI. Therefore, TSET will likely remain limited to major academic centers specializing in the treatment of lymphomas.

## 24.4 Ocular Tumors

Ocular tumors, predominantly ocular melanomas and retinoblastomas, are tumors of the eye arising in the uveal layer. Larger tumors are treated using surgical enucleation of the eye, but smaller tumors are often irradiated first to preserve the eye and as much functional vision as possible. Because of the small size of ocular tumors and their immediate proximity to critical structures of the optical apparatus, treatments have to achieve high dose conformality and steep dose gradients typically associated with stereotactic radiosurgery (SRS) or brachytherapy. In 2003, the American Brachytherapy Society (ABS) published clinical recommendations for the treatment of uveal melanomas.[6] In ophthalmology, digital photography ultrasound are typically used to identify the position of ocular tumors and measure their dimension. This may be supplemented by a magnetic resonance imaging (MRI) or computed tomography (CT) study.

Brachytherapy in the form of eye plaques has been used successfully for many decades in the treatment of ocular melanomas, based on the large randomized COMS trial (Collaborative Ocular Melanoma Study), which examined enucleation versus irradiation.[7,8] An alternative is proton beam radiotherapy. Proton beams of up to 80 MeV are ideal for irradiation because of their dose characteristics and the much less invasive aspects of the procedure. Clinical trials indicate proton beams are most useful for large and/or posteriorly located tumors, but use of proton beams had historically been very limited due to the very limited availability of clinical proton beams. With the recent proliferation of clinical proton facilities, an increasing number of patients will likely be treated using this modality. Similarly, the wider accessibility to dedicated SRS treatment machines has led to the development of single-day, single-fraction SRS treatments using the Gamma Knife[9-11] or CyberKnife.[12,13] Immobilization of the tumor for proton and SRS treatments can be achieved through two methods:

1. Requiring the patient to gaze toward a defined point in the treatment room. This requires patient cooperation; eye positioning can be verified using an x-ray system to identify fiducial markers sewn onto the orbit.
2. Paralyzing the ocular musculature by locally injecting anesthesia. The medication acts as a bolus and shifts the position of the eye slightly; simulation imaging, treatment planning, and

treatment delivery have to be performed before the anesthesia agent is resorbed into the body, typically within 2 to 3 hours.

The joint ABS/AAPM TG-129[14] covers the dosimetry of $^{125}$I and $^{103}$Pd COMS eye plaques for intraocular tumors. Typical prescriptions deliver 85 Gy to a point 5 mm deep. The diameter of the eye plaque to be used is determined by the maximum diameter of the tumor. Eye plaques consist of a round or oval metal template (8 to 20 mm in diameter) with gold alloy backing to provide shielding of normal tissue. The eye plaques have standard or customizable Silastic inserts for the radioactive seeds. The seeds are glued into place in specifically designed slots, then covered with gold backing and sterilized before being sewn onto the back of the orbit for the duration of the treatment. In tumors that are close to or abut the optic nerve a "notched" plaque is used (the notch fitting in around the optic nerve). The eye plaque is sewn in in the OR and left in typically for 3 to 7 days[15] while the patient is an inpatient and then is removed surgically. Both $^{125}$I and $^{103}$Pd (and more rarely $^{131}$Cs) are used as low dose rate sources.

The location of the seeds, seed strength, and duration of treatment are determined during the treatment planning process. The depth of the tumor is an important parameter. The COMS protocol specifies a 5 mm depth, but for some larger tumors this should be modified. Though the COMS protocol specifies a 3 mm basal margin, recent calculations indicate a 5 mm margin is needed to achieve sufficient tumor coverage.[16] Because of the low energy, dose calculations are highly sensitive to seed model, plaque design, and heterogeneities. Dose calculations using the AAPM TG-43[17] algorithm for point sources and line sources in homogeneous media agree within a few percentage points of dose to the central axis. However, when heterogeneity is accounted for in the dose calculations either through MC modeling or ray tracing techniques, large differences of 37% or more have been noted between the methods. In light of rapid developments of improved brachytherapy dose calculation methods, AAPM TG-129, Dosimetry of $^{125}$I and $^{103}$Pd COMS Eye Plaques for Intraocular Tumors, recommends:

> *In anticipation of brachytherapy TPS allowing heterogeneous dose calculations, e.g., semi-analytic path length correction, MC, collapsed cone, discrete ordinates, or other approaches, the AAPM and ABS recommend performing a parallel dose calculation or estimation to include the effects of plaque material heterogeneities when these brachytherapy TPS become available. At a minimum, heterogeneity-corrected dose to the prescription point should be obtained, but preferably a 2D dose distribution.*[14]

For commissioning of a brachytherapy-based plaque program using a 3D treatment planning system, the existing guidelines for image-guided systems used in treatment planning based on ultrasound,[18] CT,[19] or MRI should be followed. The calibration and assay of low dose rate brachytherapy seeds are described in the AAPM working group report.[20]

## 24.5 Microspheres

Microsphere brachytherapy using the beta emission of $^{90}$Y is used in the treatment of hepatic malignancies. Formulations package the $^{90}$Y in small glass microspheres 20 to 60 μm in diameter, which are injected into the hepatic artery. Most treatments take place in interventional radiology departments with the support of nuclear medicine physics or health physics. In smaller clinics, the therapy physicist might need to cover this procedure; we therefore introduce a short summary of guidance documents in this text. As with all special procedures, it is recommended to either proctor with an experienced physicist and/or get dedicated vendor training on the application of microspheres.

As radioactive by-product material, the use of $^{90}$Y brachytherapy microspheres is regulated in 10 CFR 35 for agreement states in the United States. The Nuclear Regulatory Commission

(NRC) also provides additional guidance material on its website at http://www.nrc.gov/materials/miau/med-use-toolkit.html#other.

Microsphere brachytherapy makes use of the dual blood supply of the liver through the hepatic artery and portal vein. Metastatic and hepatocellular carcinoma liver tumors larger than 3 mm in diameter receive 80% to 90% of their blood supply from the hepatic artery, whereas the portal vein supplies ≈80% of the normal liver tissue. Therefore, radiation emitting sources administered through the hepatic artery will primarily target the liver malignancies, with relatively small doses being deposited in normal liver tissue. The $^{90}$Y is packaged in either glass or biocompatible resin microspheres of 20 to 60 μm diameter in a solution of sterile water. The administration of microspheres causes both an embolization of the tumor blood supply and delivery of localized radiation, combining ischemic and radiation damage to the tumor.

AAPM TG-144 on dosimetry, imaging, and QA of $^{90}$Y microsphere brachytherapy in the treatment of hepatic malignancies[21] provides a good introduction on the rationale, commercially available sources, imaging protocols, and regulatory aspects. The ACR-ASTRO-SIR practice guideline for radioembolization with microsphere brachytherapy device (RMBD) for treatment of liver malignancies covers qualifications of staff, procedural guidelines regarding activity, and administration, as well as personnel safety issues.[22] Furthermore, the Radioembolization Brachytherapy Oncology Consortium has published a consensus panel report[21] containing 14 recommendations summarizing the current state-of-the-art knowledge on the safety and efficacy of microsphere brachytherapy.

A major challenge in all liver therapy, including microsphere brachytherapy, is liver imaging. The complexity of the organ and its high vascularization requires well-developed imaging protocols to ensure accurate diagnosis of the tumor burden. In most cases, a triphasic CT (i.e., a noncontrast CT followed by a contrast CT at two defined time intervals) is often supplemented by a positron emission tomography (PET)/CT and, if available, an MRI study. In combination, these studies will provide the tumor volume needed for treatment planning. A pretreatment angiography is needed in addition to the simulation imaging to determine hepatic blood flow and catheter path for the procedure. At the same time of this pretreatment angiogram, an embolization of extrahepatic vessels is performed to avoid microsphere deposits outside the liver. This is followed by an administration of $^{99m}$Tc-MAA (albumin aggregated), which can be imaged using a gamma camera to predict microsphere dose delivery. The albumin aggregated is intended as a surrogate for the biodistribution of the microsphere and the $^{99m}$Tc-MAA imaging results determine the amount of dose shunted to the lungs.

Dosimetry of microsphere brachytherapy is based on the assumption of uniform uptake in liver and tumor tissue, minus the dose shunted to the lungs as determined by the pretreatment SPECT imaging. The dosimetry standard for microsphere brachytherapy was developed by the Medical Internal Radiation Dose (MIRD) Committee of the Nuclear Medicine Society.[23] These simpler dose calculation models have been recently supplemented by the availability of image-based 3D dose modeling using kernel convolution dosimetry, with the dose kernel determined by Monte Carlo (MC) simulation. Planar or SPECT imaging during the procedure can provide confirmation of localization of dose delivery.

There is currently no National Institute of Standards and Technology (NIST)-traceable standard for $^{90}$Y microsphere brachytherapy. The assay of the $^{90}$Y activity therefore will follow the respective vendor protocol and use a vendor-provided reference activity sample. The activity readings in nuclear medicine dose calibrators are very sensitive to geometric location of the source within the calibrator and distribution of microspheres within their respective delivery containers. It is therefore necessary to closely follow vendor recommendations on dose measurement and establish a consistent activity measurement protocol within the institution. After the procedure is completed, a second measurement on the remaining microspheres is performed to confirm the amount of delivered radiation dose. AAPM TG-144 gives the current overall uncertainty in delivered dose for $^{90}$Y microsphere brachytherapy as 20%.

Microsphere brachytherapy was developed because the low dose tolerance of liver parenchyma did not allow delivery of tumoricidal dose with the standard 1.8 Gy fractionation scheme in external beam radiotherapy. In recent years, clinical studies on liver stereotactic body radiation therapy (SBRT)[24-27] have shown good local control with acceptably low toxicity in select patients. Given the residual uncertainty of dose delivery with microspheres and the radiation exposure to staff during shipping, handling, and the invasive procedure, it remains to be seen if microsphere brachytherapy will be sustainable in the long term.

# 24.6 Intravascular Brachytherapy

Intravascular brachytherapy (IVBT) is used for the prevention of restenosis after angioplasty of a coronary or peripheral artery obstruction. The development of drug-eluting stents has reduced the number of IVBT procedures considerably. However, recent reports on in-stent restenosis of the medicated stents indicate that IVBT might make a recurrence as repeat/salvage therapy. In the United States, IVBT is Food and Drug Administration (FDA) approved only for treating in-stent restenosis, but not for de novo treatments. Dose prescriptions range from 15 to 30 Gy delivered to 1.5 mm or 2 mm depth in one fraction. AAPM TG-60, Intravascular Brachytherapy Physics,[28] provides the medical background for IVBT as well as an overview of commercially available IVBT systems and procedures. AAPM TG-149, Dose Calculation Formalisms and Consensus Dosimetry Parameters for Intravascular Brachytherapy Dosimetry,[29] provides an updated summary on the procedure, the three commercially available isotopes at the time of publication ($^{192}$Ir, $^{90}$Sr/$^{90}$Y, and $^{32}$P), and dose calculation methods.

The system currently on the market (Beta-Cath, Novoste Inc.) is a $^{90}$Sr/$^{90}$Y system consisting of a string of seeds which is remotely placed using manual controls of a hydraulic delivery system. $^{90}$Sr decays to $^{90}$Y with the emission of a 0.54 MeV beta particle (half-life 28.5 yrs) and then to $^{90}$Zr (beta 2.25 MeV $T_{1/2}$ 64 hrs). These beta particles have a range of ≈3 mm in tissue. The source train is introduced into the catheter via a handheld hydraulic transfer device. Other systems have included the Guidant system and $^{192}$Ir source for IVBT consisting of a ribbon that needs to be manually advanced through the catheter to the target location by the radiation oncologist. Of the two beta emitters, the $^{32}$P system is technically designed to be very similar to high dose rate (HDR) brachytherapy units.

The dosimetry of IVBT is more challenging than for traditional brachytherapy applications because the treatment target is very close to the source. Point source approximations cannot be used to simplify the calculation. Several Monte Carlo codes have been used to study IVBT sources; however, modeling dose on the millimeter and submillimeter scale is a challenging endeavor. In addition to Monte Carlo, experimental measurements are also used to determine dose distributions of IVBT sources. The majority of these measurements are made with GaF chromic film, which provides high spatial resolution and near water equivalency at IVBT source energies. Other detectors used are small volume scintillators and ultra-thin TLDs.

For single-seed dosimetry data, AAPM TG-149 deviates from the recommendations in AAPM TG-43[30] by selecting one set of MC calculations as the consensus value. The selection was based on completeness and resolution of the radial and anisotropy functions as well as comparison with experimental data. For line sources, the spherical AAPM TG-43 formalism is not appropriate and must be replaced with a formalism based on cylindrical coordinates. Both measurements and MC calculations were used to create averaged along and away tables for line sources.

AAPM TG-149 recommends that the source strength calibration for single-seed gamma-emitting IVBT sources follow the formalism used in conventional brachytherapy as described in AAPM TG-43. The reference absorbed dose rate of a beta-emitting source is calibrated at primary laboratories and distributed to secondary laboratories and vendors, from where the calibration is transferred using well chambers.

# 24.7 Pregnant Patients

In most Radiation Oncology clinics, women about to undergo radiation treatments are given a pregnancy test or asked if there is any chance that they might be or might become pregnant during the duration of their treatment. The ASRT radiation therapy clinical performance standards call for the radiation therapist to "verify the patient's pregnancy status."[31] ACR practice guidelines Appendix I[32] suggests that for substantial risk procedures (of which radiotherapy is one) a urine hCG test should be obtained.

Nevertheless, on occasion a patient discovers a pregnancy during her radiation treatment. A far rarer situation of encountering pregnancy in Radiation Oncology is when a pregnant woman is diagnosed with a life-threatening cancer requiring radiation treatments. In both situations, the medical physicist should be prepared to consult with the patient and her treating physician(s) on the amount of radiation dose likely to be received by the fetus and the probability and possible consequences of the fetus receiving radiation.

## DOSE ESTIMATES

AAPM TG-36, Fetal Dose from Radiotherapy with Photon Beams,[33] covers fetal dose from radiotherapy with photon beams. Figure 2 in that report provides information on the height of the fundus as a function of week of pregnancy. This information is used to determine the minimum distance to the treatment field edge if the uterus is outside the radiation field. Figures 18 through 23 in AAPM TG-36 give data on absorbed dose as a function of distance to field edge for a variety of photon energy and field sizes. Though these data provide good estimates for 3D conformal treatments, AAPM TG-36 was published before the implementation of IMRT and therefore does not contain data for IMRT out-of-field doses. Performing dose measurements in an anthropomorphic phantom emulating the actual clinical treatment as closely as possible is currently the best method to get a dose estimate for the fetus. The measurement result should be cross-checked with the out-of-field dose calculation from the treatment planning system (see Chapter 5). In case the location of the fundus is beyond the inferior or superior border of the treatment planning CT scan, most treatment planning systems allow a virtual extension by copying the last scanned slice until the desired distance is reached. Even though this method increases the uncertainty of the dose calculation, it will provide an order of magnitude estimate for the dose.

## BIOLOGICAL EFFECTS OF RADIATION ON THE FETUS

The biological effects of radiation on fetal health are not well understood. Data are sparse, mostly relying on exposures of pregnant women from the nuclear bomb explosions in Hiroshima and Nagasaki and exposure to radioactive fallout from the Chernobyl accident. Determining an accurate dose to the fetus in each of these cases is difficult and has large uncertainties associated with it. In addition, the timing and energy of the radiation are considerably different from the fractionated radiation delivery in Radiation Oncology. More recent population studies in people affected by the Chernobyl accidents also revealed that the psychological effects of trauma may lead to a higher incidence of unhealthy lifestyle choices in survivors, which in turn increases health risks such as cancer incidence and fetal health.

It is important to distinguish between radiation to an embryo (<13 weeks of gestational age) and a fetus (>13 weeks of gestational age). In the embryonic phase of development, radiation damage affects organogenesis, resulting in more severe biological effects. With the completion of organogenesis and the start of the fetal stage in the second trimester, the fetal development is dominated by maturation of existing organs, and therefore the fetus is less sensitive to radiation.

Biological effects on the fetus depend strongly on the gestational age at which the radiation was received. As a general rule of thumb, the risk of adverse effects decreases with gestational age. AAPM TG-36 offers an in-depth discussion about risks of fetal irradiation. Updated data can be found in Chapter 12 of *Radiobiology for the Radiologist*[34] and the review article by Martin.[35] Similar to the difficulty of determining increased cancer risk due to radiation because of the natural cancer incidence rate, studying the biological effects of fetal irradiation has to consider the natural incidence of each effect. AAPM TG-36 Table VI notes a significant risk of damage above 10 cGy in the first trimester and above 50 cGy in all trimesters.

The main biological effects are:

- **Lethality:** The actual risk as function of dose is difficult to quantify because of the relatively large incidence of embryonic loss by other causes in the first trimester.
- **Anatomic malformations:** The dose-response curve for anatomic malformations is generally sigmoidal; severity is in general a function of dose.
- **Severe mental retardation:** Studies in atomic bomb survivors established the highest risk to fetuses between 8 and 15 weeks of gestational age, when the majority of organogenesis of the central nervous system (CNS) occurs. The risk was confirmed for doses >0.5 Gy, but no statistically significant drop in IQ was seen at doses <0.1 Gy.
- **Growth retardation:** Growth retardation was observed for doses >0.25 Gy for the fetal stage of development for Hiroshima bomb victims.
- **Sterility:** Sterility has been observed from irradiation both in the embryonal and fetal stages of development.
- **Cancer induction:** Several studies have been performed on the increase of childhood cancer incidence for children exposed in utero. Findings range from 55 to 640 additional cancer cases per 10,000 people per Gy.
- **Genetic effects:** The International Commission on Radiological Protection (ICRP) has adopted a risk estimate of 1% per Gy for the doubling dose of genetic aberrations for low dose, low LET (linear energy transfer) radiation.

## TREATMENT PLANNING FOR PREGNANT PATIENTS

In the rare case of a pregnant patient deciding to proceed with radiation treatment after careful discussion with her physician of the medical and ethical consequences, careful attention must be paid to the design of the treatment plan. Few medical centers have access to or can construct shielding devices as discussed in AAPM TG-36 to limit the leakage and scatter. Collimator scatter is dominant closer to the field edge, while leakage becomes the dominant component at greater distances from the field edge. Internal scatter within the patient cannot be shielded. Therefore, the treatment planning strategy must aim to minimize scatter and leakage as much as feasible (e.g., using segments instead of wedges). For linacs with a flattening filter free beam, a half-split beam can approximate a wedge without the associated additional scatter. Plans should also aim for a high dose/MU ratio (i.e., using the lowest possible modulation for IMRT or VMAT plans). Before treatment start, the out-of-field dose predicted by the planning system should be cross-checked with a measurement in an anthropomorphic phantom.

Although there is no safe dose within the linear-no-threshold model of radiation damage, dose thresholds established for pregnant radiation workers (see Chapter 10) can be used as guidance on what might be considered an acceptable risk in a situation where the risks of treating a life-threatening disease have to be weighed against the risk of not providing treatment.

TABLE 24.1 ▦ Special Procedures in Radiotherapy and Issues That Require Special Attention

| Special Procedure | Issues of Particular Concern |
|---|---|
| TBI | Dose rate: Most TBI is delivered at a low dose rate (5-15 cGy/min) to minimize toxicity. The extended SSD typically required for adults can often bring the dose rate into this range, but special tuning of the linac might be needed, especially for pediatric patients. |
| | Dose and fractionation: Most TBI patients are treated on clinical protocols that specify a TBI dose and fractionation, and these must be adhered to per protocol. Typical doses are 2 Gy for nonmyeloablative ("mini") TBI and 12 Gy for myeloablative TBI. |
| | Scheduling: Because TBI is given as part of the conditioning regimen for transplant, there is often little to no room for error regarding timing of treatments. Therefore, all TBI must be closely coordinated with medical oncology. |
| | Blocking: Tolerance dose for normal organs such as lung must be respected, and blocks are typically used for higher dose TBI (such as myeloablative protocols). |
| TSET | Complexity of TSET and rarity of its use means this treatment is best delivered at larger centers that deliver TSET on a regular basis. A good TSET program requires significant resources to develop. |
| | In-vivo dosimetry: Areas parallel to beam angle can be underdosed and require boosting (such as scalp, chin, perineum, and soles of feet). Skin folds must also be minimized due to the same principle (such as inframammary folds or abdominal pannus). |
| Ocular tumors | Brachytherapy: For plaque therapy, seed strengths, locations, and treatment duration are all calculated during treatment planning. Dose calculations are highly sensitive to seed model, plaque design, and heterogeneities. |
| | Immobilization: If patients are treated with external beam therapy (protons or SRS), tumor immobilization is critical. This can be done with patient cooperation alone or with local anesthesia. |
| Microspheres | Guidelines: Multiple guidelines exist from AAPM, ACR-ASTRO-SIR, and the Radioembolization Brachytherapy Oncology Consortium |
| | Dosimetry: Prior to treatment, lung shunting is determined with $^{99m}$Tc-MAA administration. Dosimetry has historically assumed uniform uptake in liver and tumor tissues, minus lung shunting. However, with more sophisticated imaging techniques, better dose localization is possible. |
| | Assays: Without a NIST standard, vendor protocols must be followed for $^{90}$Y activity assays. |
| IVBT | Accurate localization of source position is critical for proper treatment. |
| | Dosimetry is also more challenging than traditional brachytherapy due to close proximity of source and target; therefore point source approximations cannot be applied. |
| Pregnant patient | Pregnancy state should be assessed before treatment in applicable patients. |
| | If treatment is absolutely necessary, dose can be estimated, and biological effects depend on timing during pregnancy. |
| | Special considerations must be made during treatment planning to evaluate the use of shielding and minimize scatter and leakage. |

**FOR THE PHYSICIAN**

The special procedures described in this chapter are characterized by complex techniques used on a relatively low percentage of patients. The clinical implementation of any special procedure requires a comparatively large amount of time and financial investment. The low number of patients means that none of these procedures is likely to become routine with regard to the number of staff involved or the maturation of clinical processes. They are therefore subject to increased risk of error because of infrequency of treatment, unfamiliarity with rare procedures, and treatment complexity.

Because of these factors, it is extremely important that clear policies and procedures are written for each technique used in the clinic. Prior to implementing a new technique, it is important to obtain benchmark data wherever possible and receive training from individuals who are experienced in that technique. Due to the low frequency of treatments, it may be advisable to have a dedicated team for each technique rather than training all staff for every procedure.

Table 24.1 shows the list of special procedures discussed in this chapter and the issues that deserve special attention.

## *References*

1. Wolden SL, Rabinovitch RA, Bittner NH, et al. American College of Radiology (ACR) and American Society for Radiation Oncology (ASTRO) practice guideline for the performance of total body irradiation (TBI). Am J Clin Oncol 2013;36:97–101.
2. Van Dyk J, Galvin J, Glasgow G, et al. The physical aspects of total and half body photon irradiation: A report of Task Group 29, Radiation Therapy Committee Association of Physicists in Medicine. New York: American Association of Physicists in Medicine; 1986.
3. Almond PR, Biggs PJ, Coursey BM, et al. AAPM's TG-51 protocol for clinical reference dosimetry of high-energy photon and electron beams. Med Phys 1999;2:1847–70.
4. Bloemen-van Gurp EJ, Mijnheer BJ, Verschueren TA, et al. Total body irradiation, toward optimal individual delivery: Dose evaluation with metal oxide field effect transistors, thermoluminescence detectors, and a treatment planning system. Int J Radiat Oncol Biol Phys 2007;69:1297–304.
5. Karzmark CJ, Anderson J, Buffa A, et al. Total skin electron therapy: Technique and dosimetry. AAPM Task Group 30. New York: American Institute of Physics; 1987.
6. Nag S, Quivey JM, Earle JD, et al. The American Brachytherapy Society recommendations for brachytherapy of uveal melanomas. Int J Radiat Oncol Biol Phys 2003;56:544–55.
7. Berry JL, Dandapani SV, Stevanovic M, et al. Outcomes of choroidal melanomas treated with eye physics: A 20-year review. JAMA Ophthalmol 2013;131:1435–42.
8. Hawkins BS. Collaborative Ocular Melanoma Study randomized trial of $^{125}$I brachytherapy. Clin Trials 2011;8:661–73.
9. Fakiris AJ, Lo SS, Henderson MA, et al. Gamma-knife-based stereotactic radiosurgery for uveal melanoma. Stereotactic Func Neurosurg 2007;85:106–12.
10. Marchini G, Gerosa M, Piovan E, et al. Gamma Knife stereotactic radiosurgery for uveal melanoma: Clinical results after 2 years. Stereotactic Func Neurosurg 1996;66:208–13.
11. Mueller AJ, Talies S, Schaller UC, et al. Stereotactic radiosurgery of large uveal melanomas with the gamma-knife. Ophthalmol 2000;107:1381–7.
12. Daftari IK, Petti PL, Larson DA, et al. A noninvasive eye fixation monitoring system for CyberKnife radiotherapy of choroidal and orbital tumors. Med Phys 2009;36:719–24.
13. Hirschbein MJ, Collins S, Jean WC, et al. Treatment of intraorbital lesions using the Accuray CyberKnife system. Orbit 2008;27:97–105.
14. Chiu-Tsao S-T, Astrahan MA, Finger PT, et al. Dosimetry of $^{125}$I and $^{103}$Pd COMS eye plaques for intraocular tumors: Report of Task Group 129 by the AAPM and ABS. Med Phys 2012;39: 6161–84.
15. Gagne NL, Leonard KL, Rivard MJ. Radiobiology for eye plaque brachytherapy and evaluation of implant duration and radionuclide choice using an objective function. Med Phys 2012;39:3332–42.
16. Gagne NL, Rivard MJ. Quantifying the dosimetric influences of radiation coverage and brachytherapy implant placement uncertainty on eye plaque size selection. Brachyther 2013;12:508–20.
17. Rivard MJ, Coursey BM, DeWerd LA, et al. Update of AAPM Task Group No. 43 Report: A revised AAPM protocol for brachytherapy dose calculations. Medical Phys 2004;31:633–74.
18. ACR technical standard for diagnostic medical physics performance monitoring of real time ultrasound equipment. American College of Radiology; 2011.
19. Mutic S, Palta JR, Butker EK, et al. Quality assurance for computed-tomography simulators and the computed-tomography-simulation process: Report of the AAPM Radiation Therapy Committee Task Group No. 66. Med Phys 2003;30:2762–92.

20. Butler WM, Bice WS Jr, DeWerd LA, et al. Third-party brachytherapy source calibrations and physicist responsibilities: Report of the AAPM Low Energy Brachytherapy Source Calibration Working Group. Med Phys 2008;35:3860–5.
21. Kennedy A, Nag S, Salem R, et al. Recommendations for radioembolization of hepatic malignancies using yttrium-90 microsphere brachytherapy: A consensus panel report from the radioembolization brachytherapy oncology consortium. Int J Radiat Oncol Biol Phys 2007;68:13–23.
22. <http://www.acr.org/~/media/d8086059b5f541e9b64e55d68a71693b.pdf>.
23. Loevinger R, Budinger T, Watson E. MIRD primer for absorbed dose calculations Rev Sub ed. Society of Nuclear Medicine; 1991.
24. Goodman KA, Wiegner EA, Maturen KE, et al. Dose-escalation study of single-fraction stereotactic body radiotherapy for liver malignancies. Int J Radiat Oncol Biol Phys 2010;78:486–93.
25. Høyer M, Swaminath A, Bydder S, et al. Radiotherapy for liver metastases: A review of evidence. Int J Radiat Oncol Biol Phys 2012;82:1047–57.
26. Rusthoven KE, Kavanagh BD, Cardenes H, et al. Multi-institutional phase I/II trial of stereotactic body radiation therapy for liver metastases. J Clin Oncol 2009;27:1572–8.
27. Schefter TE, Kavanagh BD, Timmerman RD, et al. A phase I trial of stereotactic body radiation therapy (SBRT) for liver metastases. Int J Radiat Oncol Biol Phys 2005;62:1371–8.
28. Nath R, Amols H, Coffey C, et al. Intravascular brachytherapy physics: Report of the AAPM Radiation Therapy Committee Task Group No. 60. Med Phys 1999;26:119–52.
29. Chiu-Tsao S-T, Schaart DR, Soares CG, et al. Dose calculation formalisms and consensus dosimetry parameters for intravascular brachytherapy dosimetry: Recommendations of the AAPM Therapy Physics Committee Task Group No. 149. Med Phys 2007;34:4126–57.
30. Meigooni AS. Dosimetry of interstitial brachytherapy sources: Recommendations. Med Phys 1995; 22:2.
31. <http://media.asrt.org/pdf/governance/practicestandards/ps_rad.pdf>.
32. <http://www.acr.org/Quality-Safety/Standards-Guidelines/Practice-Guidelines-by-Modality/Radiation-Oncology>.
33. Nath R, Anderson LL, Meli JA, et al. Code of practice for brachytherapy physics: Report of the AAPM Radiation Therapy Committee Task Group No. 56. Med Phys 1997;24:1557–98.
34. Hall EJ, Giaccia AJ. Radiobiology for the radiologist. Philadelphia: Lippincott Williams & Wilkins; 2006.
35. Martin DD. Review of radiation therapy in the pregnant cancer patient. Clin Obstet Gynecol 2011;54:591–601.

# Resource Documents

| Report | Brief Title | Year | Topics | Reference |
|--------|-------------|------|--------|-----------|
| **Commissioning and Routine QA[i]** | | | | |
| AAPM TG-142 | QA for linear accelerators | 2006 | Recommendations for routine QA of linear accelerators including daily, monthly, and annual tests and associated tolerances | [1] |
| AAPM TG-135 | QA of robotic radiosurgery (CyberKnife) | 2011 | Description of the CyberKnife system and QA recommendations | [2] |
| AAPM TG-148 | QA for helical TomoTherapy | 2010 | Overview of TomoTherapy system, description of unique QA considerations, recommendations for treatment and imaging QA | [3] |
| AAPM TG-106 | Accelerator commissioning equipment and procedures | 2008 | Physical and practical aspects of commissioning a linear accelerator; guidelines on selection of phantoms, detectors, scanning systems, and best practices for commissioning | [4] |
| AAPM TG-40 | Comprehensive QA for Radiation Oncology | 1994 | Recommended components for a quality management program, including QA of EBRT equipment, brachytherapy equipment, TPS, and the planning process and patient plans. Professional roles and responsibilities. Specific QA tests and tolerances are now mostly supplanted in other reports. | [5] |

---

[i]Information on commissioning and QA for brachytherapy is listed separately in the brachytherapy section.

| Report | Brief Title | Year | Topics | Reference |
|---|---|---|---|---|
| AAPM TETA Working Group | Flattening filter-free accelerators | 2015 | Consensus guidelines for implementation of technology. Recommendations for acceptance testing, commissioning, quality assurance, radiation safety and facility planning. | [5a] |
| AAPM TG-45 | Code of practice for radiotherapy accelerators | 1994 | General recommendations for facility design, acceptance testing, commissioning, QA, and special procedures | [6] |
| AAPM TG-50 | MLC | 2001 | Overview of MLC designs, techniques for acceptance testing commissioning, and QA | [7] |
| AAPM TG-58 | Clinical use of electronic portal imaging | 2001 | Physics of megavoltage planar imaging, early technology, clinical use scenarios, QA considerations | [8] |
| IAEA Review of Radiation Oncology physics | Chapter 10, Acceptance testing and commissioning | 2005 | Overview of techniques and tests for acceptance testing and commissioning | [9] |
| IAEA Review of Radiation Oncology physics | Chapter 12, Quality assurance of external beam radiotherapy | 2005 | Overview of quality assurance and management program with reference to AAPM TG-40 | [9] |
| CAPCA Standards: kV x-ray radiotherapy | kV x-ray radiotherapy machines from Canadian Partnership for Quality Radiotherapy (CPQR) | 2013 | Acceptance testing, commissioning, and QA of superficial kilovoltage x-ray radiotherapy devices | [10] |
| IPEM Report 81 on QC | Physics aspects of QC in radiotherapy from the UK Institute of Physics and Engineering in Medicine (IPEM) | 1999 | Extensive review of quality control, ISO9000 standards, equipment in EBRT and brachytherapy, TPS, QA tests, in-vivo dosimetry | [11] |
| *Reference Dosimetry* | | | | |
| AAPM TG-51 | Clinical reference dosimetry for high-energy photon and electron beams | 1999 | Standard dosimetry protocol from AAPM based on dose to water; guidelines for procedures and worksheets | [12] |

| Report | Brief Title | Year | Topics | Reference |
|--------|-------------|------|--------|-----------|
| AAPM TG-51 addendum | Clinical reference dosimetry for high-energy photon and electron beams | 2014 | Addendum to AAPM TG-51 provides updated kQ values for photon beams and other guidance | [13] |
| TRS-398 IAEA | Absorbed dose determination in external beam radiotherapy | 2004 | A dose to water-based protocol. Applies to high and low energy photon beams, electron, proton, and heavy ion beams. | [14] |
| AAPM TG-70 | Electron beam dosimetry | 2009 | Reference dosimetry protocol for electrons. A supplement to AAPM TG-25 that makes the protocol consistent with the AAPM TG-51 dose to water approach. | [15] |
| AAPM TG-61 | Dosimetry for 40-300 kV x-ray beams | 2001 | Formalism, technique, equipment, and protocol for reference dosimetry of kV beams | [16] |
| IPEMB Report: kV dosimetrry | kV dosimetry from the UK Institute of Physics and Engineering in Medicine and Biology (IPEMB) | 1996 | Absorbed dose determination for beams <300 kV. Theoretical background, instrumentation, beam quality measurements. Recommendations for new correction factors. | [17] |
| AAPM TG-155 | Small field and non-equilibrium condition photon dosimetry | In progress | Reviews issues with small field and non-equilibrium dosimetry, perturbation factors, and algorithms. Provides guidelines for accurate dosimetry. | Das et al. |
| | | **SRS and SBRT** | | |
| AAPM TG-101 | Stereotactic body radiotherapy | 2010 | Reviews history and rationale for SBRT, discuss procedures and best practices for simulation, planning, dosimetry, and clinical implementation including commissioning and QA | [18] |
| ACR-ASTRO guidelines for SBRT | Practice guidelines for SBRT | 2014 | Summarizes professional responsibilities, procedures, and quality control tasks | [19] |
| ACR-ASTRO guidelines for SRS | Practice guidelines for SRS | 2014 | Brief summary of professional responsibilities and QA recommendations | [20] |

| Report | Brief Title | Year | Topics | Reference |
|---|---|---|---|---|
| CARO Guidelines for SRS | Scope of practice guidelines for SRS from the Canadian Association of Radiation Oncology | 2009 | Historical review of SRS. Outline of professional roles and responsibilities. Brief overview of technical aspects of SRS. | [21] |
| CARO Guidelines for SBRT | Scope of practice guidelines for lung, liver, and spine SBRT from the Canadian Association of Radiation Oncology | 2012 | Overview of SBRT, clinical indications, and technical aspects. Recommendations for safe practices by site. Technical and process QA. Professional responsibilities. | [22] |
| ASTRO Safety white paper on SBRT | Safety considerations in SBRT | 2012 | Review of safety-critical aspects in SBRT including professional considerations, technical considerations, commissioning, and QA program | [23] |
| AAPM TG-68 | Intracranial stereotactic positioning systems | 2005 | Review of devices, recommendations on performance reporting, and testing | [24] |
| AAPM TG-42 | Stereotactic radiosurgery | 1995 | Overview of frame-based (cranial) stereotactic radiosurgery | [25] |
| *Imaging and IGRT* | | | | |
| AAPM TG-179 | Quality assurance for image-guided radiation therapy utilizing CT-based technologies | 2012 | Brief review of available systems, background on image quality and dose consideration, QA recommendations, commissioning | [26] |
| AAPM MPPG 2 | QA and commissioning of x-ray-based IGRT systems | 2014 | AAPM Medical physics practice guideline (AAPM MPPG): Minimum acceptable standards for QA and commissioning of gantry-mounted kV and MV systems | [27] |
| AAPM TG-104 | In-room kV x-ray imaging for patient setup and target localization | 2009 | Planar and volumetric CT, description of systems circa 2009, acceptance testing, commissioning, QA, and clinical use | [28] |
| AAPM TG-75 | The management of imaging dose during image-guided radiotherapy | 2007 | Description of systems circa 2007, methodology for calculating dose, typical dose values, methods of limiting dose, effective dose, and challenges | [29] |

| Report | Brief Title | Year | Topics | Reference |
|---|---|---|---|---|
| ACR-ASTRO Guidelines on IGRT | Practice guidelines for IGRT | 2014 | Summarizes professional responsibilities, types of IGRT, implementation, documentation, and quality control | [30] |
| ASTRO Safety white paper on IGRT | Safety considerations in IGRT | 2013 | Overview of IGRT, 10-point recommendations for foundations for safe use of IGRT. Recommended activities for various professional groups and stakeholders. | [31] |
| AAPM TG-66 | QA of CT simulators | 2003 | Tests and specification for QA of CT simulators | [32] |
| CAPCA QC standards: CT simulators | QA of CT simulators | 2007 | Tests and specification for QA of CT simulators | [33] |
| AAPM TG-132 | Image registration and data fusion | In progress | Review existing registration algorithms and issues in clinical implementation, assessment of accuracy, acceptance testing, and QA | Brock et al. |
| AAPM TG-58 | Clinical use of electronic portal imaging | 2001 | Physics of megavoltage planar imaging, early technology, clinical use scenarios, QA considerations | [8] |
| CAPCA QC standards: EPID | Standards for quality control: EPIDs from Canadian Association of Provincial Cancer Agencies (CAPCA) | 2005 | Quality control recommendations for electronic portal imaging devices (EPID) | [34] |
| IAEA PET/CT report | QA of PET and PET/CT | 2009 | Background on PET, acceptance testing, and QA recommendations | [35] |
| AAPM Report 100 | Acceptance testing and QA for MR | 2010 | Recommendations for acceptance testing, QA procedures, and equipment and phantoms | [36] |
| AAPM TG-154 | QA of ultrasound (US)-guided EBRT for prostate cancer | 2011 | Challenges in US localization, a primer on US physics, clinical workflow, training requirements, QA recommendations | [37] |
| AAPM TG-147 | QA for nonradiographic localization and positioning systems | 2012 | Describes surface and marker-based localization systems, principles of operation, acceptance testing, commissioning, and QA | [38] |

| Report | Brief Title | Year | Topics | Reference |
|--------|-------------|------|--------|-----------|
| *Brachytherapy* | | | | |
| AAPM TG-43 | Dosimetry of interstitial brachytherapy sources | 1995 | Formalism for dose calculations for brachytherapy seeds. See updates below. | [39] |
| AAPM TG-43 update (AAPM TG-43U1) | Update to AAPM TG-43 brachytherapy protocol | 2004 | Minor changes in dose calculation formalism. Consensus data sets on common seeds with some major changes. | [40] |
| AAPM TG-43 supplement | Supplement to the 2004 update of AAPM TG-43 | 2007 | Update providing data for eight new seed models | [41] |
| AAPM TG-43U1 impact | Impact of 2004 AAPM TG-43 update | 2005 | Impact of implementing 2004 AAPM TG-43 on dose prescription for $^{125}$I and $^{103}$Pd seed implants | [42] |
| AAPM ESTRO Report: dosimetry of brachytherapy | Dose calculations for photon-emitting sources higher than 50 keV | 2012 | Consensus data sets for commercial sources. Recommendations for dosimetry calculation and measurement methods. Uses AAPM TG-43U1 formalism. | [43] |
| AAPM TG-56 | Code of practice for brachytherapy physics | 1997 | QA, seed assays, implant procedures, and evaluation. Considers both LDR and HDR. | [44] |
| AAPM TG-64 | LDR prostate brachytherapy | 1999 | Review of techniques, dosimetry, and recommendations for equipment, assays, planning, and postimplant analysis | [45] |
| ACR-ASTRO Guidelines for the practice of LDR brachytherapy | LDR brachytherapy guidelines | 2010 | Review of treatment sites, procedures. General recommendations on personnel, equipment, and QC. | [46] |
| CAPCA QC standards: LDR prostate brachytherapy | Standards for quality control: LDR prostate brachytherapy from Canadian Association of Provincial Cancer Agencies (CAPCA) | 2007 | QA in LDR prostate brachytherapy with reference to AAPM TG-43, AAPM TG-64 | [47] |
| ABS Guidelines for LDR prostate implants | Consensus guidelines for US-guided LDR prostate implants from American Brachytherapy Society | 2012 | Comprehensive clinical discussion including indications, description of procedures and planning, dose prescriptions, postimplant evaluation, and professional responsibilities | [48] |

| Report | Brief Title | Year | Topics | Reference |
|--------|-------------|------|--------|-----------|
| ICRU-38 | Dose and volume specification for reporting intracavitary therapy in gynecology | 1985 | Description of techniques used, recommendations for reporting dose and volumes. Defines the ICRU reference points for reporting dose. | [49] |
| ICRU-58 | Dose and volume specification for reporting interstitial therapy | 1997 | Definitions and recommendations for reporting dose and volumes. Practical applications. | [50] |
| AAPM TG-59 | HDR brachytherapy | 1998 | Design of an HDR program, procedures, QA, staffing, and emergency training | [51] |
| AAPM TG-41 | Remote afterloading technology | 1993 | Review of remote afterloaders for HDR, QA, and source calibration | [51A] |
| ABS guidelines for HDR prostate implants | Consensus guidelines for HDR prostate implants from American Brachytherapy Society | 2012 | Comprehensive clinical discussion including review of experience, indications, description of procedures and planning, dose prescriptions, normal tissue constraints, and professional responsibilities | [52] |
| ABS Guidelines for cervix | Consensus guidelines for locally advanced carcinoma of the cervix from American Brachytherapy Society | 2012 | Three reports: part I: general principles; part II: HDR; part III: LDR | [53-55] |
| ABS Guidelines for vaginal cuff | Consensus recommendations for vaginal cuff brachytherapy after hysterectomy from American Brachytherapy Society | 2012 | Comprehensive clinical discussion including review of experience, indications, techniques, applicators, dose fractionation, dosimetry, and QA | [56] |
| ABS Guidelines for interstitial brachytherapy for vaginal cancer | Consensus recommendations for interstitial brachytherapy of vaginal cancer from American Brachytherapy Society | 2012 | Comprehensive clinical discussion including indications, techniques, treatment planning, and QA | [57] |

| Report | Brief Title | Year | Topics | Reference |
|--------|-------------|------|--------|-----------|
| ABS Guideline for brachytherapy of esophageal cancer | Consensus recommendations for brachytherapy of esophageal cancer from the American Brachytherapy Society | 1997 | Clinical and technical recommendations for treatment | [58] |
| ABS Guidelines for eye plaques | Consensus recommendations for brachytherapy of uveal melanoma and retinoblastoma from American Brachytherapy Society | 2014 | Indications, prescription, treatment plan, plaque selection, surgery, and follow-up | [59] |
| AAPM TG-129 | Dosimetry of $^{125}$I and $^{103}$Pd COMS eye plaques for intraocular tumors | 2012 | Review of eye plaque therapy including clinical aspects. Recommendations for dose calculation formalism and parameters, commissioning, QA, and the perioperative environment | [60] |
| AAPM TG-222 | Interstitial lung brachytherapy | In progress | Review of procedures, treatment planning, dosimetry. Recommendations for specifying and evaluating treatment, quality management, and medical events. | Thomason et al. |
| AAPM TG-186 | Model-based dose calculation in brachytherapy | 2012 | Early recommendations for MBDC to model radiation transport through non-water material (e.g., tissue and applicators) with the goal of achieving more accurate dose distributions | [61] |
| ACR-ASTRO Guidelines for the practice of HDR brachytherapy | HDR brachytherapy practice guidelines | 2014 | Review of treatment sites, procedures. General recommendations on personnel, equipment, and QC. | [62, 63] |
| ASTRO Safety white paper on HDR brachytherapy | Safety considerations in HDR brachytherapy | 2014 | Reviews applications and guidance documents from ABS and other sources, QA recommendations. Lists common error scenarios. Provides seven safety recommendations. | [64] |

| Report | Brief Title | Year | Topics | Reference |
|---|---|---|---|---|
| ESTRO Booklet No. 8 | A practical guide to quality control of brachytherapy equipment | 2004 | Extensive report including calibration, safety, QC of procedures, QA of equipment and TPS, audits. Applies to HDR, PDR, and LDR. | [65] |
| AAPM TG-128 | QA for prostate brachytherapy ultrasound systems | 2008 | Review of ultrasound principles, prostate brachytherapy templates, and recommendations for QA | [66] |
| AAPM Report No. 152 | Recommendations for electronic brachytherapy | 2009 | Bullet-point recommendations on electronic brachytherapy requirements. Report in response to CRCPD regulators. | [67] |
| AAPM TG-182 | Electronic brachytherapy | In progress | Quality management for electronic brachytherapy, including risk-based recommendations on QA, training, and other issues | Thomadsen et al. |
| **EBRT Treatment Planning** | | | | |
| AAPM TG-176 | Dosimetric effects of couch tops and immobilization devices | 2014 | Review of literature and recommendations concerning effects of common immobilization devices and table tops on external beams | [68] |
| AAPM TG-53 | QA for treatment planning | 1998 | Acceptance testing, commissioning, and QA of treatment planning systems | [69] |
| AAPM TG-244 (AAPM MPPG #5) | AAPM MPPG on commissioning and QA of TPS | In progress | Update to AAPM TG-53 | Smilowitz et al. |
| IAEA TECDOC-1540 | Acceptance testing of treatment planning systems | 2007 | Recommendations on acceptance and testing of TPS including an extensive checklist | [70] |
| IAEA TECDOC-1583 | Commissioning and testing of EBRT treatment planning systems | 2008 | Test cases for commissioning, techniques, and phantoms | [71] |
| AAPM TG-166 | Biologically related models for treatment planning | 2012 | Biology-related models in treatment planning including TCP, L-Q models, NTCP, and EUD. Recommendations on acceptance testing and QA. | [72] |

| Report | Brief Title | Year | Topics | Reference |
|--------|-------------|------|--------|-----------|
| AAPM TG-65 | Tissue inhomogeneity corrections | 2004 | Review of dose effects in inhomogeneous media, issues with charged particle equilibrium, dose calculation methods, and correction factors | [73] |
| AAPM TG-63 | Hip prostheses | 2003 | Overview of hip prostheses, effect on beam, and recommendations | [74] |
| AAPM TG-71 | MU calculations | 2014 | Formalism for MU calculations in photon and electron beams | [75] |
| AAPM TG-74 | In-air output ratio, $S_c$ | 2009 | Role of $S_c$ in MU calculations. Methods for measuring $S_c$. | [76] |
| ESTRO Booklet No. 6 | MU calculations | 2001 | Formalism for MU calculations in photon beams including example data and problems | [77] |
| AAPM TG-114 | Verification of MU calculations for non-IMRT radiotherapy | 2011 | Recommendations for MU verification methods and action levels | [78] |
| AAPM TG-105 | Monte Carlo | 2007 | Review of Monte Carlo methods, specific treatment planning implementations circa 2007, issues with simulating linac beams | [79] |
| QUANTEC | Quantitative analysis of normal tissue effects in the clinic | 2010 | Review of data on normal tissue dose tolerance levels and modeling on a site-by-site basis. Special issue of the Red Journal. Accessible via AAPM website. | [83, 84] |
| ICRU-50 | Prescribing, recording, and reporting photon beam therapy | 1993 | Nomenclature for planning and prescription. Defines target volumes (e.g., GTV, CTV, PTV, OAR, etc.). Defines an ICRU reference point for prescription. | [85] |
| ICRU-62 | Prescribing, recording, and reporting photon beam therapy | 1999 | Update to ICRU-50. Includes concept of ITV, PRV, and conformity index. | [86] |

| Report | Brief Title | Year | Topics | Reference |
|---|---|---|---|---|
| ICRU-83 | Prescribing, recording, and reporting dose in IMRT | 2005 | Review of IMRT planning and technology. Margin recipes. Target volume nomenclature, prescription, and dose reporting. Advocates DVH-based reporting of dose. | [87] |
| ASTRO Safety white paper on IMRT | Safety considerations in IMRT | 2011 | Technical and environmental considerations for safe delivery of IMRT. Table of 14 recommended tests or procedures. | [88] |
| AAPM TG-119 | IMRT dosimetry | 2009 | Multi-institutional comparison of IMRT using phantom measurements. Recommendations for QA program. Downloadable cases for benchmarking. | [89] |
| ASTRO IMRT report | Recommendations for documenting IMRT treatments | 2009 | Recommendations for prescribing and documenting IMRT treatment. Especially relevant for physician practice. | [90] |
| ACR-ASTRO Guidelines for 3D EBRT | Practice guidelines for 3DCRT | 2011 | Professional responsibilities, QA of TPS, recommendations for implementation at the general level | [91] |
| ACR-ASTRO Guidelines for IMRT | Practice guidelines for IMRT | 2011 | Professional responsibilities, QA of TPS, recommendations for implementation, QA of system, and patient-specific QA | [92] |
| AAPM TG-263 | Standardizing nomenclature for radiation therapy | In progress | Nomenclature standards for structure names, elements of dose volume histograms. Develops templates for clinical trials groups and users of specific TPS systems. | Mayo et al. |

| Report | Brief Title | Year | Topics | Reference |
|--------|-------------|------|--------|-----------|
| AAPM TG-70 | Electron beam dosimetry | 2009 | Discussion of clinical applications, recommendations for reporting dose, and a library of clinical examples. Also includes a protocol for reference dosimetry (update of AAPM TG-25). | [15] |
| IAEA Review of Radiation Oncology physics | Chapter 8: Electron beams, physical and clinical aspects | 2005 | Review of dosimetric parameters, clinical considerations including isodose curves, small fields, bolus, and effects and inhomogeneity | [9] |
| AAPM TG-76 | Respiratory motion | 2006 | Measurement of respiratory motion. Techniques for managing motion during EBRT treatment. Recommendations for personnel, treatment planning, and QA. | [93] |
| **Detectors and Devices** | | | | |
| AAPM TG-62 | In-vivo dosimetry using diodes | 2005 | Physics of diodes, acceptance testing, calibration, correction factors, QA. Special considerations for use with TBI. | [80] |
| ESTRO In-vivo dosimetry booklet | Methods for in-vivo dosimetry | 2008 | Diodes, TLDs, and other detectors. Basic characteristics, calibrations, and clinical use. | [81] |
| IAEA Report No. 8 on in-vivo dosimetry | Development of procedures for in-vivo dosimetry in radiotherapy | 2013 | Basic principles of TLDs, diodes, MOSFETs, and OSLDs. Calibration procedures and correction factors. Recommendations for establishing a program. Includes measurement data from participating institutions. | [82] |

| Report | Brief Title | Year | Topics | Reference |
|--------|-------------|------|--------|-----------|
| AAPM TG-235 | Radiochromic Film Dosimetry | 2015 | Report in progress as of 5-27-15. TG charge:<br>• To review and assess the literature on RCF dosimetry, for various film models used for various clinical applications in radiation therapy since TG-55<br>• To review and assess the literature on the densitometers/scanners used for digitizing RCF, including their features and limitations and QC since TG-55<br>• To outline the procedures to achieve accurate and precise dosimetry with a RCF dosimetry system and to evaluate measurement uncertainties<br>• To provide comprehensive guidelines on the use of RCF dosimetry for clinical radiation therapy applications | Chiu-Tsao et al. |
| AAPM TG-191 | Recommendations on the Clinical Use of Luminescent Dosimeters | 2015 | Report in progress as of 5-27-15. TG Charge:<br>• To review the variety of TLD/OSL materials available, including features and limitations of each<br>• To outline the optimal steps to achieve accurate and precise dosimetry with luminescent detectors and to evaluate the uncertainty induced when less rigorous procedures are used<br>• To develop consensus guidelines on the optimal use of luminescent dosimeters for clinical practice<br>• To develop guidelines for some special medically relevant uses of TLDs/OSLs (e.g., mixed field i.e. photon/neutron dosimetry, particle beam dosimetry, skin dosimetry) | Kry et al. |

| Report | Brief Title | Year | Topics | Reference |
|---|---|---|---|---|
| **Special Procedures & Patient Considerations** | | | | |
| AAPM TG-29 | Total body irradiation | 1986 | Review of physics, dosimetry, and commissioning in TBI. The main definitive report. | [94] |
| ACR-ASTRO Guidelines for TBI | Practice guidelines for TBI | 2011 | Description of procedure. Professional responsibilities and QA requirements. | [95] |
| AAPM TG-30 | Total skin electron therapy (TSET) | 1987 | Techniques and commissioning of TSET | [96] |
| AAPM TG-72 | IORT with mobile linear accelerators | 2006 | Review of IOERT technologies, procedures, and QA using the Mobetron and other mobile linacs | [97] |
| AAPM TG-144 | $^{90}Y$ microsphere brachytherapy for hepatic malignancies | 2011 | Rationale, commercially available sources, imaging protocols, and regulatory aspects. Recommendations for dosimetry, imaging, and QA. | [98] |
| ACR-ASTRO-SIR Practice guideline for microsphere brachytherapy | Practice guideline for radioembolization with microsphere brachytherapy device (RMBD) for treatment of liver malignancies | 2014 | Indications, review of procedure, professional responsibilities, general comments on QA, and safety | [99] |
| AAPM TG-60 | Intravascular brachytherapy physics | 1999 | Clinical background, overview of procedures, dosimetry, recommendations for dose specification. Updated by AAPM TG-149. | [100] |
| AAPM TG-149 | Dosimetry for intravascular brachytherapy | 2007 | Dose calculation formalisms and consensus dosimetry parameters | [101] |
| AAPM TG-203 | Management of patients with implanted cardiac pacemakers and defibrillators | In progress | Review of published literature and background on possible radiation damage. Recommendations for managing patients with implanted devices triaged by dose level. Will replace the outdated AAPM TG-34 (1994). | Miften et al. |

| Report | Brief Title | Year | Topics | Reference |
|---|---|---|---|---|
| AAPM TG-36 | Fetal dose from radiotherapy with photon beams | 1995 | Review of radiation risk to embryo or fetus. Techniques to estimate and limit dose during radiotherapy of pregnant patients. | [102] |
| **Proton Radiotherapy** | | | | |
| ICRU-78 | Prescribing and reporting dose in proton radiotherapy | 2007 | Extensive background of proton radiotherapy, technology, and planning considerations | [103] |
| AAPM TG-185 | Clinical commissioning of proton therapy systems | In progress | Guidance for scattered/collimated, uniform scanning, and modulated beam delivery systems | Farr et al. |
| AAPM TG-224 | Proton machine QA | In progress | Comprehensive QA procedures for proton therapy systems including tolerances | Arjomandy et al. |
| **Patient Safety and Quality** | | | | |
| AAPM TG-40 | Comprehensive QA for Radiation Oncology | 1994 | Recommended components for a quality management program, including QA of EBRT equipment, brachytherapy equipment, TPS, and the planning process and patient plans. Professional roles and responsibilities. Specific QA tests and tolerances are now mostly supplanted in other reports. | [5] |
| AAPM TG-100 | Risk assessment and reduction | In press | Formalism for risk-based assessment of hazards in clinical processes including Failure mode and effects analysis (FMEA) | [104] |
| ACR Practice guideline for RO | Practice guidelines for Radiation Oncology | 2014 | Outlines key features of the process of care, professional responsibilities, educational program, equipment requirements, and QA | [105] |
| ACR Technical guidelines for EBRT | Technical guidelines for EBRT | 2010 | Professional responsibilities, equipment needs, requirements for quality management, QA, documentation, and peer review in physics | [106] |

| Report | Brief Title | Year | Topics | Reference |
|---|---|---|---|---|
| AAPM White paper on incident learning | Structure of incident learning systems | 2012 | Review of incident learning in Radiation Oncology. Consensus recommendations for the structure and operation of incident learning systems. | [107] |
| ASTRO Safety white paper on IMRT | Safety considerations in IMRT | 2011 | Technical and environmental considerations for safe delivery of IMRT. Table of 14 recommended tests or procedures. | [88] |
| ASTRO Safety white paper on IGRT | Safety considerations in IGRT | 2013 | Overview of IGRT, 10-point recommendations for foundations for safe use of IGRT. Recommended activities for various professional groups and stakeholders. | [31] |
| ASTRO Safety white paper on peer-review | Case-oriented peer-review | 2014 | Value of physician peer review in its various forms | [108] |
| AAPM TG-103 | Peer-review between physicists | 2005 | Lists elements of physicist peer review including: independent check of machine outputs, audit of charts, review of QM program and documentation, professional development, on-site coverage, and service agreements. | [109] |
| AAPM MPPG-3 | Development, implementation, use and maintenance of safety checklists | 2015 | AAPM Medical Physics Practice Guideline (AAPM MPPG): Reviews role and impact of checklists in medicine, best practices for the design, development, and maintenance of effective checklists | [110] |
| AAPM MPPG-3 | Levels of supervision for medical physicists in clinical training | 2015 | Defines supervision levels, roles of trainees, responsibility of the supervisor, supervision plan, and safety recommendations. | [110a] |
| *Shielding* | | | | |
| NCRP-151 | Structural shielding design and evaluation for megavoltage x- and gamma-ray radiotherapy facilities | 2005 | Describes shielding methodology for linear accelerators and other high energy sources | [111] |

| Report | Brief Title | Year | Topics | Reference |
|---|---|---|---|---|
| NCRP-147 | Structural shielding design for medical x-ray imaging facilities | 2004 (rev. 2005) | Describes shielding methodology for kV imaging devices | [112] |
| IAEA Safety reports Series No. 47 | Radiation protection in the design of radiotherapy facilities | 2006 | Describes shielding methodology for megavoltage units, simulators, brachytherapy rooms, and orthovoltage units | [113] |
| AAPM Report 108 | PET and PET/CT shielding requirements | 2006 | Describes shielding for PET and PET/CT facilities including the scanning room, the patient holding area, and the facility as a whole | [114] |
| *Informatics* | | | | |
| ACR-AAPM-SIIM Report on IT security | Practice parameter for electronic medical information privacy and security | 2014 | IT systems management recommendations including the definition of responsibilities, risk analysis, backup, storage, and system downtime/recovery planning | [115] |
| AAPM TG-201 (preliminary report) | QA of external beam data transfer | 2009 | The preliminary report (cited) gives an overview of IT resource management and related issues in Radiation Oncology | [116] |
| AAPM TG-262 | Electronic charting of radiation therapy planning and treatment | In progress | Guidance on electronic charting, safe clinical practices for transitioning to electronic charting, implementation in the context of other IT systems (e.g., hospital EMR), and common pitfalls | Mechalakos et al. |
| *Website Resources* | | | | |
| AAPM task group reports | | | https://www.aapm.org/pubs/reports/ | |
| ASTRO Safety white papers | | | https://www.astro.org/Clinical-Practice/White-Papers/Index.aspx (includes the journal article executive summary as well as the full report) | |
| ACR-ASTRO practice guidelines | | | http://www.acr.org/Quality-Safety/Standards-Guidelines/Practice-Guidelines-by-Modality/Radiation-Oncology | |
| American Brachytherapy Society Guidelines | | | http://www.americanbrachytherapy.org/guidelines/ | |
| IAEA RPOP (Radiation Protection of Patients) | | | https://rpop.iaea.org/RPoP/RPoP/Content/index.htm | |

| Report | Brief Title | Year | Topics | Reference |
|---|---|---|---|---|
| IROC, Imaging and Radiation Oncology Core (formerly RPC) | | | http://www.irocqa.org/ http://rpc.mdanderson.org/RPC/ home.htm | |
| Journal of Applied Clinical Medical Physics | | | www.jacmp.org | |
| National Council on Radiation Protection (NCRP) reports | | | Note that as of 2015 all NCRP reports are available to AAPM members at: http:// www.aapm.org/pubs/NCRP/ | |

## Other Reports and Resources

AAPM TG-25 (1991). Electron beam dosimetry. Now supplanted by AAPM TG-70 (2009). Includes a valuable overview of electron beam characteristics.[117]

AAPM TG-28 (1987). Radiotherapy portal imaging quality. Now mainly of historical interest, this report describes image quality and visualization of MV port films using film cassettes.[118]

AAPM TG-69 (2007). Radiographic film for megavoltage beam dosimetry.[119]

AAPM TG-55 (1998). Radiochromic film. Provides background but protocols and film used are somewhat outdated.[120] This report will be supplanted by the forthcoming AAPM TG-235.

AAPM TG-2 (1993). Specification and acceptance testing of CT scanners. Now largely supplanted by AAPM TG-66 for radiotherapy applications.[121]

AAPM TG-8 (1990). Protocol for exposure measurements from diagnostic x-rays. Covers skin dose from radiographic procedures.[122]

AAPM TG-7 (1990). Equipment and techniques in mammography.[123]

AAPM TG-21 (1983). Reference dosimetry protocol for high energy photon and electron beams. Now outdated by AAPM TG-51, AAPM TG-21 protocol used an in-air protocol for dose calibration which applied various correction factors to account for the ionization chamber response.[124]

AAPM TG-48 (1995). IORT with linear accelerators. Now supplanted by AAPM TG-72 (2006).[125]

## References

1. Klein EE, Hanley J, Yin F-F, et al. Task group 142 report: Quality assurance of medical accelerators. Med Phys 2009;36(9):4197–212.
2. Dieterich S, Cavedon C, Chuang CF, et al. Report of AAPM TG 135: Quality assurance for robotic radiosurgery. Med Phys 2011;38(6):2914–36.
3. Langen KM, Papanikolaou N, Balog J, et al. QA for helical TomoTherapy: Report of the AAPM Task Group 148. Med Phys 2010;37(9):4817–53.
4. Das IJ, Cheng C-W, Watts RJ, et al. Accelerator beam data commissioning equipment and procedures: Report of the TG-106 of the Therapy Physics Committee of the AAPM. Med Phys 2008;35(9):4186–215.
5. Kutcher GJ, Coia L, Gillin M, et al. Comprehensive QA for Radiation Oncology: Report of AAPM Radiation Therapy Committee Task Group 40. Medical Phys 1994;21(4):581–618.
5a. Xiao Ying, et al. Flattening filter-free accelerators: a report from the AAPM Therapy Emerging Technology Assessment Work Group. J Appl Clin Med Phys 2015;16(3).
6. Nath R, Anderson LL, Meli JA, et al. AAPM code of practice for radiotherapy accelerators: Report of AAPM Radiation Therapy Task Group No. 45. Med Phys 1994;21(7):1093–121.
7. Boyer AL, Biggs P, Galvin J, et al. Basic applications of multileaf collimators: Report of Task Group No. 50. Med Phys, Madison, WI: 2001.
8. Herman MG, Balter JM, Jaffray DA, et al. Clinical use of electronic portal imaging: Report of AAPM radiation therapy committee Task Group 58. Med Phys 2001;28(5):712–37.

9. Podgorsak EB, editor. Radiation Oncology physics: A handbook for teachers and students. Vienna, Austria: International Atomic Energy Agency (IAEA); 2005.

10. Furstoss C. Kilovoltage x-ray radiotherapy machines, in Technical Quality Control Guidelines for Canadian Radiation Treatment Centres. Alberta. CA: Canadian Partnership for Quality Radiotherapy; 2013.

11. Mayles WPM, Lake R, McKanzie EM, et al. Physics aspects of quality control in radiotherapy. York, England: Institute of Physics and Engineering in Medicine; 1999.

12. Almond PR, Biggs PJ, Coursey BM, et al. AAPM's TG-51 protocol for clinical reference dosimetry of high-energy photon and electron beams. Med Phys 1999;26(9):1847–70.

13. McEwen M, DeWerd L, Ibbott G, et al. Addendum to the AAPM's TG-51 protocol for clinical reference dosimetry of high-energy photon beams. Med Phys 2014;41(4):041501.

14. IAEA. Absorbed dose determination in external beam radiotherapy: An international code of practice for dosimetry based on standards of absorbed dose to water. Vienna, Austria: IAEA; 2004.

15. Gerbi BJ, Antolak JA, Deibel FC, et al. Recommendations for clinical electron beam dosimetry: Supplement to the recommendations of Task Group 25. Med Phys 2009;36(7):3239–79.

16. Ma CM, Coffey CW, DeWerd LA, et al. AAPM protocol for 40-300 kV x-ray beam dosimetry in radiotherapy and radiobiology. Med Phys 2001;28(6):868–93.

17. Klevenhagen SC, Aukett RJ, Harrison RM, et al. The IPEMB code of practice for the determination of absorbed dose for x-rays below 300 kV generating potential (0.035 mm Al-4 mm Cu HVL; 10-300 kV generating potential). Phys Med Biol 1996;41(12):2605–25.

18. Benedict SH, Yenice KM, Followill D, et al. Stereotactic body radiation therapy: The report of AAPM Task Group 101. Med Phys 2010;37(8):4078–101.

19. ACR–ASTRO Practice parameter for the performance of stereotactic body radiation therapy. Reston, VA: American College of Radiology; 2014.

20. ACR–ASTRO practice parameter for the performance of stereotactic radiosurgery. Reston, VA: American College of Radiology; 2014.

21. Roberge D, Ménard C, Bauman G, et al. Radiosurgery scope of practice in Canada. Canadian Association of Radiation Oncology (CARO); 2009. <http://www.caro-acro.ca/Assets/Radiosurgery+Scope+of+Practice+in+Canada.pdf?method=1>.

22. Sahgal A, Roberge D, Schellenberg D, et al. The Canadian Association of Radiation Oncology scope of practice guidelines for lung, liver and spine stereotactic body radiotherapy. Clin Oncol (R Coll Radiol) 2012;24(9):629–39.

23. Solberg T, Balter JM, Stanley H, et al. Quality and safety considerations in stereotactic radiosurgery and stereotactic body radiotherapy: Executive summary. Pract Radiat Oncol 2012;2:2–9.

24. Lightstone AW, Benedict SH, Bova FJ, et al. Intracranial stereotactic positioning systems: Report of the American Association of Physicists in Medicine Radiation Therapy Committee Task Group no. 68. Med Phys 2005;32(7):2380–98.

25. Schell MC, Bova FJ, Larson DA, et al. Stereotactic radiosurgery: A report of AAPM Task Group 42. Woodbury, NY: American Institute of Phyics; 1995.

26. Bissonnette JP, Balter PA, Dong L, et al. Quality assurance for image-guided radiation therapy utilizing CT-based technologies: A report of the AAPM TG-179. Med Phys 2012;39(4):1946–63.

27. Fontenot JD, Alkhatib H, Garrett JA, et al. AAPM Medical Physics Practice Guideline 2.a: Commissioning and quality assurance of X-ray-based image-guided radiotherapy systems. J Appl Clin Med Phys 2014;15(1):4528. <http://www.jacmp.org/index.php/jacmp/article/view/4528/html_1>.

28. Yin F, Wong J. The role of in-room kV x-ray imaging for patient setup and target localization: Report of Task Group 104. College Park, MD: AAPM; 2009.

29. Murphy MJ, Balter J, Balter S, et al. The management of imaging dose during image-guided radiotherapy: Report of the AAPM Task Group 75. Med Phys 2007;34(10):4041–63.

30. ACR–ASTRO practice guidelines for image-guided radiation therapy (IGRT). Reston, VA: American College of Radiology; 2014.

31. Jaffray D, Langen KM, Mageras G, et al. Safety considerations for IGRT: Executive summary. Pract Radiat Oncol 2013;3(3):167–70.

32. Mutic S, Palta JR, Butker EK, et al. Quality assurance for computed-tomography simulators and the computed-tomography-simulation process: Report of the AAPM Radiation Therapy Committee Task Group No. 66. Med Phys 2003;30(10):2762–92.

33. Arsenault C, et al. Standa. In: rds for Quality Control at Canadian Radiation Treatment Centres: CT Simulators, in Standards for Quality Control at Canadian Radiation Treatment Centres. 2007. <https://www.medphys.ca/content.php?doc=58>.

34. Arsenault C, et al. Standards for Quality Control at Canadian Radiation Treatment Centres: Electronic Portal Imaging. In: Devices, in Standards for Quality Control at Canadian Radiation Treatment Centres. 2005. <https://www.medphys.ca/content.php?doc=58>.

35. IAEA. Quality assurance for PET and PET/CT systems. IAEA Human Health Series. Vol. No. 1. Vienna, Austria: International Atomic Energy Agency; 2009.

36. Jackson EF, et al. Acceptance testing and quality assurance procedures for magnetic resonance imaging facilities. College Park, MD: 2010. <http://www.aapm.org/pubs/reports/RPT_100.pdf>.

37. Molloy JA, Chan G, Markovic A, et al. Quality assurance of US-guided external beam radiotherapy for prostate cancer: Report of AAPM Task Group 154. Med Phys 2011;38(2):857–71.

38. Willoughby T, Lehmann J, Bencomo JA, et al. Quality assurance for nonradiographic radiotherapy localization and positioning systems: Report of Task Group 147. Med Phys 2012;39(4):1728–47.

39. Nath R, Anderson LL, Luxton G, et al. Dosimetry of interstitial brachytherapy sources: Recommendations of the AAPM Radiation Therapy Committee Task Group No. 43. American Association of Physicists in Medicine. Med Phys 1995;22(2):209–34.

40. Rivard MJ, Coursey BM, DeWerd LA, et al. Update of AAPM task group No. 43 report: A revised AAPM protocol for brachytherapy dose calculations (vol 31, pg 633, 2004). Med Phys 2004;31(12):3532–3.

41. Rivard MJ, Butler WM, DeWerd LA, et al. Supplement to the 2004 update of the AAPM Task Group No. 43 Report. Med Phys 2007;34(6):2187–205.

42. Williamson JF, et al. Recommendations of the American Association of Physicists in Medicine regarding the impact of implementing the 2004 Task Group 43 report on dose specification for $^{103}$Pd and $^{125}$I interstitial brachytherapy. Med Phys 2005;32(5):1424–39.

43. Perez-Calatayud J, Ballester F, Das RK, et al. Dose calculation for photon-emitting brachytherapy sources with average energy higher than 50 keV: Report of the AAPM and ESTRO. Med Phys 2012;39(5):2904–29.

44. Nath R, Anderson LL, Meli JA, et al. Code of practice for brachytherapy physics: Report of the AAPM Radiation Therapy Committee Task Group No. 56. Med Phys 1997;24(10):1557–98.

45. Yu Y, Anderson LL, Li Z, et al. Permanent prostate seed implant brachytherapy: Report of the American Association of Physicists in Medicine Task Group No. 64. Med Phys 1999;26(10):2054–76.

46. ACR–ASTRO practice guideline for the performance of low-dose-rate brachytherapy. Reston, VA: American College of Radiology; 2010.

47. Arsenault C, et al. Standards for quality control at canadian radiation treatment centres: Low Dose Rate Prostate Brachytherapy, in Standards for Quality Control at Canadian Radiation Treatment Centres. 2007. <https://www.medphys.ca/content.php?doc=58>.

48. Davis BJ, Horwitz EM, Lee WR, et al. American Brachytherapy Society consensus guidelines for transrectal ultrasound-guided permanent prostate brachytherapy. Brachyther 2012;11(1):6–19.

49. ICRU. Dose and volume specification for reporting intracavitary therapy in gynecology. ICRU Report 38. Bethesda, MD: International Commission on Radiation Units and Measurements; 1985.

50. ICRU. Dose and volume specification for reporting intracavitary therapy in gynecology. ICRU Report 58. Bethesda, MD: International Commission on Radiation Units and Measurements; 1997.

51. Kubo HD, Glasgow GP, Pethel TD, et al. High dose-rate brachytherapy treatment delivery: Report of the AAPM Radiation Therapy Committee Task Group No. 59. Med Phys 1998;25(4):375–403.

51A. Glasgow G, Bourland JD, Grigsby PW, et al. Weaver, Remote Afterloading Technology: Report of AAPM Task Group No. 41. New York, NY: Pub: American Institute of Physics Inc; 1993, ISBNL 1-56396-240-3, <http://www.aapm.org/pubs/reports/RPT_41.pdf>.

52. Yamada Y, Rogers L, Demanes DJ, et al. American Brachytherapy Society consensus guidelines for high-dose-rate prostate brachytherapy. Brachyther 2012;11(1):20–32.

53. Viswanathan AN, Thomadsen B. American Brachytherapy Society consensus guidelines for locally advanced carcinoma of the cervix. Part I: General principles. Brachyther 2012;11(1):33–46.

54. Lee LJ, Das IJ, Higgins SA, et al. American Brachytherapy Society consensus guidelines for locally advanced carcinoma of the cervix. Part III: Low-dose-rate and pulsed-dose-rate brachytherapy. Brachyther 2012;11(1):53–7.

55. Viswanathan AN, Beriwal S, De Los Santos JF, et al. American Brachytherapy Society consensus guidelines for locally advanced carcinoma of the cervix. Part II: High-dose-rate brachytherapy. Brachyther 2012;11(1):47–52.

56. Small W, Beriwal S, Demanes DJ, et al. American Brachytherapy Society consensus guidelines for adjuvant vaginal cuff brachytherapy after hysterectomy. Brachyther 2012;11(1):58–67.

57. Beriwal S, Demanes DJ, Erickson B, et al. American Brachytherapy Society consensus guidelines for interstitial brachytherapy for vaginal cancer. Brachyther 2012;11(1):68–75.

58. Gaspar LE, Nag S, Herskovic A, et al. American Brachytherapy Society (ABS) consensus guidelines for brachytherapy of esophageal cancer. Clinical Research Committee, American Brachytherapy Society, Philadelphia, PA. Int J Radiat Oncol Biol Phys 1997;38(1):127–32.

59. Simpson ER, Gallie B, Laperrierre N, et al. The American Brachytherapy Society consensus guidelines for plaque brachytherapy of uveal melanoma and retinoblastoma. Brachyther 2014;13(1):1–14.

60. Chiu-Tsao ST, Astrahan MA, Finger PT, et al. Dosimetry of $^{125}$I and $^{103}$Pd COMS eye plaques for intraocular tumors: Report of Task Group 129 by the AAPM and ABS. Med Phys 2012;39(10): 6161–84.

61. Beaulieu L, Carlsson Tedgren A, Carrier JF, et al. Report of the Task Group 186 on model-based dose calculation methods in brachytherapy beyond the TG-43 formalism: Current status and recommendations for clinical implementation. Med Phys 2012;39(10):6208–36.

62. Erickson BA, Demanes DJ, Ibbott GS, et al. American Society for Radiation Oncology (ASTRO) and American College of Radiology (ACR) practice guideline for the performance of high-dose-rate brachytherapy. Int J Radiat Oncol Biol Phys 2011;79(3):641–9.

63. ACR–ASTRO practice guideline for the performance of high-dose-rate brachytherapy. Reston, VA: American College of Radiology; 2014.

64. Thomadsen BR, Beth A. A review of safety, quality management, and practice guidelines for high-dose-rate brachytherapy: Executive summary. Pract Radiat Oncol 2014;4(2):65–70.

65. Venselaar J, Perez-Calatayud J, editors. A practical guide to quality control of brachytherapy equipment, in European guidelines for quality assurance in radiotherapy. Brussels, Belgium: 2004.

66. Pfeiffer D, Sutlief S, Feng W, et al. AAPM Task Group 128: Quality assurance tests for prostate brachytherapy ultrasound systems. Med Phys 2008;35(12):5471–89.

67. Thomadsen B, Biggs PJ, DeWerd LA, et al. The 2007 AAPM response to the CRCPD request for recommendations for the CRCPD's model regulations for electronic brachytherapy. College Park, MD: American Association of Physicists in Medicine; 2009.

68. Olch AJ, Gerig L, Li H, et al. Dosimetric effects caused by couch tops and immobilization devices: Report of AAPM Task Group 176. Med Phys 2014;41(6):061501-1–061501-30.

69. Fraass B, Doppke K, Hunt M, et al. American Association of Physicists in Medicine Radiation Therapy Committee Task Group 53: Quality assurance for clinical radiotherapy treatment planning. Med Phys 1998;25(10):1773–829.

70. IAEA. Specification and acceptance testing of radiotherapy treatment planning systems. Vienna, Austria: International Atomic Energy Agency (IAEA); 2007.

71. IAEA. Commissioning of radiotherapy treatment planning systems: Testing for typical external beam treatment techniques. Vienna, Austria: International Atomic Energy Agency (IAEA); 2008.

72. Li XA, Albr M, Deasy JO, et al. The use and QA of biologically related models for treatment planning: Short report of the TG-166 of the Therapy Physics Committee of the AAPM(a). Med Phys 2012;39(3):1386–409.

73. Papanikolaou N, Battista JJ, Boyer AL, et al. Tissue inhomogeneity correction for megavoltage beams: Report of Task Group 65, 2004. Madison, WI: American Association of Physicists in Medicine; 2004.

74. Reft C, Alecu R, Das IJ, et al. Dosimetric considerations for patients with HIP prostheses undergoing pelvic irradiation. Report of the AAPM Radiation Therapy Committee Task Group 63. Med Phys 2003;30(6):1162–82.

75. Gibbons JP, Antolak JA, Followill DS, et al. Monitor unit calculations for external photon and electron beams: Report of the AAPM Therapy Physics Committee Task Group No. 71. Med Phys 2014;41(3):031501.

76. Zhu TC, Bjärngard BE, Xiao Y, et al. Report of AAPM Therapy Physics Committee Task Group 74: In-air output ratio, S-c, for megavoltage photon beams. Med Phys 2009;36(11):5261–91.

77. Mijnheer B, et al. Monitor unit calculations for high energy photon beams: Practical examples, in Physics for clinical radiotherapy. ESTRO Booklet No. 6. Brussels, Belgium: 2001. <http://www.estro

.org/binaries/content/assets/estro/school/publications/booklet-6—monitor-unit-calculation-for-high-energy-photon-beams—practical-examples.pdf>.

78. Stern RL, Heaton R, Fraser MW, et al. Verification of monitor unit calculations for non-IMRT clinical radiotherapy: Report of AAPM Task Group 114. Med Phys 2011;38(1):504–30.

79. Chetty IJ, Curran B, Cygler JE, et al. Report of the AAPM Task Group No. 105: Issues associated with clinical implementation of Monte Carlo-based photon and electron external beam treatment planning. Med Phys 2007;34(12):4818–53.

80. Yorke E, et al. Diode in-vivo dosimetry for patients receiving external beam radiation therapy: Report of AAPM Task Group-62. Madison, WI: 1991. <http://www.aapm.org/pubs/reports/RPT_87.pdf>.

81. Van Dam J, Marinello G. Methods for in vivo dosimetry in external radiotherapy. Brussels, Belgium: ESTRO; 2006.

82. IAEA. Development of procedures for in vivo dosimetry in radiotherapy. IAEA Human Health Reports. Vol. No. 8. Vienna, Austria: International Atomic Energy Agency (IAEA); 2013.

83. Marks LB, Ten Haken RK, Martel MK. Guest editor's introduction to QUANTEC: A users guide. Int J Radiat Oncol Biol Phys 2010;76(3 Suppl.):S1–2.

84. Quantitative Analysis of Normal Tissue Effects in the Clinic (QUANTEC). 2010; Available from: http://aapm.org/pubs/QUANTEC.asp.

85. ICRU. Prescribing, recording and reporting photon beam therapy. ICRU Report 50. Bethesda, MD: International Commission on Radiation Units and Measurements; 1993.

86. ICRU. Prescribing, recording and reporting photon beam therapy (supplement to ICRU Report 50). ICRU Report 62. Bethesda, MD: International Commission on Radiation Units and Measurements; 1999.

87. Gregoire V, Mackie TR. ICRU committee on volume and dose specification for prescribing, recording and reporting special techniques in external photon beam therapy: Conformal and IMRT. Radiother Oncol 2005;76:S71.

88. Moran JM, Dempsey M, Eisbruch A, et al. Safety considerations for IMRT: Executive summary. Pract Radiat Oncol 2011;1(3):190–5.

89. Ezzell GA, Burmeister JW, Dogan N, et al. IMRT commissioning: Multiple institution planning and dosimetry comparisons, a report from AAPM Task Group 119. Med Phys 2009;36(11):5359–73.

90. Holmes T, Das R, Low D, et al. American Society of Radiation Oncology recommendations for documenting intensity-modulated radiation therapy treatments. Int J Radiat Oncol Biol Phys 2009;74(5): 1311–18.

91. ACR–ASTRO practice guideline for 3d external beam radiation planning and conformal therapy. Reston, VA: American College of Radiology; 2011.

92. ACR–ASTRO practice guideline for intensity modulated radiation therapy (IMRT). Reston, VA: American College of Radiology; 2011.

93. Keall PJ, Mageras GS, Balter JM, et al. The management of respiratory motion in Radiation Oncology: Report of AAPM Task Group 76. Med Phys 2006;33(10):3874.

94. van Dyk J, Galvin JM, Glasgow GP, et al. The physical aspects of total and half body photon irradiation: A report of AAPM Task Group 29. American Association of Physicists in Medicine. New York 1986.

95. ACR–ASTRO practice guideline for the performance of total body irradiation. Reston, VA: American College of Radiology; 2011.

96. Karzmark CJ, Anderson J, Buffa A, et al. Total skin electron therapy: Technique and dosimetry: Report of Task Group 30. New York: American Institute of Physics; 1987.

97. Beddar AS, Biggs PJ, Chang S, et al. Intraoperative radiation therapy using mobile electron linear accelerators: Report of AAPM Radiation Therapy Committee Task Group no. 72. Med Phys 2006;33(5): 1476–89.

98. Dezarn WA, Cessna JT, DeWerd LA, et al. Recommendations of the American Association of Physicists in Medicine on dosimetry, imaging, and quality assurance procedures for Y-90 microsphere brachytherapy in the treatment of hepatic malignancies. Med Phys 2011;38(8):4824–45.

99. ACR–SIR practice parameter for radioembolization with microsphere brachytherapy devices (RMBD) for treatment of liver malignancies. Reston, VA: American College of Radiology; 2014.

100. Nath R, Amols H, Coffey C, et al. Intravascular brachytherapy physics: Report of the AAPM Radiation Therapy Committee Task Group no. 60. American Association of Physicists in Medicine. Med Phys 1999;26(2):119–52.

101. Chiu-Tsao ST, Schaart DR, Soares CG, et al. Dose calculation formalisms and consensus dosimetry parameters for intravascular brachytherapy dosimetry: Recommendations of the AAPM Therapy Physics Committee Task Group No. 149. Med Phys 2007;34(11):4126–57.
102. Stovall M, Blackwell CR, Cundiff J, et al. Fetal dose from radiotherapy with photon beams: Report of AAPM-Radiation-Therapy-Committee Task Group No-36. Med Phys 1995;22(1):63–82.
103. ICRU Report 78. Prescribing, recording and reporting proton-beam therapy. Oxford, UK: ICRU; 2007. p. 210.
104. Huq MS, et al. Application of risk analysis methods to radiation therapy quality management: Report of AAPM Task Group 100. Med Phys 2014.
105. ACR–ASTRO practice parameter for Radiation Oncology. Reston, VA: American College of Radiology; 2014.
106. ACR practice guidelines and technical standards: Radiation Oncology. Reston, VA: American College of Radiology; 2011.
107. Ford EC, Fong de Los Santos L, Pawlicki T, et al. Consensus recommendations for incident learning database structures in Radiation Oncology. Med Phys 2012;39(12):7272–90.
108. Marks LB, Adams RD, Pawlicki T, et al. Enhancing the role of case-oriented peer review to improve quality and safety in Radiation Oncology: Executive summary. Pract Radiat Oncol 2013;3(3): 149–56.
109. Halvorsen PH, Das IJ, Fraser M, et al. AAPM Task Group 103 report on peer review in clinical Radiation Oncology physics. J Appl Clin Med Phys/Ame Coll Med Phys 2005;6(4):50–64.
110. Fong de Los Santos L, et al. Medical Physics Practice Guideline Task Group 3.a: Development, implementation, use and maintenance of safety checklists. J Clin Med Phys 2015; in press.
110a. Seibert JA, et al. AAPM Medical Physics Practice Guideline 3. a: Levels of supervision for medical physicists in clinical training. J Appl Clin Med Phys 2015;16(3).
111. NCRP. NCRP Report No. 151, Structural shielding design and evaluation for megavoltage X- and Gamma-ray radiotherapy facilities. Bethesda, MD: National Council on Radiation Protection and Measurements (NCRP); 2005.
112. NCRP. Structural shielding design for medical X-ray imaging facilities. Bethesda, MD: National Council on Radiation Protection and Measurements (NCRP); 2004.
113. IAEA. Radiation protection in the design of radiotherapy facilities. IAEA Safety Report Series. Vol. No. 47. Vienna, Austria: International Atomic Energy Agency (IAEA); 2006.
114. Madsen MT, Anderson JA, Halama JR, et al. AAPM Task Group 108: PET and PET/CT shielding requirements. Med Phys 2006;33(1):4–15.
115. ACR–AAPM–SIIM practice parameter for electronic medical information privacy and security. Reston, VA: American College of Radiology; 2014.
116. Siochi RA, Balter P, Bloch C, et al. Information technology resource management in Radiation Oncology. J Appl Clin Med Phys 2009;10(4):16–35.
117. Kahn FM, Doppke KP, Hogstrom KR, et al. Clinical electron-beam dosimetry: Report of AAPM Task Group-25. Colchester, VT: American Institute of Physics; 1991.
118. Reinstein L, Amols HI, Biggs PJ, et al. Radiotherapy portal imaging quality: Report of AAPM Task Group-28. American Association of Physicists in Medicine. New York, NY; 1987.
119. Pai S, Das IJ, Dempsey JF, et al. TG-69: Radiographic film for megavoltage beam dosimetry. Med Phys 2007;34(6):2228–58.
120. Niroomand-Rad A, Blackwell CR, Coursey BM, et al. Radiochromic film dosimetry: Recommendations of AAPM Radiation Therapy Committee Task Group 55. Med Phys 1998;25(11):2093–115.
121. Lin PJ, Beck TJ, Borras C, et al. Specification and acceptance testing of computed tomography scanners: Report of AAPM Task Group-2. New York, NY: American Institute of Physics; 1993.
122. Chu RYL, Fisher J, Archer BR, et al. Standardized methods for measuring diagnostic x-ray exposures: Report of AAPM Task Group-8. Colchester, VT: American Institute of Physics; 1990.
123. Yaffe MJ, Barnes GT, Conway BJ, et al. Equipment requirements and quality control for mammography: Report of AAPM Task Group-7. New York, NY: American Institute of Physics; 1990.
124. A protocol for the determination of absorbed dose from high-energy photon and electron-beams: Report of AAPM TG-21. Med Phys 1983;10(6):741–71.
125. Palta JR, Biggs PJ, Hazle JD, et al. Intraoperative electron beam radiation therapy: Technique, dosimetry, and dose specification: Report of task force 48 of the Radiation Therapy Committee, American Association of Physicists in Medicine. Int J Radiat Oncol Biol Phys 1995;33(3):725–46.

# Glossary

## Professional Societies and Organizations

| | | |
|---|---|---|
| AAPM | American Association of Physicists in Medicine | http://www.aapm.org |
| ABR | American Board of Radiology | http://www.theabr.org |
| ABS | American Brachytherapy Society | http://www.americanbrachytherapy.org |
| ACGME | Accreditation Council for Graduate Medical Education | https://www.acgme.org/acgmeweb/ |
| ACR | American College of Radiology | http://www.acr.org |
| AHRQ | Agency for Healthcare Research and Quality | http://www.ahrq.gov/ |
| ASTRO | American Society of Therapeutic Radiation Oncology | http://www.astro.org |
| CAMPEP | Commission on Accreditation of Medical Physics Education Programs | http://www.campep.org/ |
| CAPCA | Canadian Association of Provincial Cancer Agencies | http://www.capca.ca/ |
| CARO | Canadian Association of Radiation Oncology | http://www.caro-acro.ca/ |
| COMP | Canadian Organization of Medical Physicists | http://www.medphys.ca/ |
| CRCPD | Council of Radiation Control Program Directors | http://www.crcpd.org/ |
| DICOM | Digital Imaging and Communications in Medicine | http://dicom.nema.org/ |
| DIN | Deutsche Institut fur Normung | http://www.din.de |
| ESTRO | European Society of Therapeutic Radiation Oncology | http://www.estro.org |
| IAEA | International Atomic Energy Agency | http://www.iaea.org |
| ICRP | International Commission on Radiological Protection | http://www.icrp.org/ |
| ICRU | International Commission on Radiation Units & Measurements | http://www.icru.org/ |
| IEC | International Electrotechnical Commission | http://www.iec.ch/ |
| IHE-RO | Integrating the Healthcare Enterprise—Radiation Oncology | http://www.ihe-ro.org/ |
| IPEM | Institute of Physics and Engineering in Medicine | http://www.ipem.ac.uk/ |
| IROC | Imaging and Radiation Oncology Core | http://rpc.mdanderson.org/rpc/ |
| NCCN | National Comprehensive Cancer Network | http://www.nccn.org/default.aspx |
| NPSF | National Patient Safety Foundation | http://www.npsf.org/ |
| NRC | Nuclear Regulatory Commission | http://www.nrc.gov |
| NCRP | National Council on Radiation Protection & Measurements | http://www.ncrponline.org |
| NRG | A coalition of cancer trials groups | http://www.nrgoncology.org/ |
| PTCOG | Particle Therapy Cooperative Group | http://www.ptcog.ch/ |
| RTOG | Radiation Therapy Oncology Group | http://www.rtog.org/ |

## Acronyms

| | |
|---|---|
| 4DCT | Four-dimensional Computed Tomography (*aka* Respiration-correlated CT) |
| ABC | Active Breathing Coordinator |
| ALARA | As Low As Reasonably Achievable |

| | |
|---|---|
| APBI | Accelerated Partial Breast Irradiation |
| APeX | Accreditation Program for Excellence (from ASTRO) |
| ART | Adaptive Radiation Therapy |
| AV | Audio-visual |
| BB | Ball Bearing |
| BED | Biologically Equivalent Dose |
| BEIR | Biological Effects of Ionizing Radiation (committee of the National Academies of Sciences) |
| BID | "bis in die" (twice per day) |
| CARS | Center for Assessment of Radiological Sciences |
| CAX | Central Axis |
| CBCT | Cone-beam CT |
| CFR | Code of Federal Regulations (United States) |
| CGE | Cobalt-Gray Equivalent |
| CI | Conformity Index |
| CK | CyberKnife |
| CME | Continuing Medical Education |
| CNS | Central Nervous System |
| CSI | Craniospinal Irradiation |
| CT | Computed Tomography |
| CTDI | CT Dose Index |
| CTV | Clinical Target Volume |
| DICOM | Digital Imaging and Communications in Medicine |
| DLP | Dose-length Product |
| DQA | Delivery Quality Assurance |
| DOT | Department of Transportation (in U.S.) |
| DRR | Digitally Reconstructed Radiograph |
| DVH | Dose Volume Histogram |
| EBRT | External Beam Radiation Therapy |
| EHR | Electronic Health Record |
| EMR | Electronic Medical Record |
| EPID | Electronic Portal Imaging Device |
| EUD | Equivalent Uniform Dose |
| FDA | Food and Drug Administration (in U.S.) |
| FDG | Fluorodeoxyglucose |
| FFF | Flattening Filter Free |
| FMEA | Failure Mode and Effects Analysis |
| FOV | Field of View |
| FWHM | Full Width at Half Maximum |
| gEUD | Generalized Equivalent Uniform Dose |
| GTV | Gross Tumor Volume |
| GK | GammaKnife |
| Gy | Gray |
| GyE | Gray Equivalent (or GY(E)) |
| HDR | High Dose Rate |
| HI | Homogeneity Index |
| H&N | Head and Neck |
| HVL | Half-value Layer |
| IDR | Instantaneous Dose Rate |
| IGRT | Image-guided Radiation Therapy |
| ILS | Incident Learning System |

| | |
|---|---|
| IMPT | Intensity Modulated Proton Radiotherapy |
| IMRT | Intensity Modulated Radiation Therapy |
| IORT | Intraoperative Radiotherapy |
| IOERT | Intraoperative Electron Radiotherapy |
| IRAK | Integrated Reference Air Kerma |
| IT | Information Technology |
| ITV | Internal Target Volume |
| IVBT | Intra-vascular Brachytherapy |
| kV | Kilovoltage |
| kVp | Kilovoltage at Peak |
| LDR | Low Dose Rate |
| LET | Linear Energy Transfer |
| LNT | Linear No-Threshold (model for radiation risk) |
| LQ | Linear Quadratic (biological effect model) |
| MC | Monte Carlo |
| MIP | Maximum Intensity Projection |
| MinIP | Minimum Intensity Projection |
| MLC | Multileaf Collimator |
| MOC | Maintenance of Certification (in ABR system) |
| MOSFET | Metal Oxide Semiconductor Field-Effect Transistor |
| MPPG | Medical Physics Practice Guideline (from AAPM) |
| MRI (or MR) | Magnetic Resonance Imaging |
| MU | Monitor Unit |
| MV | Megavoltage |
| NIST | National Institutes of Standards and Technology (in U.S.) |
| NRC | (U.S.) Nuclear Regulatory Commission |
| NTCP | Normal Tissue Complication Probability |
| OAR | Organ at Risk |
| OF | Output Factor |
| OR | Operating Room |
| OSLD | Optically Stimulated Luminescence Dosimeter |
| PACS | Picture Archiving and Communication System |
| PDD | Percent Depth Dose |
| PDR | Pulsed Dose Rate |
| PET | Positron Emission Tomography |
| PHI | Protected Healthcare Information |
| PRV | Planning Risk Volume |
| PSI | Prostate Seed Implant |
| PSO | Patient Safety Organization (in U.S.) |
| PTV | Planning Target Volume |
| P&P | Policies and Procedures |
| QA | Quality Assurance |
| QUANTEC | Quantitative Analysis for Normal Tissue Effects in the Clinic |
| QC | Quality Control |
| QI | Quality Improvement |
| QM | Quality Management |
| QMP | Qualified Medical Physicist |
| RBE | Relative Biological Effect |
| RCA | Root Cause Analysis |
| RCT | Randomized Controlled Trial |
| RECIST | Response Evaluation Criteria for Solid Tumors |

| | |
|---|---|
| rem | Roentgen Equivalent Man |
| RO | Radiation Oncology |
| ROI | Region of Interest |
| ROILS | Radiation Oncology Incident Learning System |
| ROSIS | Radiation Oncology Safety Information System |
| RT | Radiation Therapy |
| RTT | Radiation Therapy Technologist ("Radiographer" in UK) |
| RVR | Remaining Volume at Risk |
| R&V | Record & Verify |
| SABR | Stereotactic Ablative Radiotherapy |
| SAD | Source to Axis Distance |
| SAFRON | Safety in Radiation Oncology (system from IAEA) |
| SBRT | Stereotactic Body Radiotherapy |
| SSD | Source to Surface Distance |
| SOBP | Spread-out Bragg Peak |
| SPA | Safety Profile Assessment (from AAPM) |
| SPC | Statistical Process Control |
| SPECT | Single Photon Emission Tomography |
| SRS | Stereotactic Radiosurgery |
| SUV | Standard Uptake Value |
| Sv | Sievert |
| TBI | Total Body Irradiation |
| TCP | Tissue Complication Probability |
| TG | Task Group (of AAPM) |
| TJC | The Joint Commission (U.S., formerly JCAHO) |
| TLD | Thermoluminescent Dosimeter |
| TPS | Treatment Planning System |
| TRAK | Total Reference Air Kerma |
| TRUS | Trans-rectal Ultrasound |
| TSET | Total Skin Electron Treatment |
| TV | Treated Volume |
| TVL | Tenth Value Layer |
| T&O | Tandem and Ovoid |
| T&R | Tandem and Ring |
| VMAT | Volumetric Modulated Arc Therapy |
| WF | Wedge Factor |

## Definitions

Absorbed dose—Energy absorbed per unit mass at a given point by ionizing radiation.
Air kerma—The sum of kinetic energy of all charged particles liberated per unit mass.
I50—Depth of 50% ionization as measured by an ion chamber.
R50—Depth of 50% dose as measured by any dosimeter.
Linac—Linear accelerator abbreviation.
Point of measurement—The reference point of a dosimeter.
Reference air kerma—Air kerma rate at a reference point of 1 cm or 1 m.
Reference depth—The depth at which a calibration measurement is taken.

# INDEX

Page numbers followed by "*f*" indicate figures, "*t*" indicate tables, and "*b*" indicate boxes.